Similarity and analogical reasoning

Similarity and analogical reasoning

Edited by

STELLA VOSNIADOU
ANDREW ORTONY

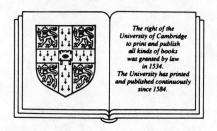

The right of the
University of Cambridge
to print and publish
all kinds of books
was granted by law
in 1534.
The University has printed
and published continuously
since 1584.

CAMBRIDGE UNIVERSITY PRESS

Cambridge
New York   New Rochelle   Melbourne   Sydney

Published by the Press Syndicate of the University of Cambridge
The Pitt Building, Trumpington Street, Cambridge CB2 1RP
32 East 57th Street, New York, NY 10022, USA
10 Stamford Road, Oakleigh, Melbourne 3166, Australia

First published 1989

Printed in the United States of America

Library of Congress Cataloging-in-Publication Data
Similarity and analogical reasoning.
"Papers delivered at a Workshop on Similarity and
Analogy held at the Allerton House of the University of
Illinois, Urbana-Champaign, in June 1986" – Pref.
1. Comparison (Psychology) – Congresses.
2. Similarity (Psychology) – Congresses. 3. Analogy –
Psychological aspects – Congresses. 4. Reasoning
(Psychology) – Congresses. 5. Learning, Psychology of –
Congresses. I. Vosniadou, Stella. II. Ortony, Andrew,
1942–   . III. Workshop on Similarity and Analogy
(1986 : Allerton House)
BF446.S56 1989   153.4'3   88–11813

British Library Cataloguing in Publication Data
Similarity and analogical reasoning.
1. Analogical reasoning.
I. Vosniadou, Stella   II. Ortony, Andrew
153'.4'3

ISBN 0-521-36295-4 hard covers
ISBN 0-521-38935-6 paperback

Contents

v

Preface

The contributions to this volume are extensively revised versions of papers delivered at a Workshop on Similarity and Analogy held at the Allerton House of the University of Illinois, Urbana-Champaign, in June 1986. The purpose of the workshop was to bring together scientists working on similarity and analogy to explore current theoretical developments in this area and to consider the practical implications of this work for learning and instruction. The group was interdisciplinary in character and included scientists looking at similarity and analogy from psychological, computational, and educational points of view. The workshop was exciting, enjoyable, and rewarding, and we would like to take this opportunity to thank all the participants for helping to make it so.

Much of the workshop's original structure survived in the transition to this edited volume. The contributions in the first part deal with the issue of similarity. The second part includes the contributions dealing with analogical reasoning. Because analogies are fundamentally concerned with similarity at the level of representational structure, the chapters in the second part provide a theoretical context for those dealing with analogical reasoning by examining a number of questions about the nature of similarity and its relation to conceptual structure. The contributions in the third part discuss analogical reasoning in relation to learning and instruction. All three parts end with one or more chapters that offer commentaries, providing quite detailed discussions of most, although not all, of the other chapters in the book.

The Workshop on Similarity and Analogy was made possible by a grant from the Army Research Institute and was also supported in part by the Center for the Study of Reading. To these we would like to express our thanks. We would like to express our particular thanks to Judith Orasanu from ARI for her enthusiasm for this project and for her support throughout all phases of the workshop. The workshop, and as a result this book, would not have been possible without the assistance of many of our colleagues in the Department of Psychology and the Center for the Study of Reading. In particular, Doug Medin, Dedre Gentner, and Brian Ross joined us in forming a steering committee that organized the workshop, and were instrumental in shaping its character and contents. We would also like to acknowledge the help of Marlo Schommer, Ala Samarapungavan, Sue Wyatt, and, particularly, Delores Plowman, whose expert secretarial skills greatly facilitated the preparation of the manuscript. Finally, our thanks go to Katharita Lamoza of Cambridge University Press for her patience and cooperativeness as production editor for this book.

Stella Vosniadou
Andrew Ortony

Contributors

DANIEL K. ANDERSON School of Medicine, Southern Illinois University

JOHN R. ANDERSON Department of Psychology, Carnegie-Mellon University

LAWRENCE W. BARSALOU School of Psychology, Georgia Institute of Technology

JOHN D. BRANSFORD Department of Psychology, Vanderbilt University

WILLIAM F. BREWER Department of Psychology, University of Illinois at Urbana-Champaign

ANN L. BROWN Center for the Study of Reading, University of Illinois at Urbana-Champaign

MARK BURSTEIN Bolt, Beranek & Newman, Inc.

ALLAN COLLINS Bolt, Beranek & Newman, Inc.

RICHARD L. COULSON School of Medicine, Southern Illinois University

GERALD DEJONG Coordinated Science Laboratory, University of Illinois at Urbana-Champaign

PAUL J. FELTOVICH School of Medicine, Southern Illinois University

JEFFERY J. FRANKS Department of Psychology, Vanderbilt University

DEDRE GENTNER Department of Psychology, University of Illinois at Urbana-Champaign

KEITH J. HOLYOAK Department of Psychology, University of California at Los Angeles

PHILIP N. JOHNSON-LAIRD MRC Applied Psychology Unit, Cambridge, England

DOUGLAS MEDIN Department of Psychology, University of Illinois at Urbana-Champaign

RYSZARD S. MICHALSKI Department of Computer Science, George Mason University

ANDREW ORTONY Beckman Institute, University of Illinois at Urbana-Champaign

xiii

DANIEL N. OSHERSON Department of Psychology, Massachusetts Institute of Technology

STEPHEN E. PALMER Department of Psychology, University of California at Berkeley

LANCE J. RIPS Department of Behavioral Sciences, University of Chicago

BRIAN H. ROSS Department of Psychology, University of Illinois at Urbana-Champaign

DAVID E. RUMELHART Department of Psychology, Stanford University

ROBERT D. SHERWOOD Department of Teaching and Learning, Vanderbilt University

EDWARD E. SMITH Department of Psychology, University of Michigan

LINDA B. SMITH Department of Psychology, Indiana University

RAND J. SPIRO Center for the Study of Reading, University of Illinois at Urbana-Champaign

PAUL R. THAGARD Cognitive Science Laboratory, Princeton University

ROSS THOMPSON Department of Psychology, Carnegie-Mellon University

STELLA VOSNIADOU Center for the Study of Reading, University of Illinois at Urbana-Champaign, and Aristotelian University of Thessaloniki, Greece

NANCY J. VYE Department of Psychology, Vanderbilt University

Similarity and analogical reasoning: a synthesis

STELLA VOSNIADOU and
ANDREW ORTONY

The ability to perceive similarities and analogies is one of the most fundamental aspects of human cognition. It is crucial for recognition, classification, and learning, and it plays an important role in scientific discovery and creativity. In recent years, similarity and analogy have received increasing attention from cognitive scientists. This growth of interest is related to the realization that human reasoning does not always operate on the basis of content-free general inference rules but, rather, is often tied to particular bodies of knowledge and is greatly influenced by the context in which it occurs. In a reasoning system of this kind, learning does not get accomplished by merely adding new facts and applying the same inference rules to them. Rather, successful learning often depends on the ability to identify the most relevant bodies of knowledge that already exist in memory so that this knowledge can be used as the starting point for learning something new.

All the chapters in this volume have something to say about the role that similarity and analogy play in this process, although they often do so from radically different points of view. This is not surprising since the contributors of this volume come from related but nevertheless distinct disciplines. For some, the focus is on the psychological processes involved in reasoning by similarity and analogy and on how these processes develop. Others are interested in solving the computational problems involved in simulating analogical processing in problem-solving situations. Finally, some researchers, particularly those interested in educational issues, are concerned about the conditions that promote the application of analogical reasoning.

We value this diversity because we believe that an understanding of the role that similarity and analogy play in cognition is most likely to come about by integrating knowledge from diverse specialized do-

1

mains. Beyond the interdisciplinary character of the contributions to this volume, however, the differences we find in the treatment of similarity and analogy are also representative of the state of the art in cognitive science today. Because similarity judgments and analogical reasoning are based on people's representation of entities, even the most superficial treatment of these topics requires some assumptions about how knowledge is represented and how these representations change. Although some authors deal with the question of knowledge representation more explicitly than others, this is an issue that runs through most of the chapters in this volume, coloring the treatment of similarity and analogy and accounting for a lot of the diversity we observe.

The purpose of this synthesis is to provide a roadmap to the book, making connections, pointing out similarities and differences, integrating some of the material, and raising some questions that need to be pursued in future research. In an attempt to structure this introduction to correspond roughly to the major groupings of the chapters, we shall discuss first issues having to do with similarity and the structure of concepts; we shall then turn to the nature of analogical reasoning; and finally we shall discuss the implications of existing theories of similarity and analogy for learning and instruction.

Similarity and the structure of concepts

Two important issues pertaining to similarity emerge from the collection as a whole, and particularly from the chapters in Part I, Similarity and the Structure of Concepts. The first of these concerns the question of what kinds of similarity there are. Is there only one kind, or are there more? If there is more than one kind of similarity, what distinguishes them? The second issue has to do with the relation between conceptual systems and similarity. Here, the key questions are whether perceived similarity determines the nature of our concepts, whether the nature of our concepts determines what we perceive as similar, or whether there is a mutual interdependence between conceptual structures and perceived similarity.

Kinds of similarity

On the question of how many kinds of similarity there are, two basic approaches can be found – approaches that are by no means mutually exclusive. The most widespread of these is based on the explicit or implicit assumption, held by many of the contributors, that there is a fundamental difference between something that might be called *sur-face* similarity and *deep* similarity. The second approach, which is discussed explicitly only by Linda Smith, is to distinguish between *global* and *dimensional* similarity. This distinction essentially focuses on the fact that one can perceive two things as being similar in terms of some holistic perception of them or, in a more constrained way, by viewing them as being similar only along certain discriminable dimensions. In either case, according to Smith, the proper theoretical account has to be in terms of a complex relational system of similarity kinds, rather than in terms of some idealized "pure" similarity.

The contact between the notion of dimensional similarity and the more widespread distinction between surface and deep similarity is that the latter distinction, insofar as it can be clarified sufficiently to be theoretically useful, appears to apply readily to dimensional similarity but to bear no relation to the notion of global similarity. If two things just seem to be similar in general, without reference to any particular dimensions, then the question of whether this perceived similarity is based on surface or deep aspects of the objects does not arise. It arises only when one comes to consider the respects in which two things are similar, for then one can argue that they are similar either in terms of readily accessible dimensions that are apparent on the "surface" or in terms of "deeper" underlying properties that are not.

A clear commitment to the surface/deep distinction can be found in the chapter by Lance Rips. According to Rips, perceptual (i.e, surface) similarity is cognitively primitive and well defined and therefore can be used as a construct to explain other psychological functions, such as categorization. Similarity based on underlying properties is, however, too vague to be useful for such purposes.

In contrast to Rips, Smith is less comfortable with the idea that perceptual similarity is well defined. She argues that there are major shifts with development in the way in which perceptual similarity is distinguished. Early in development children understand the similarities in the way objects look only in terms of global, syncretic resemblances. With development, the relational similarity system becomes differentiated into distinct and interrelated kinds of similarity based on dimensions such as part identify, color, and size, the relations of greater-than, less-than, and so on.

Yet another basis for distinguishing different kinds of similarity emerges from Dedre Gentner's chapter. Gentner makes a distinction between object attributes (one-place predicates characterizing simple descriptions of objects) and relations (two-or-more-place predicates characterizing relations). She then goes on to argue that surface similarity is based on shared object attributes, whereas structural similarity is similarity at the level of relational structure.

Finally, Stella Vosniadou argues that information that may be considered as object attributes can be quite difficult to access (e.g., the spherical shape of the earth, the solidity of the moon, etc.) whereas some relations (e.g., movement) can be readily accessible. Vosniadou proposes using the term *salient similarity* instead of *surface similarity* to refer to similarity grounded in easily retrievable aspects of representations, regardless of whether or not they represent descriptive or relational, perceptual or conceptual properties. According to this account, the surface/deep similarity distinction is a dynamic one because in the process of knowledge acquisition the properties of people's underlying representations, which are salient and therefore easy to retrieve, may change.

Douglas Medin and Andrew Ortony also focus on how the distinction between surface and deep similarity might be operationalized, and on what the connection between deep and surface similarity might be. They present the distinction in terms of knowledge representations, suggesting that surface similarities can be thought of as those based on readily accessible components of concepts (of the kind that people describe when asked to list the properties of objects), and deep similarity as similarity with respect to more central, core properties of concepts. One of their main claims is that there is a nonarbitrary, casual relation between surface and central properties, such that the latter constrain and sometimes even generate the former. Medin and Ortony believe that organisms are sensitive to just those kinds of surface similarities that lead them toward the more central properties, a point also made by Ann Brown.

According to Brown, infants come predisposed to seek casual explanations for events (particularly with respect to physical and personal casuality), and these predispositions constrain what is selected from the range of available perceptual attributes to form categories. Children seem to be sensitive to certain perceptual properties of objects that have the possibility of leading to the deeper, more central properties. For example, infants pay particular attention to the movement of objects, noticing very rapidly that some objects need to be pushed or pulled in order to move, whereas other objects do not. This early sensitivity to movement leads infants to differentiate animate from inanimate objects and to continue further differentiating these two categories into finer and finer distinctions as their knowledge of biology and physics increases.

Similarity and conceptual structure

Because similarity judgments are based on people's representations of entities, a theory of similarity has to be concerned with the nature of these representations and how they change in the process of knowledge acquisition. A number of contributors address this issue quite directly. Lawrence Barsalou argues that there is great variability in the concepts that represent categories and that the resulting instability of concepts affects both within-category and across-category similarity. He argues that careful analyses of how individuals represent specific concepts are needed before one can understand how concepts in general are structured.

An example of such an analysis is provided by Ryszard Michalski. Michalski agrees that concepts have flexible meanings and offers some ideas as to how such flexibility might be achieved. He proposes a two-tiered representation for concepts, according to which the concept meaning is distributed between a base concept representation and an inferential concept interpretation. The base representation contains the "core" of the concept's meaning (the easily explainable concept meaning). Inference processes of all sorts (deductive, inductive, and analogical) operate to relate observations to this base concept representation. Michalski's proposal brings up the question of what the criteria are for distinguishing between the base concept representation and the inferential component, a challenge that is raised, although not resolved, by Gerald DeJong.

An important theoretical issue concerns the question of whether perceived similarity helps shape the nature of concepts or vice versa. A strong denial of the first of these possibilities, that perceived similarity determines the nature of our concepts, is presented in the chapter by Rips. There it is argued that similarity cannot explain how people make category judgments and that resemblance models of categorization (e.g., exemplar and prototype models) may work well for artificial categories but not for richer categories that people know a lot about. Rips presents the results of several experiments suggesting that it is possible to alter similarity judgments without affecting category performance and to alter category judgments without affecting similarity. He concludes that category decisions are better viewed as being based on inferences to the best explanation rather than on similarity of putative members to category prototypes.

Judgments of category membership clearly are pivotal in the creation and maintenance of concepts. The suggestion by Rips that such judgments are perhaps not grounded in similarity is something of a radical departure from the prevailing view in cognitive psychology. If similarity is not a crucial component in category judgments, one might wonder whether there are any general psychological processes in which it plays an important role. In the chapter by Edward Smith and Daniel Osherson, an important class of such processes is identified, and a provocative analysis of the role of similarity in decision making is proposed. Thus one might view this chapter by Smith and Osherson as going some way toward restoring confidence in the potential that theories of similarity might have as explanatory mechanisms in important psychological processes. These authors propose a model of decision making according to which a person estimates the probability that an object belongs to a class by relying on the similarity that the object bears to the prototype of the class (e.g., they judge the probability that "Linda" is "a feminist bank teller" by computing the similarity between Linda and their prototype of a feminist bank teller). Smith and Osherson argue that such a model can explain why people often violate certain principles of probability and statistical theory (such as the conjunction rule and Bayes's theorem) as uncovered by Kahneman and Tversky (e.g., 1972, 1973; Tversky & Kahneman, 1982, 1983).

Comparing what might be considered the rather pessimistic view of the significance of similarity as an explanatory construct presented by Rips with the relatively optimistic view presented by Smith and Osherson leads to the possibility that the truth lies somewhere between the two. This is the position that Medin and Ortony take. They argue that similarity may not be as powerful as Smith and Osherson want it to be, although it may play a greater role in categorization than Rips argues for. They acknowledge that the results of Rip's experiments are quite damaging to a theory of categorization that is restricted to similarity in terms only of surface properties, but they see no reason why category judgments cannot in principle be made with respect to similarity of more central aspects of concepts.

Analogical reasoning

There is general agreement that analogical reasoning involves the transfer of relational information from a domain that already exists in memory (usually referred to as the *source* or *base* domain) to the domain to be explained (referred to as the *target* domain). Similarity is implicated in this process because a successful, useful analogy depends upon there being some sort of similarity between the source domain and the target domain and because the perception of similarity is likely to play a major role in some of the key processes associated with analogical reasoning.

Three such processes appear to be critical, and discussions of one or more of them surface in virtually every chapter in Parts II and III. These processes are, first, gaining access to an (appropriate) analog; second, mapping some part of the information associated with that analog onto the target domain; and third, the side effects of analogical reasoning in terms of the production of more general rules and representations. In this section, we shall discuss these issues in greater detail while indicating how they relate to a fourth general issue, namely, one having to do with the relation between two distinct kinds of analogies.

The two kinds of analogies we have in mind are those in which the analogically related items are drawn from conceptually different or remote domains and those in which the items are drawn from the same domain, or at least from conceptually very close domains. The first kind might be called *between-domain* (or metaphorical) analogies, and the second we shall refer to as *within-domain* (or literal) analogies. Some of the chapters (e.g., John Anderson and Ross Thompson; Brian Ross) deal exclusively with within-domain analogies, focusing on the use of old problems to solve new ones in the same domain. Others (e.g., Keith Holyoak and Paul Thagard; Gentner; Philip Johnson-Laird) concentrate primarily on between-domain analogical reasoning. We think it is important not to lose sight of the distinction between the two kinds of analogies, because it is possible that somewhat different processes might be involved in the two cases. A discussion of some of these issues can be found in the chapter by Vosniadou.

Similarity and the problem of analogical access

One major way in which similarity is implicated in analogical reasoning is that a theory of analogical reasoning must explain how an analog is retrieved in the first place. In order to access an appropriate analog when constructing an analogy, people must perceive some similarity between the target domain and a source domain. It appears relatively easy to construct a plausible model of the access mechanism in the case of within-domain analogies, which usually exhibit some similarity between target and source domains with respect to both their surface properties and their relational structure. Many empirical findings show that the likelihood of retrieving an analog increases when the surface similarity (similarity in simple, descriptive properties) between the source and the target is increased (Gentner & Landers, 1985; Holyoak & Koh, 1986; Ross, 1984). Understanding exactly what role surface similarity plays in accessing an analog is complicated, however, by equivocation over exactly what surface similarity is.

The real challenge about access, however, arises in cases where the source domain is remote from the target domain. This is because the likelihood of similarity in surface properties triggering access decreases as the remoteness of the domains increases. One solution for how to account for access when the source domain is very remote from the target domain might be *plan-based indexing*. This is the view that, when a problem cannot be solved with reference to an existing general rule or schema, people start searching for an analog that can provide a solution to the problem that satisfies the problem's goals without violating the target's solution constraints. This proposal was originally suggested by Carbonell (1983), and a modified version of it is utilized in the "processes of induction" (PI), the computer model described by Keith Holyoak and Paul Thagard. In PI there is no explicit search for an analog. Instead, possible analogs can be retrieved as a side effect of the general rule, and concept activation can be generated in the context of the problem-solving activity.

Although plans and goals may play an important role in access, there is doubt that they can account for access completely. Empirical work in analogical problem solving has shown that both adults and children have great difficulty retrieving a remote analog that can satisfy the target problem's goals, even in experimental situations in which such a potential analog has just been provided (e.g., Gick & Holyoak, 1980, 1983). The problem often lies in the fact that neither children nor adults represent the problems at a level abstract (content-free) enough for the plan-based indexing solution to succeed. Furthermore, when they do, they sometimes have access to a specific higher-order schema or concept, which makes the application of analogical reasoning unnecessary. If a specific general schema for solving a problem already exists in memory, why not use that schema instead of reasoning by analogy? This issue is discussed by DeJong in his criticism of the various computational approaches to analogical reasoning.

Another solution is proposed by Vosniadou, who argues that sometimes access to an analog for a between-domain analogy can be based on the identification of some *salient* similarity in the properties of the source and the target. Unlike surface similarity, salient similarity is defined only with respect to the status that it has with respect to people's underlying representations and not on the basis of whether it represents simple, descriptive properties.

One interesting finding is that for between-domain analogies access appears to be less of a problem for adults and experts than for children and novices (Brown, this volume; Gentner, this volume; Novick, 1988). What is it about development and knowledge acquisition that allows easier access to analogs from remote domains? One possibility is that adults and experts are more likely to notice and use similarity with respect to relational as opposed to nonrelational properties – that there is what Gentner calls, an "attribute-to-relations shift" with development and with the acquisition of knowledge. Another possibility is that the ability to notice and use similarity in relations is available to children and novices but that children's and novices' knowledge representations do not contain the relational information that is needed when it is needed. This is the position taken by Brown. Yet a third possibility, not inconsistent with the last one, is that access is determined by salient similarity in the properties of the source and target, but what is *salient* similarity may change as people's conceptual representations become reorganized with the acquisition of knowledge (as discussed by Vosniadou). As a result, what may be considered deep properties in the conceptual representations of novices may come to be salient and thus easily accessible to experts (see Carey, 1985; Chi, Feltovich, & Glaser, 1981; Vosniadou & Brewer, 1987).

Research on analogical access has important implications for training and instruction, some of which will be discussed in greater detail later. However, two illustrations of this are worth mentioning now. Brian Ross's suggestion to enhance surface similarity among problems of the same problem type in order to increase the probability that they are placed in the same general category has its source in the finding that surface similarity is an important determinant of access. Similarly, the proposal in the chapter by John Bransford and his collaborators that new material be presented in a problem-solving format is supported by the plan-based indexing view of memory retrieval. In other words, information stored as a problem solution may be more likely to be accessed and used in similar problem-solving situations.

Analogical mapping

Analogical mapping involves setting up correspondences between properties in the two domains and transferring a relational structure that embodies some of the relations between these properties. Curiously, however, none of the contributors discusses the conditions under which mapping is required. In many instances of analogy comprehension, transfer of the relational structure is not needed because the relational structure already exists in the target domain.

Analogical reasoning and attendant subprocesses such as access and mapping involve the dynamic interplay of many interrelated systems. For this reason, a number of different computational approaches to analogical reasoning have been developed. Relative to the more traditional techniques of experimental psychology, computer modeling and artificial intelligence techniques provide powerful alternative ways of exploring and testing ideas about analogical reasoning. It should be noted, however, that the adoption of computer modeling techniques in no way eliminates the need for and usefulness of traditional experimental techniques. The present collection includes four different computational approaches to analogical reasoning, or aspects of it, but in almost all cases these models are influenced by experimental data and suggest further experiments. This interaction between computer modeling and psychological experiments is characteristic of the cognitive science approach to dealing with complex information-processing problems. Although there is no doubt that this is a positive development, care needs to be exercised in distinguishing descriptions of computer programs designed to model particular processes from the underlying theories of those processes.

An important difference of opinion in the area of analogical mapping, one discussed in some detail by Philip Johnson-Laird, is whether the emphasis is placed on structural as opposed to pragmatic factors (i.e., ones based on the reasoner's plans and goals). An example of the structure-mapping approach is provided by Gentner. She proposes a structure-mapping process that relies on structural/relational commonalities as opposed to specific prior content and that is not influenced by the system's problem-solving goals, except to the extent that these goals affect the current representation of the domain. In her chapter, Gentner describes how a theory of this kind can be implemented in a computer model that searches for potential local and global matches between the source and target systems, evaluates them on the basis of the depth of the relational match, and selects the deepest, the most systematic, and the most consistent mappable structure.

In contrast to this structure-mapping approach, a more pragmatic approach is possible. For example, Holyoak and Thagard describe a computer model called PI. The basic design of PI involves a bidirectional search in which rules become active as a result of both a forward search from the problem situation to possible actions and a backward search from the goal to possible actions and preconditions that could achieve it (the subgoal transfer mechanism). Analogical mapping is used when an activated source analog provides a more efficient solution procedure than a known rule. If a source analog is found, the mapping process (a) maps identical relations, (b) postulates that the relational goals of the two problems are analogous and proceeds from there to map the corresponding arguments of these relations, and (c) hypothesizes an analogical solution to the problem. In this model, the selection of a source analog is a side effect of rule activity directed toward solving the target problem. Holyoak and Thagard consider this to be an advantage over most systems that evade serious examination of the question of when analogies are invoked. PI does not base its selection of source elements to be transferred on structural criteria. Rather, the subgoal transfer mechanism insures that what are transferred are applicable elements of the source problem with functional relevance to a solution.

We have already emphasized the need for a distinction between within-domain analogies and between-domain analogies. Both the Gentner model and Holyoak and Thagard's model are computer models that attempt to handle between-domain analogies, the former by design and the latter by side effect. Within-domain models tend to focus on problem-solving tasks in which the problems to be solved are all of the same general kind (e.g., problems in computer programming or statistics). John Anderson and Ross Thompson describe a computer model (known as PUPS) designed to handle within-domain analogies of this kind, using a production system architecture. The key to their approach lies in the structure of the knowledge representation that they employ. Knowledge is organized in schema-like structures consisting of function and form slots. Analogy is a mechanism for achieving form–function relationships in domains where skills for doing so have not yet been acquired. Analogy does this by finding a source domain that achieves an analogous function (or form) that has the corresponding form (or function) filled. This is achieved by looking for a source in which the first element in the function slot is identical to the corresponding element in the target. The remaining elements are put into correspondence. The system uses various inductive inferences in the mapping.

The computational approaches that we have discussed so far all lie within the symbolic representation paradigm. Knowledge structures and rules for operating on them are explicitly represented in symbolic form. During the last ten years or so, an alternative computational approach known as *connectionism* has become increasingly influential. Connectionism eschews the idea of explicit symbolic representations. It is based on the idea that representations are not localized and symbolically represented but are emergent properties of memory and learning systems that are composed of a very large number of computationally very simple (neuronlike) elements. Such systems have been developed to perform a wide array of relatively low-level tasks (such as letter and word recognition), but they have not yet reached the point of being able to deal with high-level, complex tasks such as analogical reasoning. Nevertheless, it is important to consider how such parallel distributed processing systems might, in principle, be able to approach such problems. A speculative account of how this might be done can be found in the chapter by David Rumelhart. Rumelhart describes such a distributed memory system in which collections of elements, which he calls microfeatures, could represent both the physical characteristics of a situation and its more relational aspects. Depending on how familiar it is, when an input enters the memory system it is either recognized and assimilated to stored patterns, or rejected by the system (at this point the activity of the memory system is shut down). Analogical reasoning would occur in situations in which the information stored in memory provided no close match.

It is clear that accounts of the computational approaches of the kind we have been discussing represent powerful ways of exploring some of the complex issues surrounding the problem of analogical reasoning and mapping. However, they raise some problems that are not easy to resolve. One of these concerns the question of how to choose among competing accounts. The difficulty here lies in the fact that most implemented models have unavoidable limitations of scope that make it almost impossible to undertake fair and objective comparisons of performance. Another, emphasized by Johnson-Laird, concerns the possibility that computational models of analogy are in principle limited to cases of what he calls *expository* analogies, but that *profound* analogies, which he believes involve genuine creativity, are computationally intractable.

Analogy and generalization

For most researchers who work in the area of problem solving, analogical reasoning (mainly within-domain analogical reasoning) is a mechanism used primarily by novices who lack general rules or schemata. There is reason to believe that young children (who also lack general rules and expertise in domains) use analogical reasoning as a primary problem-solving and knowledge acquisition mechanism. Given that novices often use analogical reasoning in problem solving, one important question with serious implications for learning is whether the successful application of analogical reasoning helps novices learn general rules and build schemata they lack. Many researchers believe so, although the question of how and when such generalizations are made is far from clear (as discussed by Allan Collins and Mark Burstein in the final chapter).

According to Anderson and Thompson, analogy is used only at the beginning stages of problem solving. In PUPS, every time an analogy is used, the abstract implicational structure is extracted and a rule is formed. This prevents the system from having to use an analogy a second time. Overgeneralization is prevented by adding heuristic constraints based on empirical cases.

For Holyoak and Thagard, analogy is seen as a trigger for induction. A generalized rule is induced after the analogy is used to form an abstract problem schema. It could also be argued (as it is by Ross, for example) that the process of analogical reminding itself may force certain very conservative generalizations, which nevertheless can lead students to learn about problem types. Such a process may be one means by which novices go from superficial similarities to structural similarities, given that the two are related. The use of surface or salient similarity as a means for discovering, transferring, and generalizing a casual mechanism by young children is also discussed by Brown and by Vosniadou in the context of discussing the developmental literature on analogical reasoning.

Finally, Rand Spiro and his colleagues in considering the use of explicit, instructional, between-domain analogies in ill-structured domains give a number of examples of people's tendency to overgeneralize on the basis of single analogies. The problem here is that, whereas analogies help novices gain a preliminary grasp of difficult concepts, they may later become impediments to fuller or more correct understandings.

Implications for instruction

A major challenge facing research on learning and instruction is the question of how to liberate "inert" knowledge. The issue here is not that the problem solver lacks the knowledge to solve the problem but rather that the problem solver cannot recruit that knowledge as and when it is needed. This problem is a major theme in Part III. Starting with the premise that knowledge is often isolated and context-bound and that this makes the noticing of similarity and the spontaneous application of analogical reasoning difficult, some researchers (e.g., Bransford et al.; Brown) focus on how the knowledge base can become more flexible and discuss certain instructional techniques for making it so. Others (e.g., Ross; Vosniadou; Spiro et al.) think that reasoning by similarity and analogy itself can make the knowledge base more flexible and facilitate the learning of general rules and the acquisition of new schemata (see also the discussion above on analogy and generalization).

Bransford and his colleagues think that the problem of inert knowledge is related to the way people are taught. Often, instruction involves teaching facts that can be recalled but cannot be used in new situations. Experiments show that instructional procedures that result in learning (in the sense of being able to recall relevant information) provide no guarantee that people will use this information later on. Bransford et al. suggest that this problem can be solved by teaching people in problem-oriented learning environments rather than by the mere presentation of factual information.

Bransford and his colleagues also discuss how instruction can facilitate the noticing of relevant features of problem situations and how new advances in instructional technology make it possible to teach in new and more effective ways. For example, videotapes can be used to create contrasts that highlight the similarities and differences between concepts. It is also important to encourage students to take multiple perspectives on the same problem and to understand how different concepts can illuminate it (a point also made by Spiro, et al., as well as by Brown).

Like Bransford and his collaborators, Ross emphasizes the context dependence and isolation of knowledge. Ross argues that people have difficulty in transferring information not only when what has been learned needs to be transferred across remote domains, but even in the same domain. Although the phenomenon of highly contextualized knowledge may be the result of lack of expertise, much of what we believed to be accomplished by abstract processing mechanisms may be accomplished by more specific mechanisms based on highly similar materials (a point also made by Rumelhart). Surface similarity may often enhance the probability of people using analogical reminding to notice that problems belong to the same problem type.

Vosniadou suggests that similarity in salient properties between the source and target domains can lead to the discovery of a productive analogy, that is, an analogy that can produce *new* knowledge about the structure of the target system. In this respect, analogy can become an important mechanism in the acquisition of new knowledge. According to Vosniadou, children use analogical reasoning to acquire new knowledge about a domain just like adults do. What develops is not the analogical mechanism itself but the conceptual system upon which this mechanism operates.

In her chapter, Brown approaches the problem of inert knowledge by arguing for the importance of functional flexibility. A potential solution to a problem is often not seen although it is in plain sight, because it is embedded in a familiar, but currently irrelevant, context. This suggests that it is important to experiment with objects in many different ways, to look at them from different points of view. Such activities are likely to free objects from specific roles, thus rendering them more useful as tools for more varied applications. Brown's experimental findings with young children show that experiences that enhance flexibility lead to increases in transfer, whereas the habitual use of an object to perform a specific task produces a lower rate of transfer.

In considering the role of analogical reasoning in instruction, little attention has been paid to the process of understanding an explanatory analogy explicitly presented to facilitate knowledge acquisition in an unfamiliar domain. By far the lion's share of the theoretical attention has been devoted to the question of analogy creation, although Spiro and his colleagues discuss a number of issues related to the cognitive consequences of analogy comprehension. Because of their concern over the potential that analogies have for leading to false or oversimplified representations, Spiro and his collaborators focus on instructional strategies that might avoid such undesirable consequences. They recommend using explicit analogies to facilitate the process of knowledge acquisition in ill-structured domains where teaching rules is not possible (even if it were desirable) and where there is considerable conceptual load. Their technique involves the use of integrated multiple analogies to counteract missing or misleading information that a single analogy might contain.

It appears that analogical reasoning can fulfill a number of useful functions to facilitate learning. What is still lacking, however, is a systematic treatment of the differences and similarities among these various functions and of the unique problems and/or advantages each one presents.

Conclusion

The chapters in this volume advance our understanding of similarity and analogy on a number of different fronts. On the issue of similarity, they make it clear that there is a complex relational system of similarity kinds. This similarity system is not static but changes with development and the acquisition of knowledge. Furthermore, because similarity judgments are based on people's representations of entities, any developments in understanding the structure of the similarity system will be related to developments in understanding how concepts are represented and how this conceptual structure changes with knowledge acquisition.

One important issue that has emerged from the contributions to this volume is that of the distinction between surface similarity and deep similarity. Several contributors believe that there are systematic causal relations between the two and that similarity in the surface properties can be used as the basis from which to infer similarity in deeper (or more central) properties. Further progress in this area, however, depends crucially on a better understanding of what constitutes more surface versus deep similarity and how this distinction is related to conceptual structure.

The question of analogical mapping has been approached from a number of different points of view (e.g., structure-mapping, pragmatic). Also, various computational approaches to analogical mapping have been presented. It has become clear that, from the production point of view, analogical reasoning is a common mechanism used by novices and children to solve problems and answer questions. However, experts use analogical reasoning too. When they do, the main problem becomes one of access rather than one of mapping.

Explicit analogies can also be used for the purpose of instruction. Here, the question of access becomes irrelevant because the analog is given. Now, the question of mapping comes into focus, particularly in situations where the person who has to understand the analogy has a relatively impoverished structure for the target domain. In this situation, mapping is likely to result in a richer representation. It would be a mistake to suppose, however, that the communicative and instructional force of an analogy is restricted to the creation of new cognitive structures. Analogy may sometimes serve the purpose of highlighting what is already known. This highlighting could be effected either through changing the salience of the properties of the target representation or by providing a metaphorical way of labeling relations that are difficult to express using literal language.

Finally, the views presented in this volume have some important practical applications. For example, it appears that analogical learning and transfer of knowledge are facilitated when people are taught in problem-oriented learning environments as opposed to being taught facts; when the surface similarity between what is taught and the situations in which it needs to be transferred is enhanced; and when students are encouraged to take many perspectives and to look at objects from different points of view.

REFERENCES

Carbonell, J. G. (1983). Learning by analogy: Formulating and generalizing plans from past experience. In R. S. Michalski, J. G. Carbonell, & T. M. Mitchell (Eds.), *Machine learning: An artificial intelligence approach* (Vol. 1, pp. 137–161). Palo Alto, CA: Tioga.

Carey, S. (1985). *Conceptual change in childhood*. Cambridge, MA: MIT Press (Bradford Books).

Chi, M. T. H., Feltovich, P. J., & Glaser, R. (1981). Categorization and representation of physics problems by experts and novices. *Cognitive Science, 5*, 121–152.

Gentner, D., & Landers, R. (1985, November). Analogical reminding: A good match is hard to find. *Proceedings of the International Conference on Systems, Man and Cybernetics*, Tucson, AZ.

Gick, M.L., & Holyoak, K.J. (1980). Analogical problem solving. *Cognitive Psychology, 12*, 306–355.

Gick, M.L.. & Holyoak, K.J. (1983). Schema induction and analogical transfer. *Cognitive Psychology, 15*, 1–38.

Holyoak, K. J., & Koh, K. (1986). *Analogical problem solving: Effects of surface and structural similarity*. Paper presented at the annual meeting of the Midwestern Psychological Association, Chicago.

Kahneman, D., & Tversky, A. (1972). Subjective probability: A judgment of representativeness. *Cognitive Psychology, 3*, 430–454.

Kahneman, D., & Tversky, A. (1973). On the psychology of prediction. *Psychological Review, 80*, 237–251.

Novick, L. R. (1988). Analogical transfer, problem similarity, and expertise. *Journal of Experimental Psychology: Learning, Memory, and Cognition, 14*, 510–520.

Tversky, A., & Kahneman, D. (1982). Judgments of and by representativeness. In D. Kahneman, P. Slovic, & A. Tversky (Eds.), *Judgment under uncertainty: Heuristics and biases* (pp. 84–98). Cambridge: Cambridge University Press.

Tversky, A., & Kahneman, D. (1983). Extensional versus intuitive reasoning; The conjunction fallacy in probability judgment. *Psychological Review, 90*, 293–315.

Vosniadou, S., & Brewer, W. F. (1987). Theories of knowledge restructuring in development. *Review of Educational Research, 57*, 51–67.

Similarity and the structure of concepts

The contributions included in Part I have something to say either about similarity itself or about how people's conceptual representations affect similarity judgments. The papers by Lance Rips and by Edward Smith and Daniel Osherson look at similarity from the point of view of the role it plays in other psychological processes, like categorization and decision making. Rips argues that, although similarity may provide some cues to an object's category identity, it fails to provide an adequate explanation of people's category judgments. In contrast, Smith and Osherson believe that similarity plays an important role in decision making. They propose an explicit model wherein a person estimates the probability that an object belongs to a certain class by relying on the similarity the object bears to a prototype of the class. Linda Smith discusses the issue of how the complex system of similarity kinds that people use may develop.

Lawrence Barsalou's chapter deals with the question of instability (or flexibility) in people's conceptual representations and its implications for a theory of similarity. The contribution by Ryszard Michalski has been placed in Part I because it extends some of Barsalou's arguments about the flexibility of conceptual representations and offers a method for achieving such flexibility in a computer model of induction. Finally, Douglas Medin and Andrew Ortony discuss the contributions to Part I and also present their own views about similarity and, particularly, about the role that similarity might play in categorization.

1

Similarity, typicality, and categorization

LANCE J. RIPS

Here is a simple and appealing idea about the way people decide whether an object belongs to a category: The object is a member of the category if it is sufficiently similar to known category members. To put this in more cognitive terms, if you want to know whether an object is a category member, start with a representation of the object and a representation of the potential category. Then determine the similarity of the object representation to the category representation. If this similarity value is high enough, then the object belongs to the category; otherwise, it does not. For example, suppose you come across a white three-dimensional object with an elliptical profile; or suppose you read or hear a description like the one I just gave you. You can calculate a measure of the similarity between your mental representation of this object and your prior representation of categories it might fit into. Depending on the outcome of this calculation, you might decide that similarity warrants calling the object an egg, perhaps, or a turnip or a Christmas ornament.

This simple picture of categorizing seems intuitively right, especially in the context of pattern recognition. A specific egg – one you have never seen before – looks a lot like other eggs. It certainly looks more like eggs than it looks like members of most other categories. And so it is hard to escape the conclusion that something about this resemblance *makes* it an egg or, at least, makes us think it's one. In much the same way, if you happen to be a subject in a concept-learning experiment and are told that your job is to decide on each trial whether a meaningless pattern of dots is a member of Category A or of Category B, then you might be right to think that resemblance must be the key to the correct answer. You may have nothing else to go on. Or again, in the case of a child learning what things should be called *egg*, it seems very likely that perceptual similarity to previously labeled eggs – and perhaps perceptual *dis*similarity to certain kinds of noneggs – will play a big role in the developmental story. (Even for artificial categories and even for children's classification, similarity might not be the *whole* story; we shall return to this later in discussing results due to Carey, 1982; Fried & Holyoak, 1984; and Keil, 1986.)

But despite the intuitive appeal of this *resemblance* approach to categorizing, it has lately come in for some criticism. This criticism stems from philosophical discussions of similarity, particularly by Goodman (1970) and Quine (1969), but these antiresemblance views are now gaining ground in psychology too (Murphy & Medin, 1985; Oden & Lopes, 1982). For example, in a recent *Psychological Review* paper, Murphy and Medin (1985) argue that similarity is just too loose a notion to explain categorization adequately. Following Goodman (1970), they assert that similarity is highly relative and context-dependent: Our judgment of what is similar to what, according to this view, depends on the kinds of objects, properties, relations, and categories that we happen to have learned. But if that is right, then psychological similarity may depend on categorization rather than the other way around. In other words, the resemblance theory of categorization is vacuous unless we can specify how similarity is determined without begging the very questions about categorization that it is supposed to solve. But, in Murphy and Medin's view, the prospect for this is dim. They advocate an alternative approach in which concepts are taken to be minitheories about the nature of the categories they describe. Categorizing an object is then a matter of applying the relevant theory. So, on this view, everyday classification is very much like scientific classification, with the proviso that lay theories are likely to be less accurate and less detailed than those of scientists.

If this conclusion is correct, it has important implications, since it undercuts a whole class of models in cognitive psychology. In general, I think their conclusion *is* right, but I would like to try in this discussion to argue for it from a different angle. One reason for doing this is that you might question whether similarity is really as relative as Murphy and Medin make it out. True, there is evidence that similarity ratings in psychological experiments depend on context; they depend on the set of things that the subject is rating (Tversky, 1977; Tversky & Gati, 1978). But is this variation in ratings due to a change in our sense of similarity, or is it due instead to the constraints of translating this sense into a response on a one-dimensional rating scale? Murphy and Medin's arguments (as well as the arguments of their philosophical sources) have a 1950s-style New Look about them – things resemble each other because you believe they are in the same category – a view few psychologists these days wholeheartedly endorse. Second, you might also feel that the choice of theory-based models over similarity-based models is not as clear-cut as Murphy and Medin believe.

After all, does the notion of a theory really provide a firmer foundation for everyday categories? Even if similarity is as vague and variable as they claim, surely theories – especially lay theories – are not noticeably less vague or less variable. On first glance, the two types of models don't present much to choose from. Why not stick with similarity, then, where at least we have some inkling of the shape that a model would take, thanks to work by Tversky (1977) and others?[1]

In any event, what I would like to argue is this: Even if we grant that people have a stable sense of resemblance or similarity and even if we can give this sense a correct psychological description, similarity still will not be either necessary or sufficient for dealing with all object categories. As long as we stick to the ordinary meaning of similarity – the meaning that it has for nonexperts – then similarity will not be enough to explain human concepts and categories. To convince you of this, I'll present evidence from a set of experiments in which subjects were asked either to categorize an instance or to judge its similarity with respect to two potential categories. These experiments demonstrate that the favored response sometimes differs in the two tasks; that is, subjects may judge the instance more similar to Category A than to Category B but also judge the same instance more likely to be a member of Category B than Category A. On the basis of these results, I'll claim that there are factors that affect categorization but not similarity and other factors that affect similarity but not categorization. In other words, if all this goes through, there is a "double dissociation" between categorization and similarity, proving that one cannot be reduced to the other.

I'll begin by reminding you of the role that similarity plays in some well-known psychological theories of categorization, since that should make it easier to see exactly what damage would be done by undermining the resemblance theory. With this as background, I'll then describe two experiments that purport to show that similarity cannot be all there is to categorizing. That's the easy part. I'll then mention two more experiments that try to show that, for some concepts, similarity and categorization are actually independent. That's the hard part. A word of warning: None of these experiments is very high-tech. They all rely on simple ratings collected from groups of subjects. Some of them also make use of rather bizarre categories as stimuli. I'll try to head off some objections on this score in finishing up.

The role of similarity in theories of categorization

To start out, let's take a look at how similarity enters into models of categorization. Figure 1.1 lists several kinds of models, with those at

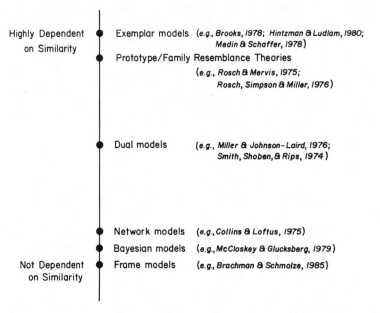

Highly Dependent
on Similarity

Exemplar models *(e.g., Brooks, 1978; Hintzman & Ludlam, 1980;*
Medin & Schaffer, 1978)
Prototype/Family Resemblance Theories
(e.g., Rosch & Mervis, 1975;
Rosch, Simpson & Miller, 1976)

Dual models   *(e.g., Miller & Johnson-Laird, 1976;*
Smith, Shoben, & Rips, 1974)

Network models   *(e.g., Collins & Loftus, 1975)*
Bayesian models   *(e.g., McCloskey & Glucksberg, 1979)*
Frame models   *(e.g., Brachman & Schmolze, 1985)*

Not Dependent
on Similarity

Figure 1.1. A summary of major approaches to categorization, arranged according to their theoretical dependence on resemblance.

the top being most dependent on similarity and those at the bottom least dependent. This list of models is far from complete, of course, and you should take it only as a very rough guide to the categorization terrain. The part that similarity plays clearly depends on what the theory takes to be the mental representation of categories; and a good rule of thumb might be that the more concrete the representation, the more dependent the theory is on similarity. In general, models at the top of the continuum assume fairly concrete representations, whereas those at the bottom are much more abstract. Beginning at the more dependent end, we have those theories that represent categories as specific instances. According to this type of approach, you mentally represent the category of eggs, say, in terms of memories of specific eggs that you have actually encountered. These exemplar theories, as they are usually called, are largely at the mercy of similarity. That is because, if your only source of knowledge about a category is a record of the exemplars you have seen, then the only way for you to decide if a new instance is also a member is to compare that instance to the remembered ones.[2]

A good example of the exemplar approach is the model proposed by Medin and Schaffer (1978), which they call the "context theory." According to Medin and Schaffer, if you have to decide whether a given instance is a member of one of several categories, you do it by retrieving from memory a category member that the target instance reminds you of. The member that you retrieve then determines the category of the new instance. For example, if the target instance happens to remind you of a particular egg – maybe the one you had for breakfast today – then you will classify this new instance as an egg too. For our purposes, the important point is that the instance you are reminded of is assumed to be entirely a function of similarity. Medin and Schaffer put it like this: "The probability of classifying exemplar i into category j is an increasing function of the similarity of exemplar i to stored category j exemplars and a decreasing function of the similarity of exemplar i to stored exemplars associated with alternative categories" (Medin & Schaffer, 1978, p. 211). This reliance on similarity is also apparent in other instance-based approaches – for example, in the MINERVA model of Hintzman and Ludlam (1980) and in work of members of the Canadian School of Nonanalytic Psychology (e.g., Brooks, 1978; Jacoby & Brooks, 1984).

Similarity also plays a crucial role in models that represent categories as prototypes or as central values of their instances. Simple versions of such models assign an instance to a category if the instance meets some criterial level of similarity to the prototype or, at least, is more similar to this prototype than to those of other categories. Within the framework of these models, it seems natural to think of the similarity between instance and prototype as the *typicality* of the instance with respect to the category: The more similar an instance is to the prototype, the more typical it is of the category, and the more likely it will be classified as a category member. This relationship among similarity, typicality, and categorization makes a tidy package, since it allows us to explain in a unified way a large portion of the data from experiments on natural concepts. Rosch and others demonstrated that subjects are more likely to produce typical members as examples of a given category, to learn them earlier, and to classify them faster than atypical members. Under the simple prototype theory, these effects, and others like them, are all consequences of the similarity between the instance and the category prototype. (Smith & Medin, 1981, is the classic review of these findings.)

However, Rosch's own ideas about categories were more complex. She believed, in fact, that a prototype was merely "a convenient grammatical fiction" (Rosch, 1978, p. 40), except in the case of certain artificially generated categories. The relative typicality of an instance, on her account, could be the result of a variety of structural principles, of which the most important is probably family resemblance of category members (Rosch & Mervis, 1975; Rosch, Simpson, & Miller, 1976). But as the term *family resemblance* implies, typicality and category membership are closely related to similarity, even in this more complicated theory. Rosch held that prototypicality is equivalent to degree of category membership; and, for any given instance, prototypicality is a function of how similar the instance is to other category members and how dissimilar it is to members of contrast categories. (Tversky, 1977, also gives an account in which the family resemblance of an instance within a category reduces to the combined similarity between that instance and other category members.)[3]

Exemplar and prototype models are tied to similarity willy-nilly; but similarity also shows up in other sorts of categorization theories in a less pure form. For instance, the *dual models* in Figure 1.1 distinguish between identification procedures that use similarity to make relatively fast, error-prone decisions and a core system that has access to deeper conceptual properties. For example, according to the feature comparison model (Smith, Shoben, & Rips, 1974), categories were supposed to be represented as sets of semantic features or attributes. We explained categorization as a two-part process, where the first part was devoted to determining the overall similarity between instance and category by comparing all of the features associated with them. The second part of this model was supposed to be more analytic, but the first part clearly committed us to the view that similarity is an important component in category decisions. What we said at the time was that the "contrast between early holistic and later analytic processing accords well with our introspections that decisions about logical matters are sometimes made quickly on a basis of similarity, while at other times decisions are the result of a more deliberative process" (Smith et al., 1974, p. 223).

Finally, at the far end of the continuum, we have network models (e.g., Collins & Loftus, 1975), frame models (Brachman & Schmolze, 1985), and Bayesian models (McCloskey & Glucksberg, 1979). All of these proposals can presumably accommodate effects of similarity on category decisions (perhaps as a by-product of other processes), but they do not give similarity a privileged role. These models are adequately described elsewhere (e.g., Rumelhart & Norman, 1988; Smith & Medin, 1981), and I will have nothing to say about them in what follows. However, their presence at the bottom of Figure 1.1 is a reminder that there are approaches to categorization other than those based on resemblance. For the rest of this discussion, then, I'll concentrate on what we can call *pure resemblance theories*, such as exemplar and prototype models, with just a word about dual models at the end.

In sum, similarity plays a key role in many of the best-known theories of concepts, and it does so in two interrelated ways: (*a*) Similarity determines the typicality of an instance with respect to a category; and (*b*) similarity determines the probability that people will classify an instance as a category member. One way to put these ideas together is to assume first that similarity accounts for typicality; that is, typicality just *is* either similarity of an instance to a prototype or average similarity of the instance to known category members. Second, typicality in turn measures the degree of category membership. And, finally, degree of membership explains categorization probability. A trout is generally similar in size, shape, and other characteristics to other fish, and it is generally dissimilar to members of contrast classes like mammals and reptiles. Subjects therefore believe trouts to be typical fish, assume that trouts enjoy a high degree of membership in the fish category, and are very likely to categorize trouts as fish. That's the resemblance theory of concepts in a nutshell. If we can show that it is wrong, then the pure resemblance models are in trouble.

Is similarity all there is to categorizing?

In its pure form, resemblance theory claims that similarity assessment is really all there is to categorizing. The probability that a subject will assign an instance to a category is solely a function of similarity, where similarity can be computed as resemblance to one or more previously classified category members, to a prototype, or to some other representative of the category. We can also allow this similarity computation to include degree of dissimilarity to other categories. However, no other factors (apart from random error) influence category decisions. In order to be sporting, we can further concede that resemblance theory applies only to categories of natural kinds and artifacts. Clearly, resemblance theory doesn't have a chance with what Barsalou (1985; this volume) calls "goal-derived" categories such as things-to-take-with-you-on-a-vacation, since there is no reason to think that bathing suits and toothbrushes belong to this category because of their similarity to each other or to other category members. Indeed, Barsalou (1985) found that, for goal-derived categories, average similarity to other category members was not a very good predictor of an instance's rated goodness of membership within the category.

Effects of variability on categorization

Obviously, one way to disconfirm the resemblance theory is to find a factor that affects categorization but not similarity. Let me suggest that one such factor might be constraints on variability among category members. In order to clarify what I mean, consider this problem: Suppose there are two categories, one of which is relatively variable and the other relatively fixed on some physical dimension. An example might be the categories of pizzas and U.S. quarters (i.e., 25-cent pieces), since pizzas are relatively variable and quarters relatively fixed in their diameters. Now suppose there is an object about which you know only that it has a 3-inch diameter, and consider two questions about it: First, is it more likely to be a pizza or a quarter? And second, is it more similar to pizzas or to quarters? The answer to the first question clearly seems to be that the object is a pizza; for even though 3 inches is much smaller than the pizzas you usually encounter it is easy to imagine making one this small. It is harder (though not impossible) to imagine how a 3-inch quarter could come about. But, now, what about the similarity question? This one is not as clear-cut, perhaps. Yet it seems in this case that limitations governing the size of quarters do not play such a crucial role. Instead, it is plausible to take into account the simple difference in size between the 3-inch object and normal quarters or pizzas, and this may lead you to say that the object is more similar to quarters. After all, it is probably closer to the diameter of an average quarter than to the diameter of an average pizza.

To see if there really is a difference in the answers to categorization and similarity questions, we ran an experiment using 36 problems similar to the one I just mentioned. We told subjects that we were about to ask them some questions about pairs of common categories and about dimensions along which these categories varied. In every case, one of these categories was relatively fixed on the dimension in question, either by official decree or by convention, whereas the other category was relatively free to vary. For example, one trial concerned the pizzas-and-quarters pair. The diameter of quarters is presumably fixed by law, but the diameter of pizzas certainly varies widely. Other examples of categories and dimensions include: the volumes of tennis balls and teapots, the number of members in the U.S. Senate and in rock groups, the heights of volleyball nets and automobiles, and the durations of basketball games and dinner parties. The first member in each of these pairs seems relatively fixed and the second relatively variable.

We also manipulated which category – the fixed or the variable one – had normally larger values on the specified dimensions. On half of the trials, the fixed category was smaller, as in the pizza–quarter example. On the other trials, we chose the categories so that the fixed category was larger. For instance, we also included a trial concerning the diameters of basketball hoops and grapefruit, in which the fixed category (basketball hoops) has the larger values.

During an individual trial the subject's first task was to estimate the value of the largest member of the small category and the smallest member of the large category that he or she could remember. In the pizza–quarter case, for example, the subject gave us the diameter of the smallest pizza and the diameter of the largest quarter. We then told the subject that we were concerned with an object with a specific value, which we had calculated to be exactly half-way between the two extreme values he or she had named. So if the subject had said that the smallest remembered pizza was 5 inches in diameter and that the largest quarter was 1 inch, we told the subject that we were thinking of an object with a diameter of 3 inches. This intermediate value was calculated separately for each subject.

In one condition, we then asked subjects to decide which of the two categories the intermediate object belonged to; in a second condition, they chose which category the intermediate object was more typical of; and in a third condition, they chose which category the object was more similar to. For pizzas and quarters, the subject had to decide for the hypothetical object whether it was a quarter or a pizza, whether it was more typical of a quarter or a pizza, or whether it was more similar to a quarter or a pizza. This task was a between-subjects variable in this experiment, so that a given subject made only category decisions, only typicality decisions, or only similarity decisions. It is important to realize that all subjects received the same information about the categories. Moreover, there was nothing in the descriptions or instructions that encouraged subjects in the Similarity group to use one sort of property as the basis of their decision and subjects in the Typicality or Categorization groups to use some other property (except, perhaps, the very words *similarity*, *typicality*, and *category membership*).

Figure 1.2 displays subjects' choices in the three tasks, plotted as the percentage of subjects who chose the fixed category. It shows as separate functions those trials in which the fixed category was smaller (as in the pizza–quarter example) and those in which the fixed category was larger (as in the case of the basketball hoop–grapefruit pair). The first thing to notice about the results is that most subjects in the

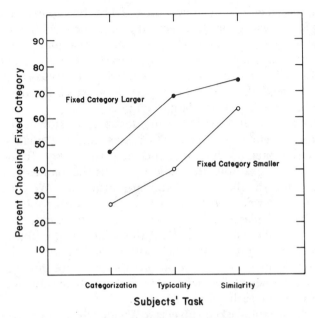

Figure 1.2. Percentage of subjects choosing the fixed category over the variable category in the Categorization, Typicality, and Similarity groups. The top function represents pairs in which the fixed category was the larger member; the bottom function represents pairs in which the fixed category was smaller.

Categorization group say that the mystery object belongs to the variable category, whereas most subjects in the Similarity group say that the object is more similar to the fixed category. The Typicality group fell in between. Over all stimulus items, 37% of the Categorization group, 54% of the Typicality group, and 69% of the Similarity group chose the fixed category. This difference is reliable, when either subjects or stimuli serve as the random variable. (This is true as well for all differences that I'll refer to as significant.)

We would expect Categorization subjects to choose the variable category if they were taking into account known constraints on the variability of these items. It may be less clear, however, why the Similarity subjects prefer the fixed category. But recall that we picked the value of the mystery item to be midway between the smallest member of the large category and the largest member of the small category. Since one of these categories is highly variable and the other fixed, the mystery instance would tend to be closer to the mean of the fixed category than to the mean of the variable category. So if the Similarity subjects were making their decision according

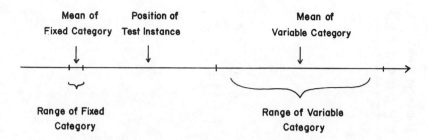

Figure 1.3. Hypothetical arrangement of fixed category, variable category, and test instance on a physical continuum.

to absolute distance between the instance and the average category value, this setup would favor the fixed category. Figure 1.3 illustrates this point. Suppose that a subject tells us that the smallest pizza is 5 inches and the largest quarter 1 inch. Then the mystery instance would be 3 inches in diameter, as mentioned earlier. Assuming that the average diameter of a pizza is 12 inches and the average diameter of a quarter is 1 inch, then the instance would be 2 inches from the average quarter but 9 inches from the average pizza.

One further fact about these data may be of interest. The distance between the two functions in Figure 1.2 shows that in all three groups subjects were biased toward choosing the larger of the two categories. Subjects were more likely to pick the fixed category given a choice between, say, basketball hoops and grapefruits than when they were given the choice between quarters and pizzas. This may be due merely to the particular categories we used as stimuli, since different category pairs appeared in these two conditions. Perhaps you could also explain this difference in terms of a Weber–Fechner function. For although the mystery item was numerically midway between the subjects' extreme values, it may have been subjectively closer to the larger category. This would have increased the chances that subjects would pick the larger category, which is the result that we obtained. A final possibility is that the difference has to do with how easy it is to imagine altering the fixedness of the fixed category. It may be intuitively easier for a fixed category to become smaller than to become larger; for example, several of the subjects in the Categorization group, when asked whether an intermediate-sized object was more likely to be a paper clip or a foot ruler, said that it was more likely to be a "broken ruler." In Kahneman and Tversky's (1982) terms, a change from large to small is a "downhill" change, whereas a change in the

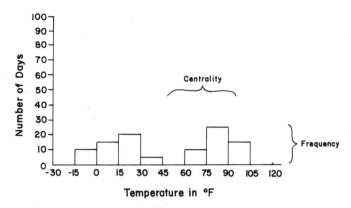

Figure 1.4. Sample histogram of the subjective distribution of daily high Chicago temperatures in January and July.

opposite direction is "uphill." If this factor enters into all three of the subjects' tasks, it could also account for the larger–smaller difference.[4]

Effects of other distributional properties

The results of the experiment just described suggest that the potential variability of category members influences categorization but has a weak impact, if any, on similarity judgments. If this is right, then it is going to be difficult to reduce categorization to similarity. Allan Collins has come up with a way to explore this relationship further, using the form of the category's density function, and it is worthwhile to report some data that Collins and I have collected (Collins & Rips, in preparation) because they provide evidence that reinforces some of the conclusions from the previous study.

To see how Collins's idea works, imagine that a meteorologist is studying daily high temperatures in Chicago, half of which occurred during the month of January and half during July. If we were to graph these temperatures, we would presumably get a bimodal distribution of values, such as the distribution in Figure 1.4. Now consider temperature readings between 45° and 60°, and ask yourself how likely it is that temperatures in this interval are among the values the meteorologist is studying, how typical they are of these temperatures, and how similar they are to the temperatures. Intuitively, the probability seems relatively low that 45°– 60° temperatures are in this set, since they fall between the peaks of the distribution. And for the same reason they may not be especially typical. The question about similarity again seems a bit more difficult to answer; but 45°–60° is fairly close to the center of the distribution, so on average the similarity may be reasonably high. The advantage of a bimodal distribution is that it allows us to separate the effect of frequency from the effect of distance to the center of the distribution. Collins's notion was that these two factors might have differential impact on judgments about categorization, typicality, and similarity.

In our preliminary work, we gave subjects 18 problems like the one about temperatures. All of these problems involved impromptu categories composed of a mixture of elements, a mixture that we hoped would convey to subjects a bimodal distribution along a particular dimension. In addition to the temperature example, we used a problem about the weights of 100 children, half of whom were 5-year-olds and half 15-year-olds. Another problem concerned hair length of 100 teenagers, half of whom were boys and half girls.

The experiment itself consisted of two sessions. In the first one, subjects rated the likelihood, typicality, or similarity of each of a set of intervals with respect to the categories defined by the problems. On one of the trials, for example, we told our Similarity subjects that a meteorologist was studying 100 daily high temperatures in Chicago, half of which were in January and half in July. We then asked them to rate the similarity of temperatures within particular intervals to the temperatures in this set. They rated the similarity of temperatures between −30° and −15° to the temperatures studied by the meteorologist, the similarity of temperatures between −15° and 0°, between 0° and 15°, and so on. There were 10 to 11 such intervals for each problem, spanning what we hoped would be the relevant range of values (see Figure 1.4). Subjects in the Typicality group received problems of the same sort, but they rated the typicality of each interval with respect to the set. Finally, subjects in the Categorization group rated the likelihood that temperatures in each interval were among the temperatures in the set. Each group contained 12 subjects. In the second session of the experiment, subjects from all three groups received a description of the same categories in a new random order. But this time we gave them graph paper and asked them to draw a histogram for these categories. For instance, one of their problems was to draw a histogram of the distribution of temperatures that the meteorologist was studying. The intervals that we marked off on the base of the histogram corresponded to the intervals they had been quizzed about in the earlier session.

For each problem and for each subject, then, we have two kinds of information: a frequency histogram and ratings of similarity, typi-

Table 1.1. *Mean standardized regression weights (β's) for ratings as a function of histogram frequency and centrality*

	Rating type		
	Categorization	Typicality	Similarity
Frequency	.47	.41	.33
Centrality	− .01	.09	.17

cality, or category likelihood. Our aim was to see whether aspects of the distribution differentially influenced the ratings, and we therefore extracted two measures from each of the distributions. One measure was simply the height of the histogram at each interval; the other was a measure of how close that interval was to the median value of the histogram.[5] I'll call the first of these measures the *frequency* of the interval and the second the *centrality* of the interval. Figure 1.4 illustrates these measures for a sample histogram of the temperature problem.

Our next step was to perform regression analyses in which the ratings served as the dependent variable and the frequency and centrality measures served as independent variables. We carried out three separate regressions, one each for the Similarity, Typicality, and Categorization groups. Table 1.1 lists the β weights (i.e., standardized regression coefficients) from these analyses. It is apparent that the categorization judgments are quite sensitive to frequency; so if an interval is near one of the peaks of the histogram, subjects tend to rate the interval as likely to be in the category. On the other hand, categorization ratings do not depend on how close the value is to the histogram's center. A value is just as likely (or unlikely) to be a category member whether it is in the middle of the distribution or is at an equally frequent point in the tails. For typicality judgments, there is a hint of a centrality effect and slightly less dependence on frequency. The similarity ratings continue this trend with a more robust centrality effect and a weakened effect of frequency. The interaction between rating type and measure (frequency or centrality) is significant in these data.

Implications

The two studies I have just described have some common properties that are worth noticing. In the first place, both experiments suggest that categorization is sensitive to distributional properties in a way that similarity decisions are not. In Study 1 this was manifest in the Categorization group's choice of the variable over the fixed category and in Study 2 by the correlation between frequency and category ratings. This evidence is also consistent with earlier experiments by Fried and Holyoak (1984), using artificial categories consisting of grids of filled and unfilled cells. They found, in particular, that subjects tended to classify test instances as members of a high-variable rather than a low-variable category, even when the instances were physically closer to the low-variable category's prototype. If category decisions, but not similarity decisions, depend on variability and like factors, then categorization cannot be equated with similarity.

A second commonality between the experiments is that similarity responses appear to depend on distance to the categories' central values. This relationship explains why the Similarity group in the first study preferred the fixed category to the variable one. It showed up again in the second study as a correlation between similarity and centrality. As we noted in the first part of this discussion, resemblance theories propose that people categorize instances in terms of distance to the categories' central tendency. It is ironic, then, that the results of the second study suggest that although centrality affects similarity judgments, it has no effect on categorization. This centrality factor also hints that we may be able to alter the similarity of an instance to a category without changing the probability that subjects will classify it as a category member. Experiments that I describe later pursue this hint.

A third common feature of these experiments is that typicality decisions appear to be a compromise between categorization and similarity. The usual story is that similarity is responsible for variations in typicality and that typicality itself is simply a measure of degree of category membership. However, the results so far suggest that although typicality may share properties with both similarity and probability of category membership it is identical with neither. As we shall see, this last conclusion will have to be reassessed in light of later results. Nevertheless, these parallels between the experiments are reassuring. Because you might object to the unnaturalness of forced choice in the first study, it is helpful to find similar results for ratings in the second. Likewise, the somewhat artificial mixture of categories in the second study is balanced by the more ordinary categories in the first.

Of course, we still need to be cautious before settling on an interpretation of these studies. One point that bears emphasis is that these data do not imply that similarity plays *no* part in category decisions. It is certainly possible that subjects' similarity judgments and their category judgments both depend on some common process. Maybe you could even call this a *similarity* or *resemblance* computation without doing too much violence to these terms. Likewise, similarity could sometimes serve as a heuristic for category assignment (as Medin & Ortony suggest in chapter 6). Neither possibility is at stake here. What I believe the studies do show, however, is that category decisions are not *solely* a matter of similarity (even in the special sense of a common underlying process): If they were, then factors like variability that affect categorization should also affect similarity judgments. Because resemblance theory is precisely the claim that categorization can be reduced to similarity alone, resemblance theory must be false.[6]

However, there is one way of salvaging resemblance theory that we need to consider carefully. This is the idea that resemblance itself may come in several varieties, one of which is responsible for categorization judgments and another for similarity judgments. For example, one explanation of the first study is that subjects in both the Categorization and the Similarity groups were computing the similarity between the mystery instance and the means (or other central values) of the two categories. However, Categorization subjects, according to this hypothesis, used normed distance, with distance to the variable category normed by the variable category's standard deviation and distance to the fixed category normed by the fixed category's standard deviation. Similarity subjects, on the other hand, used unnormed distance to the two means.

But, although this hypothesis accounts for the obtained difference, it does not accord with subjects' own view of the matter. In the first study, we asked subjects to talk aloud as they made their choice, and we recorded their responses. When Categorization subjects chose the variable category, they typically said that the mystery object *must* be a member of that category because members of the fixed category *can't* be that size. Here are some examples:

> *Subject A*: Is something with 170 members an English alphabet or a bowl of rice? "An English alphabet is restricted to 26 letters, but a bowl of rice can be any size; so it must be a bowl of rice."

> *Subject B*: Is an object that holds 1.75 cups a teapot or a tennis ball? "I'd say a teapot – a smaller teapot – because tennis balls would have to be the same size."

Is someone 20 years old a master chef or a cub scout? "I'd say he'd be a master chef, because I mean cub scouts – I mean the things like nickels [in an earlier problem] and things like that just seem real – I mean they just *can't* be outside of that age group or they're not even that thing anymore. So I can imagine a chef that's 20 years old, but it's just hard to imagine a cub scout that's that old."

Subject C: Is something 4.75 feet high a stop sign or a cereal box? "It would probably be one huge cereal box, because no one would see the stop sign if it were that small....A stop sign would have to be a certain height, and while I wouldn't expect to see a cereal box that big, it wouldn't make sense to have such a small sign."

Subject D: Is something 18.75 hours long Valentine's day or a final exam? "A final exam. I was thinking about that one and it wouldn't be a day or a Valentine's day according to any definition if it was 18 hours; so it would have to be some sadistic final exam."
    Is something with 47 members a jar of pickles or a deck of playing cards? "A jar of pickles, because if a deck of playing cards didn't have 52 or greater cards it wouldn't *be* a deck of playing cards."

Subjects' modal constructs in these examples – "it *must* be a bowl of rice"; "they just *can't* be outside of that age group or *they're not even that thing*"; "*would have to be* a certain height"; "it *wouldn't* be a day *according to any definition*" – indicate that they are engaging in a form of reasoning that goes beyond simple distance comparison. Subject C, for example, does not justify his choice on the grounds that 4.75 feet is closer to the size of a cereal box than to the size of a stop sign. Instead, he believes that something of that height simply can't be a stop sign ("it wouldn't make sense"); hence, by elimination, it must be a cereal box, which doesn't have these limitations on height. In other words, the relevant restrictions don't appear to be altering the subjects' sense of what's similar to what, but instead they act directly to rule out the very possibility that the mystery instance is a category member. For Subject C the restriction is a functional one (people would have trouble seeing such a short stop sign); in other cases it appears to be definitional (a day is defined as 24 hours long) or conventional (tennis balls have to be the same size).

Of course, it may well be true that there are multiple types of similarity that come into play at different stages of development (L. Smith, this volume) or for different purposes (Gentner, this volume); however, there is little evidence that such differences account for the above results. We will return to the multiple-similarity idea at the end of this chapter, armed with evidence from some additional studies.

The independence of similarity and category judgments

> *The Callitrices differ from the rest [of the monkeys] in nearly their whole appearance.*
>
> From a Latin bestiary (trans. White, 1954)

I have been arguing that categorizing may be more complex than resemblance theory would lead you to believe. In retrospect, it is not surprising that the purest of the pure resemblance models have been developed to account for classifying artificial categories of dot patterns, schematic faces, letter strings, and the like; subjects in these experiments have no information about the categories except what they can extract during the learning trials. But, for categories like eggs or quarters or Chicago temperatures, subjects know a lot; and some of this knowledge may simply be too abstract or too extrinsic to contribute to the categories' similarity, at least according to the meaning that subjects attach to *similarity*.

This way of viewing the issue suggests that similarity and categorization may be independent relations, in the sense that we can manipulate one of them with only minimal effects on the other. To investigate this question, we have looked for situations in which similarity could change without changing classification. And to provide a contrast we have also tried to construct cases in which an instance switches categories without a change in similarity. The first type of situation is one where an object's properties are accidentally transformed in such a way that they begin to resemble those of members of a different category. The second situation occurs when an object's properties are altered in a more essential way. Of course, *essential* in this context does not mean that the properties are necessarily true (*de re*) of the instance itself. An essential change is simply one that subjects believe is important to the instance's membership in a specified category, and an accidental change is one that is not important in this way.[7] For the sake of generality, we have carried out two experiments of this sort, one with natural kinds and the other with categories of artifacts.

Transformations on natural kinds

We tried to simulate the relevant situations for our subjects by means of a group of stories describing transformations that happen to imaginary animals. In the *Accident* condition, each story described a hypothetical animal in such a way that subjects were likely to identify it as a member of a particular category – either birds, fish, insects, reptiles, or mammals. The story then described the animal as undergoing some catastrophe that caused many of its surface properties to resemble those of one of the other categories. For example, an animal that started out as a bird might come to have some insect properties. The actual category labels *bird* and *insect*, however, did not appear in the story. The subjects were then asked to rate whether the animal was more likely to be a bird or an insect, whether it was more typical of a bird or an insect, and whether it was more similar to a bird or an insect. The subjects circled a number on a 10-point rating scale that had *bird* on one end and *insect* on the other. Each subject read and rated 10 stories, with each story corresponding to a different pair drawn from the five categories. Here, for example, is the story of the bird who became insectlike:

There was an animal called a sorp which, when it was fully grown, was like other sorps, having a diet which consisted of seeds and berries found on the ground or on plants. The sorp had two wings, two legs, and lived in a nest high in the branches of a tree. Its nest was composed of twigs and other fibrous plant material. This sorp was covered with bluish-gray feathers.

The sorp's nest happened to be not too far from a place where hazardous chemicals were buried. The chemicals contaminated the vegetation that the sorp ate, and as time went by it gradually began to change. The sorp shed its feathers and sprouted a new set of wings composed of a transparent membrane. The sorp abandoned its nest, developed a brittle iridescent outer shell, and grew two more pairs of legs. At the tip of each of the sorp's six legs an adhesive pad was formed so that it was able to hold onto smooth surfaces; for example, the sorp learned to take shelter during rainstorms by clinging upside down to the undersides of tree leaves. The sorp eventually sustained itself entirely on the nectar of flowers.

Eventually this sorp mated with a normal female sorp one spring. The female laid the fertilized eggs in her nest and incubated them for three weeks. After that time normal young sorps broke out of their shells.

We hoped that this story – besides alerting our subjects to the hazards of toxic wastes – would get them to rate the sorp more likely to be a bird but more similar to an insect. Half of the subjects in the Accident condition read the story just mentioned in which the sorp begins life with bird properties and ends with some insect properties. The other subjects read a similar story about an animal that begins with insect properties and acquires bird properties. For purposes of comparison, an Accident control group read a shortened form of the same stories, which described only the first, precatastrophe part of the animals' lives. These subjects, we felt sure, would rate the animal as uniformly more likely to be, more typical of, and more similar to the initial category. For example, we gave these control subjects the first, birdy part of the sorp description and expected them to rate the sorp as more likely to be a bird, more typical of a bird, and more similar to a bird.

In addition to the Accident condition and its control, we also included an *Essence* condition, whose purpose was to influence categorization ratings without influencing similarity. Subjects in this condition also read stories about animals that undergo some radical transformation; but this time the change was the result of maturation, similar to the change from a tadpole to a frog or from a caterpillar to a butterfly. The two halves of an animal's life were given separate names in order to mark this distinction. For example, this is the sorp's story as it appeared in the Essence condition:

> During an early stage of the doon's life it is known as a sorp. A sorp's diet mainly consists of seeds and berries found on the ground or on plants. A sorp has two wings, two legs, and lives in a nest high in the branches of a tree. Its nest is composed of twigs and other fibrous plant material. A sorp is covered with bluish-gray feathers.
>
> After a few months, the doon sheds its feathers, revealing that its wings are composed of a transparent membrane. The doon abandons its nest, develops a brittle, iridescent outer shell, and grows two more pairs of legs. At the tip of each of the doon's six legs an adhesive pad is formed so that it can hold onto smooth surfaces; for example, doons take shelter during rainstorms by clinging upside down to the undersides of tree leaves. A doon sustains itself entirely on the nectar of flowers.
>
> Doons mate in the late summer. The female doon deposits the eggs among thick vegetation where they will remain in safety until they hatch.

After reading each story, our subjects rated the similarity, typicality, and likely category membership of the animal's first stage. After the sorp/doon story, the subjects rated whether the sorp – not the doon – was more similar to a bird or an insect, more typical of a bird or an insect, and more likely to be a bird or an insect. We also included an Essence control condition, in which a new group of subjects read descriptions of only the animals' early stage and rated the same three dimensions. Each group contained 24 subjects. An individual subject always rated the dimensions in the same order; however, within a group, four subjects were assigned to each of the six permutations.

The results of this experiment are easy to relate. Let's look first at the mean ratings from the Accident condition and its control in Figure 1.5. The scale on the *y* axis is oriented in the figure so that high ratings correspond to the category of the animals' original appearance. For example, in the case of the sorp, which started off as a bird and

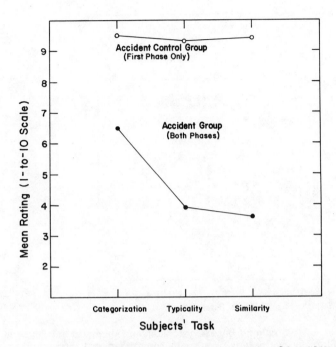

Figure 1.5. Mean ratings from Accident condition, Experiment 3. High numbers represent the category most like the animals' original appearance; low numbers, the category most like their later appearance. Top function is from Accident control subjects, and bottom function from Accident experimental subjects.

developed insect properties, high numbers indicate that subjects rated it as a bird, whereas low numbers indicate that they rated it as an insect. The control group (open circles in the figure) provides a base line in this experiment. This group read only the first-phase descriptions; and, as expected, they thought the animals similar to, typical of, and more likely to be members of this first-phase category. However, the experimental group's knowledge of the animals' later mishaps caused the ratings to shift in the direction of the alternative category, with a much greater drop for typicality and similarity ratings than for categorization ratings. Although we were unable to change similarity ratings without changing categorization at all, the interaction between groups and rating tasks is nevertheless reliable in these data. Notice, in particular, that the experimental subjects tended to think that a transformed animal is more likely to be a member of its first-phase category, but more similar to and more typical of the category whose properties it develops.

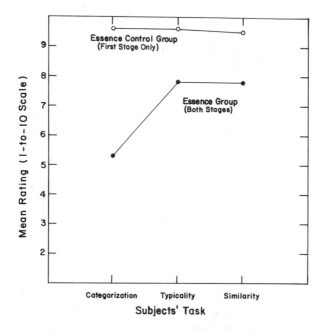

Figure 1.6. Mean ratings from Essence condition, Experiment 3. High numbers represent the category most like the animals' original appearance; low numbers, the category most like their later appearance. Top function is from Essence control subjects, and bottom function from Essence experimental subjects.

It is also worth noting that in this experiment (as well as in later ones) mean typicality is nearly equal to the similarity ratings. This differs from the results of the previous experiments in which typicality was somewhere between similarity and categorization. The change may be the result of moving from a between-subjects design to a within-subjects design on the three types of ratings. In none of the experiments, however, is typicality equivalent to category ratings, contrary to what you might expect on the assumption that typicality measures degree of category membership.

When we turn to the data from the Essence condition, we find a very different pattern of results. Figure 1.6 plots the mean ratings so that high numbers again correspond to the category most like the animals' initial description. For the birdlike sorp whose metamorphosis changed it into an insectlike doon, high numbers mean that subjects rated it as a bird and low numbers that they rated it as an insect. As before, the control group knew only about the first-stage properties, and their ratings are at ceiling. The experimental subjects learned about the animals' transformation, and this caused an obvious drop in scores. What is important, though, is that the decrease is significantly larger for categorization ratings than for either typicality or similarity ratings. In other words, facts about the animal's mature state clearly influence the way subjects classify the immature form but have much less effect on its similarity. This contrasts with the results from the Accident condition, where the big difference appeared in rated typicality and similarity. Taken together, these results give us the double dissociation that we were looking for.

Resemblance theories have trouble accounting for results from both Essence and Accident conditions; for if similarity and categorization amount to the same thing, then any increase or decrease in one should be accompanied by a like change in the other. What the results show is that similarity and category judgments are not perfectly correlated. It is certainly possible to induce relatively large effects on either type of decision with only relatively small effects on the other. Before drawing further conclusions, however, I want to mention the results from a final experiment on artifact categories like pajamas and radios. I will be brief because the design of this experiment parallels that of the animal study.

Transformations of artifacts

The distinction between essential and accidental changes seems more clear-cut in the case of natural kinds than in the case of artifacts. Natural kinds like reptiles or sugar or quasars have inner natures that can support lawlike generalizations (e.g., All reptiles are cold-blooded) and counterfactual conditionals (e.g., If Rudolph were a reptile, he'd be cold-blooded). Artifacts, on the other hand, do not have inner natures, at least on some theories of these objects (Schwartz, 1980). It is certainly unlikely that scientists would ever seriously study the nature of, say, umbrellas; and likewise, *umbrella* is hardly the kind of term that we would expect to show up in scientific laws. If subjects adopt this view of artifacts, they may conceive of all changes to these objects as accidental changes; they may believe that there simply isn't any essence to change. On the other hand, certain properties of artifacts, although perhaps not strictly necessary, are clearly important in qualifying an object as a category member. It is possible that changes to these properties may be enough to shake subjects' confidence in the object's membership status. In the protocol examples from the first study, Subject D apparently takes this attitude toward decks of playing cards, saying that collections with less than 52 cards "wouldn't *be* a deck of playing cards." Changes to properties of this sort may produce the same effects as essential changes to natural kinds.

Of course, accidental changes are easy to produce, since artifacts can undergo all sorts of surface alterations without necessarily becoming a member of a new category. To cite one of the stimulus stories, you can imagine altering an umbrella so that it looks much like a lampshade. As long as the object is still used to keep off the rain, it remains an umbrella; it has not switched categories. The actual story read like this:

> Carol Q. has an object which is a collapsible fabric dome. It consists of multicolored waterproof fabric stretched taut across six metal struts radiating from a central post in the dome. The metal struts are jointed so that they may be folded and this allows the fabric dome to be collapsed. When fully extended the dome is about three feet wide. Carol uses this object to protect her from getting wet when she is walking in the rain.
> Carol saw an article in a fashion magazine about a new style for objects such as this which she copied with her own. She added a pale pink satin covering to the outside surface, gathering it at the top and at the bottom so that it has pleats. Around the bottom edge of the object she attached a satin fringe. To the inside of the dome at the top she attached a circular frame that at its center holds a light bulb. Carol still uses this object to protect her from the rain.

As expected, it proved more difficult to come up with essential changes in an artifact while preserving its similarity to its original category. Our first thought was that we could do this by stipulating a new function for the object – for example, by describing an umbrella that someone comes to use as a lampshade. But this ploy didn't work. Subjects in a pilot study insisted that the umbrella remained an umbrella no matter how people happened to use it. Clearly, function is not the sole criterion for classifying artifacts. Eventually, it occurred to us that a better way to produce an essential change in an artifact was to specify the intentions of the designer who produced it. For example, we could describe an object that looks exactly like an umbrella; then, by telling subjects that its designer meant it as a lampshade we might be able to convince them that it was a lampshade that just happens to resemble an umbrella. Here is the umbrella/lampshade story we constructed:

> Carol Q. of CMR Manufacturing designed an object which is a collapsible fabric dome. It consists of multicolored waterproof fabric stretched taut across six metal struts radiating from a central post in the dome. The metal struts are jointed so that they may be folded and this allows the fabric dome to be collapsed. When fully extended the dome is about three feet wide.
> Carol intended for this object to be used with the inside of the dome facing

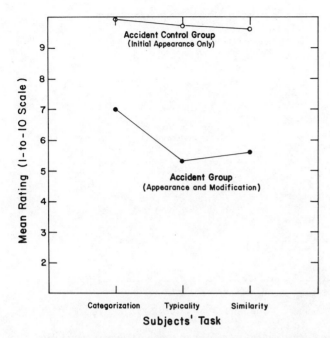

Figure 1.7. Mean ratings from accident condition, Experiment 4. High numbers represent the category most like the artifacts' original description; low numbers, the category most like their later appearance. Top function is from Accident control subjects, and bottom function from Accident experimental subjects.

up as an attachment to ceiling light fixtures. Attached in that way the multicolored fabric filters the light emanating from an overhead light fixture.

We composed 18 stories describing accidental changes, each story dealing with a different pair of common artifacts. An additional 18 stories described essential changes to the same artifact pairs. As in the previous experiment, these two sets of stories were given to separate groups of subjects, who rated similarity, typicality, and likelihood of category membership. We also tested two control groups, who received just the first parts of the object descriptions. Each of the four groups contained 12 subjects.

Mean ratings from the Accident group and its control appear in Figure 1.7, with larger values on the *y* axis again indicating ratings congruent with the instance's original category. Although the effect is not as dramatic as it was for the natural categories, we were able to decrease similarity and typicality ratings significantly more than category ratings. Carol's fashionable umbrella – decorated with satin

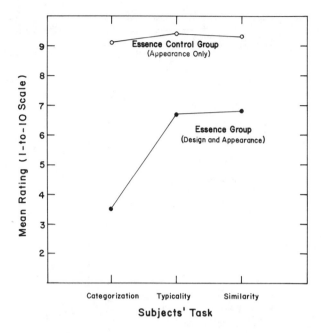

Figure 1.8. Mean ratings from Essence condition, Experiment 4. High numbers represent the category most like the artifacts' original description; low numbers, the category most like the designers' intention. Top function is from Essence control subjects, and bottom function from Essence experimental subjects.

ruffles and a light bulb – is still an umbrella but no longer especially similar to or typical of one. We can compare these results to those in Figure 1.8 from the Essence group and its control. Specifying the intentions of the object's designer completely changed the way subjects classified the object, even though the object still resembled members of the alternative category. If Carol designs an object as a lampshade, then it *is* a lampshade despite looking much like an umbrella.

Both natural kinds and artifacts, then, exhibit some independence between properties that make them resemble members of this or that category and properties that qualify them as category members. The essential properties for natural kinds apparently have to do with the mature, reproductive state of the organism, whereas the essential properties of artifacts lie in the intentions of their designers. The results for natural kinds have some precedents in the developmental literature. For example, Carey (1982) notes that 4-year-olds rate people as being more similar to toy monkeys than to (real) worms. Yet, when taught a new property about people – that they have a green thing called a spleen inside them – these children were more likely to say that worms have spleens than that toy monkeys do. Apparently, brute resemblance does not mediate generalization of specifically biological characteristics, even in young kids. In research that is closer to our own methods, Keil (1986) told his subjects about animals that undergo surgical procedures that change their surface properties to those of a different species. Keil's example is a raccoon that comes to look exactly like a skunk as the result of "cosmetic" surgery. When asked which category the animal belonged to – raccoon or skunk – most kindergarten children insisted that it had become a skunk; most fourth-graders and adults, however, classified it as a raccoon. Unfortunately, Keil did not collect similarity judgments, but it seems likely that both younger and older subjects thought the animal more similar to a skunk, especially since they saw a picture of a skunk as an illustration. If this is correct, then in Keil's experiment, too, underlying biological properties are countermanding similarity.

Where did resemblance theory go wrong?

Resemblance theory suffers two deficiencies. First, it has trouble with factors such as variability, frequency, underlying biological properties, and personal intentions that affect how an instance is classified but do not much affect the instance's similarity. These properties have a common characteristic: They are all hidden from a casual view of the instance. None are obvious parts of the instance, either because they are relational or because they are discernible only with scientific acumen. It is likely that this extrinsic or nonpart status disqualifies these properties (in our subjects' opinion) from contributing to the instance's similarity to another instance or category. The second difficulty is that resemblance theory cannot explain why aspects of an instance's appearance should affect the similarity of the instance to a category but not the probability that it is a category member. These surface features are part of the instance itself and, therefore, play a role in similarity computations; they simply are not important in determining the instance's category membership.

As noted earlier, none of this shows that similarity *never* plays a role in classifying things. In many ordinary settings, properties that make an instance similar to a category probably also furnish clues to its category membership. The point is that these clues are not definitive; they are only presumptive. They are not sufficient, since there are instances that are highly similar to a category without being members (as in the case of Carol the designer's lampshade that looks like an umbrella). And they are not necessary, since there are bona fide category members that look more like members of some other species (as in the case of Keil's surgically altered raccoon or our bird who accidentally came to look like an insect). The idea that similarity is a fallible clue or heuristic for categorization is probably the inspiration for dual models (Miller & Johnson-Laird, 1976; Smith et al., 1974), which I mentioned at the beginning of this chapter. Nothing in these data refutes models of this type, as long as the two components are loosely coupled. Likewise, similarity may well provide an important heuristic in decision making (Smith & Osherson, this volume), conceptual combination (Smith, Osherson, Rips, & Keane, in press), and other higher cognitive tasks. It's *pure* resemblance models that are the casualties of the present experiments.

Objections and responses

Before giving up pure resemblance, however, we should consider what resemblance theorists might say in their own defense. There appear to be three lines of argument, which amount to objections to the evidence I've presented here. The first is that we have considered the wrong kinds of categories, and the second, that we have looked at the wrong kind of categorization task. The third objection takes up the multiple-similarities idea that we touched on at the end of the second section.

Objection 1: two kinds of categories. One line that resemblance theorists might adopt is to deny the relevance of the stimuli. They might say, for example, that resemblance theory was never intended to account for the kinds of examples that these studies employed. They could point to the sci-fi quality of the stimuli and claim that resemblance theory need not apply to these radically contrary-to-fact categories.

It is true, of course, that many of the instances that we constructed are not ones you are likely to come across. Birdlike creatures don't transform themselves into insects, and people don't adorn their umbrellas with light bulbs. Our aim in creating these examples was to drive a wedge between resemblance and categorization and not to mimic real objects. However, I think it is possible to maintain that cases like the ones we studied are not all that rare: Although birds don't change into insects, fishlike objects do turn into frogs and wormlike ones into butterflies. There are also lots of cases in which artifacts look like members of other categories. Christmas catalogs list jewelry boxes in the form of heads of lettuce, candles that look like pieces of fruit, cameras that look like cigarette packs, and so on. Resemblance theory cannot dodge all such examples without seriously weakening its own credibility.

Objection 2: two kinds of categorization. Another objection along the same lines challenges the nature of the experimental tasks. The idea is that the most representative cases of categorization are ones that occur quite rapidly, on the order of a few hundred milliseconds. You see an object and immediately recognize it as an egg. You don't stop to consider whether it might be a Russian ornament that some clever jeweler has designed. By contrast, the studies I have described obviously call for deeper reasoning or problem solving on the subjects' part. It is quite possible that similarity is responsible for immediate categorization, even if it does not suffice for these more complex situations.

It may well be correct that immediate perceptual categorization often rests on similarity. Thus, if the categorizing situation is time-limited so that a subject has access only to the surface properties of the instance, then these surface properties will dominate the decision. Since overlap on surface properties seems to be the hallmark of similarity (given our own results), it is quite natural to think of this sort of categorization as similarity-based.

Still, we need to be careful about resemblance theory even for on-the-spot perceptual categorizing. What seems to be rapid classification based on surface properties may well turn out to involve procedures more complicated than similarity matching. For example, consider the process of assigning a visually presented object to a superordinate category (e.g., furniture) or a goal-derived category (e.g., birthday presents). Assuming that people can assign instances to these categories rapidly, they must be doing so on the basis of processes that go beyond similarity. Similarity may help them decide that something is a bunch of flowers, perhaps; but they must then make additional inferences to decide that this is a possible birthday present. Along the same lines, imagine a perceptual version of the first study, in which subjects see, for example, an outlined circle representing the mystery instance and decide whether something of this size and shape is more similar to, more typical of, or more likely to be a pizza or a quarter. There is no reason to think that the results of such a study would be any different from those we have obtained.

The real danger in this approach, however, is taking fast-paced object recognition as the archetype for categorization. Countless category decisions are not of this type. We classify people as friendly or hostile, arguments as convincing or fallacious, numbers as prime or composite, investments as safe or risky, policies as fair or biased, governments as socialist or totalitarian, cultures as advanced or primitive, religions as orthodox or heterodox, documents as authentic or forgeries, crimes as felonies or misdemeanors, diseases as chronic or acute, purchases as expensive or cheap, jokes as funny or offensive, speeches as informative or boring, jobs as rewarding or make-work, vacations as relaxing or vexing. Even if it turns out that first-glance object recognition is driven by similarity, we would need additional arguments (convincing ones) to show that this kind of classification has a privileged status that should be taken as a model for all categorizing.

Objection 3: two kinds of similarity. In discussing the first two studies, we considered the possibility that the results of the Similarity and Categorization conditions were both due to similarity but with a different metric for the two types of judgment. Of course, simple transformations of distance or similarity would not account for the results of the last two experiments, but there might be a generalization of this idea that would work. A proponent of resemblance theory might say, for example, that subjects in the Accident and Essence conditions used similarity to determine both their similarity and categorization ratings; however, for the similarity ratings they weighted surface properties especially heavily, whereas for the categorization ratings they weighted underlying properties more heavily.

It is easy to make fun of proposals of this kind, since they seem contrived to get the theory out of trouble. In other words, this objection sounds as if Resemblance theorists are trying to convince us that there are really two kinds of similarity: "categorization similarity," which is involved in classifying things, and "similarity similarity," which is involved in ordinary similarity judgments. This seems absurd, since there appears to be no justification for extending the meaning of *similarity* in this way. (It is a bit like saying that all life is a dream – but some dreams are waking dreams and some are sleeping dreams.) But perhaps we should not be too quick to dismiss this objection. I think people are tempted by this line because they believe that categorizing things and judging their similarity have some significant points in common. As discussed earlier, both processes might inspect predicates that are true of the objects in question, and both might compare these predicates in certain ways. It would be nice to have a term to refer to these shared factors, and *similarity* and *resemblance* easily come to mind.

Certainly none of the evidence that I have presented contradicts the idea that categorizing and judging similarity have some commonalities, and those who wish to use *similarity* or *resemblance* in a technical sense to mark these commonalities are free to do so. However, there are two serious problems with this way of thinking. One problem is that this technical sense of *similarity* is nearly vacuous as a psychological explanation. Consulting and comparing mental predicates takes place, not only in categorizing and in judging similarity but also in nearly every other kind of cognitive task: language comprehension, memory search, reasoning, problem solving, decision making, and so on. Until this sense of *similarity* is made more specific, it cannot shed much light on the process of categorizing, contrary to the claims of resemblance theory. The second deficiency is that this kind of similarity may be open to the sort of circularity arguments advanced by Murphy and Medin (1985) and others. If similarity is cognitively primitive and perceptually given, then you might hope to use it in order to reconstruct categorization, without worrying that category knowledge will alter similarity itself. But if similarity is simply predicate comparison, then all bets are off. For example, if you explain why people classify bats as mammals by saying that bats are similar to other mammals, you cannot simultaneously explain that similarity by invoking shared predicates such as *is a mammal*. (This is not to say, however, that all predicate-comparison theories are circular; see n. 1.)

The implication is this: On the one hand, if similarity denotes something like raw perceptual resemblance (which is what it seems to mean to most subjects), then resemblance theory is not, by itself, powerful enough to explain categorization. That is what the four studies establish. On the other hand, if similarity merely means predicate comparison, then resemblance theory risks vacuity and circularity. There may be a way of slipping through this dilemma, but it is up to the resemblance theorist to show us how this can be done.[8]

Categorization as explanation

You can get a good glimpse of what is wrong with resemblance theory by considering an example of Murphy and Medin's. Imagine a man at a party who jumps into a swimming pool with all his clothes on. You might well classify such a person as drunk, not because he is similar in some way to other drunk people or to a drunk prototype, but because drunkenness serves to explain his behavior. As Murphy and Medin point out, classification in this case is a matter of an inference about the causes of the action we witnessed.

But notice that this example generalizes easily to other category decisions. In most situations that call for categorizing, we confront some representation of an instance with our knowledge of the various categories it might belong to. If the assumption that the instance is in one of these categories provides a reasonable explanation of the information we have about it and if this explanation is better than that provided by other candidate categories, then we will infer that that instance is a member of the first category. For example, in deciding whether an object with a 3-inch diameter is a quarter or a pizza, we might consider alternative stories about how a pizza or a quarter of that size could come about. Because the pizza explanation is probably more parsimonious than the quarter explanation, we will infer that the object is indeed a pizza.[9]

The results of the last two experiments also yield to this sort of analysis. For example, if we learn about a birdlike animal that turns insectlike as the result of a chemical accident, then we might well consider the possibility that the chemicals modified the superficial appearance of the animal, leaving the genetic structure unchanged. Since this explanation seems a bit more plausible than the alternative possibility that the chemicals actually changed the genetic structure, we are likely to decide that the animal is a bird. On the other hand, suppose we are told about a birdlike creature that matures into one that is insectlike. Given what we know about biological development, it seems reasonable to suppose that the later stage is indicative of the animal's true category. Hence, the hypothesis that the creature is an insect may provide a better explanation of this instance than the hypothesis that it is a bird.

Of course, this way of thinking about categorizing is not very close to a true cognitive model. In order to fill in the details, we would need an account of how people generate explanations and how they evaluate them. Unfortunately, these problems have proved extremely difficult ones in philosophy of science (see, e.g., Achinstein, 1983), and there is no reason to think that they will be any easier within a psychological framework (Fodor, 1983). To make matters worse, this type of account may be open to problems of circularity in much the same way as the predicate-comparison idea, discussed in the preceding section. But despite these difficulties, an explanation-based approach to categorizing is worth taking seriously, partly because similar processes are required for other cognitive abilities. For example, Schank, Collins, and Hunter (1986) have argued that category learning also depends on constructing explanations. In particular, mistakes in classifying objects or events should sometimes cause us to modify our beliefs about the nature of the relevant category. It is not always easy, though, to determine exactly which beliefs led to the error, and in these situations we may have to search for a plausible explanation of how the difficulty came about. In other words, category learning is often like troubleshooting a mechanical device, requiring similar explanations and tests. But if explanation figures into the way we learn about categories, it would not be surprising if it also played a role in the categorizing process itself.

Second, explanation is also needed as part of an account of many forms of nondeductive reasoning (Harman, 1966, 1986). Scientific inference, for example, is generally a matter of accepting the truth of the hypothesis that gives the best explanation of the data at hand. Indeed, categorization and category learning are special cases of inference to the best explanation. In the Murphy–Medin example, we conclude that the partygoer is drunk because drunkenness provides a good account of why he jumped into the pool. In the pizza–quarter example, we conclude that the 3-inch object must be a pizza rather than a quarter because we can more easily explain how a pizza of that size could be created. One way to see the connection between categorization and inference to the best explanation is to notice that many inference problems can be turned into categorization problems by a minor change of wording. The question whether all material of a given type conducts electricity is equivalent to asking whether it is a member of the category of electricity-conducting objects. To answer questions like this, we typically use evidence about the underlying nature of the objects and their lawful interrelations. Mere similarity is too weak to solve these inductive problems.

The idea that categorizing is a form of inference bears an obvious kinship to other recent hypotheses about the nature of concepts. Many investigators have proposed that similarity-based heuristics cannot possibly account for all uses of concepts. As a result, these investigators have postulated concept cores that figure in language understanding (Miller & Johnson-Laird, 1976) and conceptual combination (Osherson & Smith, 1981); theoretical aspects that determine conceptual coherence (Murphy & Medin, 1985) and conceptual change (Carey, 1982, 1985); and essential aspects that help account for people's beliefs about conceptual stability (Medin & Ortony, this volume; Smith,

Medin, & Rips, 1984). Although Smith and Medin (1981) once com-
plained that conceptual cores did little to explain psychological data,
it now seems that they are pulling their weight. The present suggestion
is certainly consistent with these ideas, since cores, theories, or essences
could easily be the source of many of the explanations subjects invoke
in categorizing things. In fact, when categories have clear definitions,
we would expect the explanations to amount to little more than a
reference to the core. For example, it is natural to say that 794 is an
even number *because* it's divisible by 2 (see Armstrong, Gleitman, &
Gleitman, 1983).

However, the advantage of explanations can be seen most clearly
when category decisions involve more than a recital of core properties.
Recall, for example, Subject C's comments on why something 4.75
feet high would have to be a cereal box rather than a stop sign: "no
one would see the stop sign if it were that small. . . . A stop sign would
have to be a certain height, and while I wouldn't expect to see a cereal
box that big, it wouldn't make sense to have such a small sign." This
subject is not merely citing a core property of stop signs (as would be
the case if he had said, "By definition, all stops signs are 7.5 feet
high"). Instead, he reasons that a stop sign of that height would be
hard to see and hence would not fulfill the function that stop signs
are supposed to serve; therefore, the object probably isn't a stop sign.
Information about a stop sign's function could certainly be among its
core properties, but further inferences are. necessary to use this information in classifying the object. The subject is obviously creating
his argument on the fly to deal with the case at hand. The same can
be said, I think, of Subject B's remarks on tennis balls and teapots,
cited earlier. Of course, subjects do sometimes mention a core property and leave it at that, but this is not the only strategy available to
them. Explanations have sufficient flexibility to subsume these
strategies.

In short, resemblance theory seemed an attractive prospect: On
this theory, similarity accounts for typicality, typicality measures
degree of category membership, and degree of membership explains classification behavior. The problem is that this chain breaks
somewhere in the middle, since neither similarity nor typicality
fully accounts for degree of membership, as our subjects judge it.
The view that classification is inference to the best explanation is
not so tidy; it means that an adequate theory of categorization will
have to await (or to develop alongside) an adequate theory of
nondeductive reasoning. This may seem a disappointing state of

affairs, but at least it locates categorization in the right space of complex mental processes.

NOTES

I have benefited from comments on an earlier version of this paper from audiences at the Workshop on Similarity and Analogy at the University of Illinois, and at colloquia at the Yale AI Lab, the University of Arizona Psychology Department, the UCSB Cognition Group, and the University of Wisconsin Psychology Department. Closer to home, Reid Hastie, Greg Murphy, Eldar Shafir, and Roger Tourangeau commented on an earlier draft of the manuscript. I should also like to acknowledge the help of Marshall Abrams, Judy Florian, and Janis Handte in conducting the experiments reported here. National Institute of Mental Health Grant MH39633 supported this research. The analyses of the second experiment were carried out at the University of Arizona, thanks to the Cognitive Science Committee and its chairman, Peter Culicover.

1 Murphy and Medin (1985) have a more general version of their relativity argument, which may not be susceptible to problems with the New Look. This is that similarity is always relative to some standard or set of criteria, where this standard varies from one category to the next. Thus, there is no way of computing similarity that is independent of the particular objects or categories in question, again leading to circularity when one tries to explain categorizing via similarity. (I have heard a very similar argument from Herbert Clark in discussion.) It is not clear to me, however, that this type of variation in the way similarity is computed entails that resemblance theory is viciously circular. Let us suppose, hypothetically, that people determine the similarity of an object to a category simply by counting the number of shared predicates in their representations. In general, if object O is compared to category C, a different set of shared predicates will be relevant than if O is compared to another category C'. And one might say, in this situation, that a different standard or set of criteria was involved for the O–C than for the O–C' comparison. But although there is probably a lot that is wrong with such a theory, I do not think it would be fair to accuse it of circularity. The theory *would* be circular, of course, if it presupposed that people must know the category of which O is a member before they can carry out the similarity computation that is supposed to determine membership status. But it is hard to see why such a presupposition is necessary in our hypothetical case. In short, it seems you can have (some kinds of) relative standards without putting the resemblance theory into a loop.

2 An exception to this rule is Kahneman and Miller's (1986) norm theory. On this approach, categories are stored as remembered instances; however, the categorizing process can also make use of more abstract information that is computed from the instances (by a parallel process) at the time of the category decision. This clearly gives the model much more flexibility

56   LANCE J. RIPS

than earlier exemplar theories and makes it less dependent on resemblance. Whether it escapes the problems with exemplar models that I describe later depends on how powerful the abstraction process is. It is certainly possible that subjects can compute on the fly properties like the variance or density of a category's distribution, which play a role in Experiments 1 and 2. But it is less likely that subjects obtain theoretical information (e.g., hidden biological properties, designers' intentions) in the same way. If these properties are crucial to category decisions (as in Experiments 3 and 4), then exemplars do not provide a rich enough representation.

3 In recent work, Lakoff (1987) proposes what he calls a prototype theory for a variety of linguistic and psychological phenomena. Although this theory is supposed to account for findings like those of Rosch and others, it is clearly much broader than the prototype models just described. In particular, similarity to a prototype has no special status in the theory. Instead, the basic representational unit is an *idealized cognitive model*, which can be thought of as an elaborated frame or schema. In terms of the typology of Figure 1.1, Lakoff's approach should be grouped with frame theories at the bottom of the scale, despite its title.

4 Douglas Medin suggested the psychophysical explanation to me in conversation. One problem with both the uphill/downhill and the psychophysics hypotheses is that one might well expect such factors to interact with the type of task subjects performed. Given the account just sketched for the main effect of task, variations in fixedness should produce a bigger difference for the Categorization group than for the Similarity group, whereas variations in subjective magnitude should yield a bigger difference for the Similarity group than for the Categorization group. Figure 1.2 shows a trend in the former direction, but the interaction is not a significant one. A larger experiment might be necessary to examine these possibilities in detail.

5 To get a measure of centrality for an interval, we computed the distance between the midpoint of the interval and median of the distribution. The distances for all the intervals within a given problem were then transformed to z scores in order to correct for differences in units of measurement across problems. (Recall that one problem involved temperatures Fahrenheit, another hair length in inches, and so on.) Finally, we multiplied each z score by −1 so that larger numbers represent intervals nearer the median. This gives centrality and frequency coefficients the same polarity in Table 1.1.

6 Much the same can be said of a second suggestion of Medin and Ortony (this volume): that both the Categorization and the Similarity subjects in the first study were computing similarity but with different instantiations of the mystery instance. This explanation is unlikely to be true, given subjects' reports of their own deliberations (as discussed later in this section). But even if it were, it would not be of much help to resemblance theory. We would still need an explanation of why instructions to categorize an instance caused subjects to imagine examples that differed systematically from the ones Similarity subjects envision. By hypothesis, the factors responsible for this difference cannot themselves be reduced to similarity and hence support the major claim of this chapter. This same point also applies to the experiments that I report in the next section.

7 Some subjects may, in fact, believe in properties that are necessarily true *de re*. An example might be Subject D's comments on decks of cards, cited earlier. For other subjects, however, the properties that are necessary for category membership are probably not ones they believe are essential to the objects' continued existence.

8 Susan Goldman suggested this way of putting the matter. Notice that I am not defending the view that *similarity* always means perceptual resemblance. We can obviously talk about the similarity of entities (e.g., ideas, goals, or personalities) that do not have perceptual attributes. Nor am I criticizing any particular theories of similarity. The experiments reported here, however, convince me that people place heavy emphasis on perceptual properties in their similarity judgments when this strategy is open to them. Perceptual resemblance may therefore be a root sense or default sense of similarity. This root sense could be extended in certain ways in order to describe the similarity of more abstract objects, but extending it in an unconstrained way – so that similarity can stand for any type of property comparison – may lead to the sorts of conceptual difficulties just discussed.

9 This way of looking at categorization is probably congenial to schema or frame theorists, since one of the points of these theories has been that a schema applies to an instance if it adequately accounts for the instance's properties. See Rumelhart and Norman (1988) for a review of these theories that stresses this perspective.

REFERENCES

Achinstein, P. (1983). *The nature of explanation*. Oxford: Oxford University Press.

Armstrong, S. L., Gleitman, L. R., & Gleitman, H. (1983). What some concepts might not be. *Cognition, 13*, 263–308.

Barsalou, L. W. (1985). Ideals, central tendency, and frequency of instantiation as determinants of graded structure in categories. *Journal of Experimental Psychology: Learning, Memory, and Cognition, 11*, 629–654.

Brachman, R. J., & Schmolze, J. G. (1985). An overview of the KL-ONE knowledge representation system. *Cognitive Science, 9*, 171–216.

Brooks, L. (1978). Nonanalytic concept formation and memory for instances. In E. Rosch & B. B. Lloyd (Eds.), *Cognition and categorization* (pp. 169–211). Hillsdale, NJ: Erlbaum.

Carey, S. (1982). Semantic development: The state of the art. In E. Wanner & L. R. Gleitman (Eds.), *Language acquisition: The state of the art* (pp. 347–389). Cambridge: Cambridge University Press.

Carey, S. (1985). *Conceptual change in childhood*. Cambridge, MA: MIT Press (Bradford Books).

Collins, A. M., & Loftus, E. F. (1975). A spreading-activation theory of semantic processing. *Psychological Review, 82*, 407–428.

Collins, A., & Rips, L. J. (in preparation). *An inductive approach to categorization*.

Fodor, J. A. (1983). *The modularity of mind*. Cambridge, MA: MIT Press.

Fried, L. S., & Holyoak, K. J. (1984). Induction of category distributions: A framework for classification learning. *Journal of Experimental Psychology: Learning, Memory, and Cognition, 10,* 234–257.

✓ Goodman, N. (1970). Seven strictures on similarity. In L. Foster & J. W. Swanson (Eds.), *Experience and theory* (pp. 19–29). Amherst: University of Massachusetts Press.

Harman, G. (1966). Inference to the best explanation. *Philosophical Review, 74,* 88–95.

✓ Harman, G. (1986). *Change in view: Principles of reasoning.* Cambridge, MA: MIT Press.

Hintzman, D. L., & Ludlam, G. (1980). Differential forgetting of prototypes and old instances: Simulation by an exemplar-based classification model. *Memory & Cognition, 8,* 378–382.

Jacoby, L. L., & Brooks, L. R. (1984). Nonanalytic cognition: Memory, perception, and concept learning. In G. H. Bower (Ed.), *The psychology of learning and motivation: Advances in research and theory* (Vol. 18, pp. 1–47). New York: Academic Press.

Kahneman, D., & Miller, D. T. (1986). Norm theory: Comparing reality to its alternatives. *Psychological Review, 93,* 136–153.

✓ Kahneman, D., & Tversky, A. (1982). The simulation heuristic. In D. Kahneman, P. Slovic, & A. Tversky (Eds.), *Judgment under uncertainty: Heuristics and biases* (pp. 201–208). Cambridge: Cambridge University Press.

Keil, F. C. (1986). The acquisition of natural kind and artifact terms. In W. Demopoulos & A. Marras (Eds.), *Language learning and concept acquisition* (pp. 133–153). Norwood, NJ: Ablex.

✓ Lakoff, G. (1987). *Women, fire, and dangerous things: What categories tell us about the nature of thought.* Chicago: University of Chicago Press.

McCloskey, M., & Glucksberg, S. (1979). Decision processes in verifying category membership statements: Implications for models of semantic memory. *Cognitive Psychology, 11,* 1–37.

Medin, D. L., & Schaffer, M. M. (1978). Context theory of classification learning. *Psychological Review, 85,* 207–238.

✓ Miller, G. A., & Johnson-Laird, P. N. (1976). *Language and perception.* Cambridge, MA: Harvard University Press.

Murphy, G. L., & Medin D. L. (1985). The role of theories in conceptual coherence. *Psychological Review, 92,* 289–316.

Oden, G. C., & Lopes, L. L. (1982). On the internal structure of fuzzy subjective categories. In R. R. Yager (Ed.), *Recent developments in fuzzy set and possibility theory* (pp. 75–89). Elmsford, NY: Pergamon.

Osherson, D. N., & Smith, E. E. (1981). On the adequacy of prototype theory as a theory of concepts. *Cognition, 9,* 35–58.

Quine, W. V. O. (1969). Natural kinds. In W. V. O. Quine, *Ontological relativity and other essays* (pp. 114–138). New York: Columbia University Press.

✓ Rosch, E. (1978). Principles of categorization. In E. Rosch & B. B. Lloyd (Eds.), *Cognition and categorization* (pp. 27–48). Hillsdale, NJ: Erlbaum.

Rosch, E. & Mervis, C. B. (1975). Family resemblances: Studies in the internal structure of categories. *Cognitive Psychology, 7,* 573–605.

Rosch, E., Simpson, C., & Miller, R. S. (1976). Structural bases of typicality effects. *Journal of Experimental Psychology: Human Perception and Performance, 2,* 491–502.

Rumelhart, D. E., & Norman, D. A. (1988). Representation in memory. In

R. C. Atkinson, R. J. Herrnstein, G. Lindzey, & R. D. Luce (Eds.), *Handbook of experimental psychology* (Vol. 2, pp. 511–587). New York: Wiley.

Schank, R. C., Collins, G. C., & Hunter, L. E. (1986). Transcending inductive category formation in learning. *Behavioral and Brain Sciences, 9*, 639–686.

Schwartz, S. P. (1980). Natural kinds and nominal kinds. *Mind, 89*, 182–195.

✓ Smith, E. E. & Medin, D. L. (1981). *Categories and concepts*. Cambridge, MA: Harvard University Press.

Smith, E. E., Medin, D. L., & Rips, L. J. (1984). A psychological approach to concepts: Comments on Rey's "Concepts and stereotypes." *Cognition, 17*, 265–274.

Smith, E. E., Osherson, D. N., Rips, L. J., & Keane, M. (in press). Combining concepts: A selective modification model. *Cognitive Science*.

Smith, E. E., Shoben, E. J., & Rips, L. J. (1974). Structure and process in semantic memory: A featural model for semantic decisions. *Psychological Review, 81*, 214–241.

Tversky, A. (1977). Features of similarity. *Psychological Review, 84*, 327–352.

✓ Tversky, A., & Gati, I. (1978). Studies of similarity. In E. Rosch & B. B. Lloyd (Eds.), *Cognition and categorization* (pp. 79–98). Hillsdale, NJ: Erlbaum.

White, T. H. (1954). *The bestiary: A book of beasts, being a translation from a Latin bestiary of the 12th Century*. New York: Putnam.

2
Similarity and decision making

EDWARD E. SMITH and DANIEL N. OSHERSON

Our goal is to extend certain theoretical notions about similarity – particularly notions about similarity to prototypes – to studies of decision making and choice. For the past decade, the psychology of decision making has been dominated by the brilliant research of Daniel Kahneman and Amos Tversky. Although Kahneman and Tversky (hereafter K & T) have contributed greatly to this area, their research seems to be swimming against the strongest current in contemporary psychology in that it is not primarily concerned with issues of representation and process. We think that this neglect of a computational perspective has limited the generalizations that K & T and their followers have drawn from studies of decision making. We will support our position by showing that an explicit model of similarity and decision making promotes new generalizations and suggests new insights about some of K & T's best-known studies.

In particular, such a model will allow us to specify the factors that control the phenomena that K & T have uncovered, thereby permitting us to determine the conditions under which the reasoning illusions they describe will arise. This is in contrast to K & T's approach of simply demonstrating the phenomena, with no attempt to delineate boundary conditions. Our approach should also enable us to connect the areas of decision and choice to recent advances in the theory of knowledge representation.

Our chapter is organized as follows. First, we illustrate K & T's basic contribution to decision making by describing three of their best known cases. Second, we consider some limitations of their analyses. Third, we use a model of similarity and prototypes to specify representations and processes that are relevant to decisions based on similarity. Fourth, we show that this model provides a richer account of K & T's three cases than does their purely descriptive, noncomputational approach. Fifth and finally, we show how our account can be extended to deal with choice problems.

60

The Kahneman & Tversky approach to decision making

In the early 1970s human decision making was often understood in terms of a normative theory. People were assumed to have readily accessible intuitions that corresponded to major principles of probability and statistical theory (see, e.g., Edwards, 1968; Peterson & Beach, 1967). Two such principles are:

- The *conjunction rule*, which says that a conjunction, *A* and *B*, is never more probable than either of its constituents
- *Bayes's theorem*, which says that the probability of a hypothesis, *H*, given evidence, *E*, is given by:
  $P(H/E) = P(E/H)P(H)/P(E)$
- Thus, $P(H/E)$ should increase with both $P(E/H)$ and the prior probability of the hypothesis, $P(H)$.

Beginning in the early 1970s, K & T began to demonstrate that human judgments often violate these principles. These demonstrations undermined the conviction that normative theory could provide a qualitative idealization of human probabilistic judgment. The gist of the K & T argument is illustrated by the following three cases.

Violating the conjunction rule. When asked to estimate the probabilities that an object belongs to (a) a conjunctive category versus (b) its constituent categories, people tend to estimate the similarity of the object with respect to the categories (this is called the *representativeness heuristic*). Reliance on this heuristic can lead to a violation of the conjunction rule, that is, to a *conjunction fallacy*. To use one of K & T's examples, a hypothetical woman, Linda, described as "outspoken and concerned with issues of social justice," is judged more likely to be a *feminist bank teller* than a bank teller. This of course is impossible if people are considering true probabilities, but the fallacy is explicable if people are considering similarities, because Linda is more similar to the prototype of a feminist bank teller than to that of a bank teller (Tversky & Kahneman, 1982a; 1983).

Ignoring base rates. Contrary to Bayes's theorem, when people estimate the probability of a hypothesis given some evidence, they often ignore the prior probability of the hypothesis – the base rate – and consider only the representativeness or similarity of the evidence to the hypothesis. In one of K & T's studies, one group of subjects were told that a panel of psychologists had interviewed 30 engineers and 70 lawyers and written brief descriptions of them; the subjects were then given five randomly chosen descriptions, and, for each one, were asked to indicate the probability that the person described was an engineer. Another group of subjects were given identical instructions except that they were told there were 70 engineers and 30 lawyers. The substantial variation in base rates between the groups had very little effect: When given a description that seems prototypical of an engineer (lawyer), subjects in both groups thought there was high probability of the person being an engineer (lawyer); and when given a description that was completely neutral, subjects in both groups estimated there was a .5 probability of the person being an engineer (lawyer) (Kahneman & Tversky, 1972, 1973).

Interpreting base rates causally. Though people ignore base rates that are presented in abstract form, they use base rates that are presented in "causal" form. This difference is nicely illustrated by the "cab" problem. In the problem's abstract form, subjects are told that: (*a*) in a town with two kinds of cabs, green and blue, an accident involving a cab occurred; (*b*) a witness identified the cab as blue and was shown to be 80% accurate in discriminating blue from green cabs in such circumstances; and (*c*) 85% of all cabs are green (the base rate). Given these facts, subjects estimate that a blue cab was involved in the accident with a probability of roughly .8, which suggests that they ignore the base rate. (Bayes's theorem, in contrast, puts the probability of the offending cab being blue at .41.) The causal version of the problem differs from the above only in that subjects are now told that: (*c'*) although the two cab companies are roughly equal in size, 85% of cab accidents involve green cabs. This suggests that the drivers of green cabs are somehow responsible for their elevated accident rate. Now subjects estimate that a blue cab was involved in the accident with probability .6, indicating some impact of the base rate information (Tversky & Kahneman, 1982b).

In short, K & T have demonstrated that people often estimate probabilities by relying on similarity and causal analysis, rather than on the basic principles of probability and statistics.

Limitations of the Kahneman & Tversky approach

The pioneering work of K & T has transformed research on human decision making. Nevertheless, the approach is limited at both the empirical and the theoretical level. With regard to empirical problems, K & T's studies consist mainly of demonstrations, generally involving extreme cases, and often there is no indication of the phenomena's boundary conditions. Consider, for example, the conjunction fallacy.

The fallacy is demonstrated with cases like the Linda story mentioned above. There is no way of knowing whether such stories are of a special type leading to the conjunction fallacy or whether conjunctions in general are judged more probable than their main constituents. Similarly, there is little concern in the K & T experiments with differential magnitudes of effects. In K & T's work on the conjunction fallacy, a couple of alternative stories might be used and a fallacy demonstrated with each one, but there is no investigation of why the magnitude of the fallacy might be greater in one case than another.

In general terms, we believe that K & T's proposal that people use decision heuristics like representativeness is correct but that such a proposal is too abstract to guide systematic, experimental work. In contrast, a detailed model of the processing that leads to the conjunction fallacy would likely tell us something about the conditions under which the fallacy arises, the relative magnitude of the effect when it does occur, and the major sources of knowledge that the subject consults in reaching his or her decision. In what follows, we sketch a more explicit model of these processes.

A similarity model

The following model is intended to describe those situations wherein a person estimates the probability that an object belongs to a class by relying on the similarity that the object bears to the prototype of the class. Although similarity is not the only heuristic factor in decision making, it does seem to be the key factor in many of K & T's studies; and, as we will demonstrate, an explicit model of similarity-based reasoning sheds new light on these studies. (The model was originally proposed as an account of how people combine simple prototypes into complex ones; see Smith & Osherson, 1984; Smith, Osherson, Rips, & Keane, in press).[1]

The model has three components: (a) a frame representation for a concept's prototype, (b) procedures for modifying these prototypes, and (c) a rule for determining the similarity of an object to a prototype. Let us start with the frame representation of a concept's prototype. A bit of a frame for the prototype of *bank teller* is presented in the leftmost column of Table 2.1. Note that the frame contains slots not only for attributes that bear directly on being a bank teller – slots for salary and education level – but also for attributes that are only characteristic of the occupation – a slot for political views. Associated with each slot or attribute (we use these terms interchangeably) are the following: (*a*) the diagnosticity of the attribute, as indicated by the

Table 2.1. *Frame representation for prototype (bank teller), particular individual (Linda), and modified prototype (feminist bank teller)*

	Bank teller	Linda	Feminist bank teller
Salary	3 Salary $\left\{\begin{array}{l}\text{\$10,000–15,000—3}\\ \text{\$15,000–20,000—6}\\ \text{Over \$20,000—1}\end{array}\right.$		3 Salary $\left\{\begin{array}{l}\text{\$10,000–15,000—3}\\ \text{\$15,000–20,000—5}\\ \text{Over \$20,000—1}\end{array}\right.$
Education	3 Education $\left\{\begin{array}{l}\text{High school}\\ \text{Junior college—3}\\ \text{College—2}\end{array}\right.$	Education {College—10	3 Education $\left\{\begin{array}{l}\text{High school—5}\\ \text{Junior college—3}\\ \text{College—2}\end{array}\right.$
Politics	1 Politics $\left\{\begin{array}{l}\text{Conservative—2}\\ \text{Moderate—3}\\ \text{Liberal}\end{array}\right.$	Politics {Liberal—10	2 Politics $\left\{\begin{array}{l}\text{Conservative}\\ \text{Conservative}\\ \text{Liberal—10}\end{array}\right.$

Sim (Linda, bank teller) =
$a(3\times2+1\times1)$
$-b(3\times10+3\times8+1\times9)$
$-c(3\times8+1\times9) =$
$7a - 63b - 33c$

Sim (Linda, feminist bank teller) =
$a(3\times2+2\times10)$
$-b(3\times10+3\times8)$
$-c(3\times8) =$
$26a - 54b - 24c$

number to the attribute's left (i.e., a measure of the extent to which the attribute values predict either presence or absence of the concept in question); (*b*) a set of possible values, or slot fillers, which instances of the concept can assume (e.g., for education, the values include high school, junior college, and college), and (*c*) a function from possible values to "votes," namely, an indication of the likelihood that a given value appears in a given instance of the concept, as indicated by the number to the value's right (we refer to these numbers as "votes for the value"). The middle column of Table 2.1 illustrates a bit of a representation of a particular person, specifically Linda. The representation of an individual person does not contain information about slot diagnosticity. Also, to keep these individual representations simple, we assume in the present sketch that all votes for an attribute are on one value.[2]

Consider next a procedure for modifying a prototype so that a simple concept is turned into a conjunction. When a constituent like *bank teller* is modified by a concept like *feminist* we assume that three operations transpire. First, the attributes in the modifier select out the corresponding attributes in the constituent (e.g., the attribute of political liberalism in *feminist* selects out this attribute in *bank teller*). Second, all votes on a selected attribute are collapsed into the value specified by the modifier (e.g., liberal); and third, the diagnosticity of each selected attribute increases. This is illustrated in the rightmost column of Table 2.1, which contains a bit of the representation for *feminist bank teller*.

What remains to be specified is a rule for determining an individual's similarity to a prototype. For this purpose we use an additive version of the "contrast rule" proposed by Tversky (1977).[3] The contrast rule represents the similarity between a concept's prototype, *p*, and an individual instance, *i*, as a linear contrast of the weighted sum of three feature sets. Letting *I* and *P* designate the features associated with *i* and *p*, respectively, the three features sets are: (*a*) $I \cap P$ (the features common to *i* and *p*), (*b*) $P - I$ (the features distinct to the prototype), and (*c*) $I - P$ (the features distinct to the instance). Using this notation, the contrast model may be summarized by:

$$\text{Sim}(i, p) = a \sum_{i \in I \cap P} w_i - b \sum_{i \in P - I} w_i - c \sum_{i \in I - P} w_i \qquad (1)$$

In Equation 1, *w* is a feature-weighting function based on diagnosticity, and *a*, *b*, *c* are parameters that determine the relative contribution of the three factors to overall similarity. (Thus, the first term on the right side of Equation 1 is the sum of the weights of all common features, this sum itself being weighted by the parameter a.) Similarity is thus conceived as an increasing function of the features common to an instance and prototype and as a decreasing function of the features distinct to the prototype and distinct to the instance.

In our application of the model, each vote counts as a feature, and the weighting function assigns to each feature the diagnosticity of the associated attribute. To illustrate, consider the similarity of Linda to *bank teller* calculated on an attribute-by-attribute basis (see Table 2.1). On the education attribute, Linda shares two features with *bank teller* (two votes on college), and each of these features is weighted by 3, the diagnosticity of the education attribute. On the politics attribute, Linda shares only one feature with *bank teller* (one vote on liberal), and this feature is weighted by 1, the diagnosticity of politics. The sum of the weighted common features is therefore $3 \times 2 + 1 \times 1$, or 7, and this sum is itself multiplied by a, the weight given to common features. Similar computations apply in determining the contributions of features distinct to the prototype and of features distinct to the instances (see Table 2.1). Beneath each prototype representation in Table 2.1, we have computed its similarity to Linda; though these representations are only partials, the computations clearly suggest that Linda is more similar to *feminist bank teller* than to *bank teller*.[4]

Applications to decision making

We now consider applications of our similarity model to the three cases that we earlier used to illustrate the K & T approach. We will endeavor to show that the model permits us to go beyond the K & T analyses, establishing boundary conditions for the phenomenon of interest and pointing toward new phenomena.

Violating the conjunction rule

In presenting the model, we illustrated how Linda, being "outspoken and concerned with issues of social justice," would be judged more similar to the conjunction *feminist bank teller* than to the constituent *bank teller*. This occurs partly because Linda's political trait matches the relevant attribute of the conjunction better than it matches that of the constituent (and partly because this matching attribute has increased in diagnosticity).

We can now specify the determinants of the conjunction fallacy and state exactly when it will occur and when it will not. According to the model, the fallacy will arise to the extent that: (a) aspects of the description mismatch attributes of the constituent, and (b) these same aspects match attributes of the conjunction. Because Linda's description mismatches the political attribute of *bank teller* yet matches that attribute of *feminist bank teller*, a large conjunction fallacy should arise. The fallacy should decrease substantially, however, if we change either factor. For example, if instead of *feminist* we use *traditionalist*, Linda's description will mismatch the political attribute of the conjunction as much as it does that of the main constituent, and Linda may even be judged less likely to be a traditionalist bank teller than a bank teller. Similarly, if instead of *bank teller* we use *social worker*, Linda's description now matches the political attribute of the constituent about as well as it matches that of the conjunction, and Linda may be judged no more likely to be a feminist social worker than a social worker.

We have experimental support for the above predictions.[5] The experiment included two distinct tasks: estimating probabilities and judging typicalities. In both tasks, subjects were presented 12 items, each item consisting of a description of a person (e.g., "Linda is outspoken and concerned with issues of social justice") plus eight alternative categories of which the person might be a member (e.g., *feminist, bank teller, social worker, feminist bank teller*). One of the alternatives was a conjunction of two other alternatives, and we varied whether this conjunction involved incompatible constituents (e.g., *feminist bank teller*) or compatible constituents (e.g., *feminist social worker*). In the typicality task, subjects ranked the eight alternatives with respect to how typical the described person was of each category. In the probability task, a different group of subjects ranked the eight alternatives with respect to the probability that the described person was a member of each category. The results are presented in Table 2.2, separately for compatible and incompatible conjunctions.

Each datum in Table 2.2 is the difference between the average rank of a constituent (e.g., *bank teller*) and the average rank of the relevant conjunction (e.g., *feminist bank teller*). Since high ranks go with low numbers, the above difference will be positive whenever the conjunction is ranked higher – more typical or more probable – than the constituent. So high numbers in the probability task indicate large conjunction fallacies. Clearly, conjunction fallacies were more prevalent and more substantial with incompatible than compatible conjunctions. Averaging over all relevant items, there is a significant conjunction fallacy with incompatible conjunctions ($t = 4.06, p < .001$) but essentially no fallacy with compatible conjunctions ($t < 1$). Hence,

Table 2.2. *Differences between average ranks of constituents and conjunctions*

Items	Compatible conjunctions		Incompatible conjunctions	
	Probability	Typicality	Probability	Typicality
1	−.40	.50	.90	.70
2	1.10	.60	.50	1.00
3	.70	.90	1.40	2.00
4	−.60	1.40	1.50	1.50
5	0	−.20	.30	.40
6	.20	.50	1.20	1.00
7	−.90	.60	.20	.40
8	.50	−.40	.40	1.30
9	−1.80	1.20	.60	.40
10	1.40	−.20	.50	.80
11	−.30	.20	1.50	1.10
12	.40	−.20	.50	1.00
Mean	.03	.41	.80	.97

we have something of a boundary condition for the conjunction fallacy. Moreover, in those cases where there is a substantial fallacy, its magnitude seems to be tied to similarity factors. Specifically, for incompatible conjunctions, there is a significant correlation of .68 between the extent to which a description is judged more probable of a conjunction than its constituent (the conjunction fallacy) and the extent to which that same description is judged more typical of a conjunction than its constituent (which is called the *conjunction effect*). This suggests that whatever controls the conjunction effect also controls the conjunction fallacy. And we know from prior work that the determinants of the conjunction effect are likely those factors spelled out in our similarity model (Smith et al., in press). As promised, then, a more computational account of the conjunction fallacy leads naturally to a specification of its boundary conditions and of the factors that control its magnitude. (See Shafir, Smith, & Osherson, 1988, for further analyses of the relation between similarity and the conjunction fallacy.)

Ignoring base rates

In the engineer–lawyer study, subjects based their decision almost entirely on the similarity of the person's description to the prototypes of an engineer and a lawyer and ignored information about base rates (e.g., the fact that 70% of the people were lawyers). An analysis of this problem in terms of our model is similar to that used with the conjunction fallacy. Thus there would be frames representing the prototypes of engineers and lawyers, and the description of an individual would be matched on an attribute-by-attribute basis to their prototypes; whichever prototype resulted in the larger similarity score would be selected as the more probable category.

Interpreting base rates causally

Recall that in the noncausal version of the cab problem, an 80%-reliable witness identified the cab in an accident as blue, though 85% of the cabs are green. In terms of our model, we need to represent two classes of cabs, green and blue, and one individual cab, the one in the accident. The decision as to whether the offending cab was green or blue can then be estimated by the similarity of the individual representation to each of the class representations. The top half of Table 2.3 illustrates the representations. The individual cab has votes on two attributes, color and accident status; there are eight blue votes on the color attribute, corresponding to the witness's 80%-reliable testimony. The class representations, in contrast, have votes on the color attribute and on the frequency attribute but no information about accident status. (To simplify matters, we have assumed that the diagnosticities of all attributes are 1.0 and have suppressed these numbers.) Given these representations, the individual cab is clearly more similar to the class of blue cabs than to the class of green ones, which explains why subjects' probability estimates greatly favored blue cabs.

In the causal version of the cab problem, subjects are told that 85% of all accidents involve green cabs. Presumably, this information induces subjects to draw the inference that green cabs are accident-prone, and this information may now appear in the accident-status attribute of green cabs, as shown in the bottom half of Table 2.3. The upshot is an increase in the similarity of the individual cab to the class of green cabs, which explains why there is an increase in subjects' probability estimate that the offending cab is green. (Although this similarity account suffices to explain the phenomena of interest, it is quite speculative in that as yet we have no data that uniquely support it.)[6]

Table 2.3. *Nomcausal and causal versions of the cab problem*

	Green cabs		Individual cab		Blue cabs
Color	Green-10	Color	Green Blue-8	Color	Blue-10
Frequency	High-10 Medium Low	Accident status	Accident-10	Frequency	High Medium Low-10

	Green cabs		Individual cab		Blue cabs
Color	Green-10	Color	Green Blue-8	Color	Blue-10
Accident status	Accident-8.5 Safe	Accident status	Accident-10	Accident status	Accident Safe-8.5

Extensions of the model to choice

Our model can also be extended to studies that K & T have conducted on the topic of choice. We illustrate the nature of our approach by considering a well-known case of K & T's analysis of choice and then show how our analysis differs from theirs.

Losses loom larger than gains

A choice problem is defined by the options among which one must choose, the possible outcomes of the options, and the probabilities associated with each of these outcomes. A simple case of a choice problem arises when one of the options involves no change in state, as in:

A. A fair coin is tossed. There is a 50% chance it will come up heads, in which case you win $50; there is a 50% chance the coin will come up tails, in which case you lose $50.
B. No change.

In Option A, there are two possible outcomes, gain $50 or lose $50, and the probability associated with each is .5. In Option B, there is only one "outcome," the status quo, and of course it has probability 1.0.

Responses to the above problem reveal an important phenomenon. Though both options have the identical expected value (0), people overwhelmingly prefer Option B. That is, people refuse to accept a fair bet on a toss of a coin. Kahneman and Tversky interpret this finding as indicating that the displeasure due to losing a sum of money (say, the $50 loss in Option A) looms larger than the pleasure generated by winning the same amount (the $50 gain in Option B); consequently, the subjective value of this option is less than zero. To explain *why* losses loom larger than gains, K & T assume that the function relating subjective value to monetary value is steeper for losses than for gains. That is, the change in subjective value associated with a fixed change in monetary value is greater for losses than for gains (Kahneman & Tversky, 1979; Tversky & Kahneman, 1981). Essentially, K & T build the phenomenon of interest directly into the assumptions of the theory.

In contrast, we hold that the phenomenon of interest is deducible from the assumptions of our similarity model. Specifically, in evaluating the outcomes of an option, we assume that people determine the similarity of each outcome to their present state (roughly, the amount of spending money they presently have available). We further assume that people will prefer a risky option to the status quo only if the possible gain is at least as dissimilar from their present state as is the possible loss (essentially, only if they have at least as much to gain as to lose). These assumptions imply that losses will loom larger than gains, as becomes evident when we consider the similarity calculations for our coin-toss problem.

Let PS designate the set of features associated with one's present monetary state; to simplify the present discussion, we assume this is nothing more than the dollars one has at his or her disposal. Similarly, let GS designate the set of features associated with one's state after a gain, which again reduces to disposable dollars. Then, Equation 1 applies in the present context as follows (where $|A|$ designates the cardinality of Set A):

$$\text{Sim}(GS, PS) = a\,|PS \cap GS| - b\,|PS - GS| - c|GS - PS| \quad (2)$$
$$= a\,(PS) - b\,(0) - c\,(\text{net gain})$$

Note that because PS designates the amount of dollars one had prior to the choice, $|PS - GS|$ must be zero. That is, in a gain situation there is nothing that one had prior to the choice that one does not also have after the choice. To illustrate Equation 2, if prior to the coin-toss choice one had \$100, then Sim $(GS, PS) = a(100) - c(50)$.

In like manner, the similarity of the monetary state one is in after a loss (LS) to one's present state is given by:

$$\text{Sim}(LS, PS) = a\,|LS \cap PS| - b\,|PS - LS| - c\,|LS - PS| \quad (3)$$
$$= a\,(LS) - b\,(\text{net loss}) - c\,(0)$$

Note that $LS - PS$ must now be zero because in a loss situation there is nothing one has after the choice that one did not have before the choice. To illustrate Equation 3, if one had \$100 prior to the coin-toss choice, Sim$(LS, PS) = a(50) - b(50)$.

In comparing Equations 2 and 3, as long as the parameter c is not much greater than the parameter b (which is in keeping with the findings of Tversky & Gati, 1982), Sim(LS, PS) must be less than Sim (GS, PS) because LS is less than PS. This means that a loss of some amount is perceived as more dissimilar from one's present state than is a gain of the same amount; hence there is more to lose than to gain, and people should reject this option and choose the status quo. The phenomenon of interest thus follows naturally from the contrast rule for calculating similarity.

(Again, we note that, though our account of the phenomenon is descriptively adequate, it is speculative in that we have no data as yet that favors it over the K & T explanation.)

Other choice problems

In the preceding case, we had to consider only the amount of money gained or lost. In most choice problems, however, probability as well as amount must be represented; and some problems may require an even richer representation. We believe, however, that the representational component of our model is sufficient to handle these more difficult cases, and that the model can be used revealingly to analyze other phenomena discussed in K & T's work on choice.

NOTES

We thank Martha Gordon, Nichlos Hatsopolous, Nancy Kanwisher, Eldar Shafir, and William Salter for discussions of the ideas presented in this paper. The research reported in this paper was supported by U.S. Public Health Service Grant MH37208, National Science Foundation Grant 870544, and by the National Institute of Education under Contract no. US-HEW-C–82–0030.

1 Other heuristic factors in decision making include causal analysis and availability (see Tversky & Kahneman, 1974, for a thorough discussion). These factors, too, may lend themselves to the kind of processing account we pursue here.
2 We are talking as if the prototype for a concept is stable, e.g, as if the same frame of information is retrieved whenever a person thinks about *bank teller*. Barsalou's recent experiments (see this volume) indicate that prototypes may not be all that stable. However, these same experiments suggest that there are some properties (attribute values) that are accessed whenever the concept is operative. These "context-independent" properties would presumably give the prototype enough stability to keep our theoretical proposals viable.
3 An axiomatization for an additive version of the contrast rule is presented in Osherson, 1987.
4 A word is in order about our adopting a feature-by-feature approach to similarity. This approach runs counter to intuition, as most people report initially experiencing a global, undifferentiated similarity between an instance and a category and only subsequently becoming aware of the contributing features. This conflict between a computational approach and intuition can readily be resolved, however. As L. Smith points out (this volume), there is no need for the order of computations to be mirrored in the order of experience. In judging any kind of similarity, we may compute on a feature-by-feature basis, but the first things to enter consciousness may be whole objects.

74   EDWARD E. SMITH AND DANIEL N. OSHERSON

5 The experiment is modeled after a study of Pennington (1982).
6 An alternative explanation of the cab problem might focus on a heuristic
   other than similarity, namely, causal reasoning. Under this account the
   critical point is that the causal version of the base rate activates causal rules
   but the noncausal version does not. Specifically, the information that 85%
   of all accidents involve green cabs may trigger the rule that "If someone
   has a disproportionate number of accidents, that person is careless," which
   in turn may trigger the rule that "Carelessness leads to further accidents."
   Hence, the base rate information finds its way into people's understanding
   of the cab problem only when the information is presented in the causal
   version.

REFERENCES

Edwards, W. (1968). Conservatism in human information processing. In B.
    Kleinmuntz (Ed.,), *Formal representation of human judgment* (pp. 17–52).
    New York: Wiley.
Kahneman, D., & Tversky, A. (1972). Subjective probability: A judgment of
    representativeness. *Cognitive Psychology, 3*, 430–454.
Kahneman, D., & Tversky, A. (1973). On the psychology of prediction. *Psychological Review, 80*, 237–251.
Kahneman, D., & Tversky, A. (1979). Prospect theory: An analysis of decisions
    under risk. *Econometrica, 47*, 263–291.
Osherson, D. N. (1987). New axioms for the contrast model of similarity.
    Journal of Mathematical Psychology, 31, 93–103.
Pennington, N. (1982). *Comments on Tversky and Kahneman's "Intentional reasoning and the conjunction fallacy."* Paper presented at the annual meeting
    of the Judgment/Decision Making Conference, Minneapolis, MN.
Peterson, C. R., & Beach, L. R. (1967). Man as an intuitive statistician. *Psychological Bulletin, 68*, 29–46.
Shafir, E. B., Smith, E. E., & Osherson, D. N. (1988). *Typicality and reasoning
    fallacies.* Unpublished manuscript, University of Michigan, Ann Arbor.
Smith, E. E., & Osherson, D. N. (1984). Conceptual combination with prototype concepts. *Cognitive Science, 8*, 337–361.
Smith, E. E., Osherson, D. N., Rips, L. J., & Keane, M. (in press). Combining
    concepts: A selective modification model. *Cognitive Science.*
Tversky, A. (1977). Features of similarity. *Psychological Review, 84*, 327–352.
Tversky, A., & Gati, I. (1982). Similarity, separability, and the triangle inequality. *Psychological Review, 89*, 123–154.
Tversky, A., & Kahneman, D. (1974). Judgment under uncertainty: Heuristics
    and biases. *Science, 185*, 1124–1131.
Tversky, A., & Kahneman, D. (1981). The framing of decisions and the
    rationality of choice. *Science, 211*, 453–458.
Tversky, A., & Kahneman, D. (1982a). Judgments of and by representativeness. In D. Kahneman, P. Slovic, & A. Tversky (Eds.), *Judgment under
    uncertainty: Heuristics and biases* (pp. 84–98). Cambridge: Cambridge University Press.
Tversky, A., & Kahneman, D. (1982b). Evidential impact of base rates. In D.
    Kahneman, P. Slovic, & A. Tversky (Eds.), *Judgment under uncertainty:*

Heuristics and biases (pp. 153–162). Cambridge: Cambridge University Press.

Tversky, A., & Kahneman, D. (1983). Extensional versus intuitive reasoning. The conjunction fallacy in probability judgment. *Psychological Review, 90*, 293–315.

3

Intraconcept similarity and its implications for interconcept similarity

LAWRENCE W. BARSALOU

> A permanently existing "idea" or "Vorstellung" which makes its appearance before the footlights of consciousness at periodic intervals, is as mythological an entity as the Jack of Spades.
> William James, 1890/1950, p. 236

A central goal of cognitive science is to characterize the knowledge that underlies human intelligence. Many investigators have expended much effort toward this aim and in the process have proposed a variety of knowledge structures as the basic units of human knowledge, including definitions, prototypes, exemplars, frames, schemata, scripts, and mental models.[1] An implicit assumption in much of this work is that knowledge structures are stable: Knowledge structures are stored in long-term memory as discrete and relatively static sets of information; they are retrieved intact when relevant to current processing; different members of a population use the same basic structures; and a given individual uses the same structures across contexts. These intuitions of stability are often compelling, and it is sometimes hard to imagine how we could communicate or perform other intelligent behaviors without stable knowledge structures.

But perhaps it is important to consider the issue of stability more explicitly. Are there stable knowledge structures in long-term memory? If so, are they retrieved as static units when relevant to current processing? Do different individuals represent a given category in the same way? Does a given individual represent a category the same way across contexts? Whatever conclusions we reach should have important implications for theories of human cognition and for attempts to implement increasingly powerful forms of machine intelligence.

The first four sections of this chapter lay the groundwork for the last two. The first section reviews demonstrations of instability in category representation, and the second reviews more systematic at-

76

tempts at assessing just how unstable category representations are. The third section considers seven possible accounts of instability, and the fourth presents a retrieval-based framework for viewing the dynamic character of human knowledge. In the context of this framework, the fifth section introduces the concept of intraconcept similarity, namely, the similarity between different representations of the same category. The sixth section concludes by considering various implications of intraconcept similarity for interconcept similarity, the similarity between representations of different categories.

Demonstrations of instability

The well-known retention phenomenon of semantic encoding variability suggests that category representations are unstable (e.g., Anderson & Ortony, 1975; Anderson, Pichert, Goetz, Schallert, Stevens, & Trollip, 1976; Barclay, Bransford, Franks, McCarrell, & Nitsch, 1974; Geis & Winograd, 1975; Thompson & Tulving, 1970; Tulving & Thompson, 1973). Investigators have generally found that the cues most effective in accessing a memory trace at retrieval are those most similar to its encoding context. For example, Barclay et al. (1974) found that "something heavy" was a better cue than "something with a nice sound" for retrieving the sentence "The man lifted the piano." In contrast, "something with a nice sound" was a better cue for retrieving the sentence, "The man tuned the piano." Because *weight* was not an effective cue for the sentence about piano tuning, it must not have been incorporated in the representation of *piano*. But because *weight* was effective for the sentence about piano moving, it must have been. Rather than using an invariant knowledge structure to represent *piano* during the comprehension of the different sentences, subjects appeared to construct different representations, with the representations in different sentences focusing on *weight* and *sound*, respectively. Greenspan (1986) qualifies this result, showing that encoding variability occurs only for context-dependent and not for context-independent information, a distinction discussed later.

Numerous demonstrations of instability have been reported in the lexical priming literature. Barsalou (1982) demonstrated that certain knowledge about a category – *context-dependent information* – becomes active only if relevant in the current context. When people read *frog* in isolation, for example, *eaten by humans* typically remains inactive in memory. However, *eaten by humans* becomes active when reading about frogs in a French restaurant. Other researchers have reported similar effects in various priming tasks, including Conrad (1978) and Whitney, McKay, and Kellas (1985). Like the retention literature, this work demonstrates that different information is incorporated into the representation of a category in different situations.

Not only do category representations vary across contexts, the properties composing these representations also vary. Halff, Ortony, and Anderson (1976) found that the representation of *red* varies widely across categories such as *apple, brick, face, hair, light, soil, wine*, and so forth. Contrary to Rips and Turnbull's (1980) suggestion that absolute properties like *red* should be relatively stable, even these properties are unstable. One could argue that *red* is stable only within particular categories rather than across all categories. But *red* clearly varies across particular exemplars within each of the categories just mentioned. Even one's memory of *red* for a particular exemplar could vary, depending on various contextual cues and subsequent exemplars encoded. As discussed by Barsalou (1987), if the properties that constitute concepts and exemplars are not stable, then it is difficult to know exactly what, if anything, is stable in human knowledge. Loftus and Loftus (1980) similarly argue that subsequent experience may continually change previously acquired information.

Kahneman and Miller (1986) review numerous findings on social decision making that can be interpreted as demonstrating instability. If one's current representation of *waiter* specifies that waiters are pleasant, for example, then seeing an unpleasant waiter causes surprise. However, seeing another unpleasant waiter soon thereafter does not cause as much surprise because the value for *pleasantness* in the representation of *waiter* has decreased. Because unpleasant waiters have become less surprising, the representation of *waiter* must have changed. Kahneman and Miller consider various phenomena in which emotions, decisions, and causal attributions vary as a function of cues in the current context and the accessibility of information in memory. They conclude that people represent categories with ad hoc representations rather than with static knowledge structures.

In the personality literature, instability of behavior has been the source of a central debate for years (e.g., Buss & Craik, 1983, 1985; Epstein, 1979; Mischel, 1968, 1983; Mischel & Peake, 1982). Rather than remaining consistent according to particular traits, people's behavior appears to be heavily determined by current context. Although it is not clear what implications such instability has for the nature of category representation, it is nevertheless consistent with the view that the human cognitive system operates in a highly dynamic manner.

Systematic assessments of instability

Whereas the studies reviewed so far demonstrate instability, studies reviewed in the next three sections assess more systematically the extent to which category representations are unstable.

Graded structure

A category's graded structure is simply the ordering of its exemplars from most to least typical. In *birds*, for example, typicality is generally perceived by American subjects as decreasing from *robin* to *pigeon* to *parrot* to *ostrich*. Much recent work has demonstrated that the graded structure of a category is unstable. Depending on the population, individual, or context, the ordering of a category's exemplars by typicality can vary widely. Whereas *robin* is more typical than *swan* when Americans take their own point of view, *swan* is more more typical than *robin* when they take the point of view of the average Chinese citizen. As argued by Barsalou (1985, 1987), changes in the graded structure of a category reflect changes in its current representation. This account assumes: (a) an exemplar's typicality increases with its similarity to the current category representation; (b) changes in the category representation alter its similarities to exemplars; (c) these changes in similarity alter graded structure. Similar accounts of typicality have been proposed by Smith, Shoben, and Rips (1974), Rosch and Mervis (1975), and Hampton (1979).

In most of the studies described in this section, subjects received category names followed by the names of exemplars and judged how typical exemplars were of their category. In some experiments, subjects ranked exemplars from most to least typical; in others, subjects rated exemplars from 1 to 7 for their amount of typicality. An average graded structure, as discussed shortly, was simply the average of all the individual graded structures for a category across subjects (i.e., the typicality of each exemplar was its average typicality across subjects).

A category's graded structure can vary widely across populations. Barsalou and Sewell (1984) correlated the average graded structures of Emory University undergraduates with the average graded structures of Emory faculty for the same categories and observed an overall .2 correlation, indicating that these two populations had graded structures that were nearly unrelated. Similarly Schwanenflugel and Rey (1986) found that the average graded structures of Spanish and English monolinguals were quite different. Because a category's graded structure varies between populations, individuals in different populations appear to represent the same category differently.

Barsalou, Sewell, and Ballato (1986) explored the extent to which different individuals from the same population produce the same graded structures for a category. To assess agreement, Barsalou et. al computed the average correlation between the typicality judgments of all possible pairs of subjects for a category's exemplars. Across four experiments with American undergraduates, the average correlation was generally around .5, indicating that one subject's graded structure generally accounted for only around 25% of the variance in another subject's graded structure.

This low level of agreement was relatively unaffected by a variety of manipulations: Agreement was only slightly higher when subjects took the culturally shared point of view of the average American (.55) than when they took their own idiosyncratic points of view (.46). In another experiment, agreement was unaffected by the familiarity of the adopted point of view, with agreement being .53 for subjects' own point of view, .54 for the point of view of the average suburban housewife, and .57 for the point of view of the average country redneck.[2] Agreement was the same when subjects judged typicality (.56) versus exemplar goodness (.53). Subjects judging 16 exemplars per category (.45) showed no less agreement than subjects judging 8 exemplars per category (.42). Agreement was somewhat higher for subjects ranking exemplars (.46) than for subjects rating exemplars (.41). Agreement was relatively unaffected by category type, with common taxonomic categories only sometimes being slightly more stable than goal-derived categories (see Barsalou, 1983, 1985, and Barsalou, Usher, & Sewell, 1985, for further discussion of these category types). Similarly Fehr and Russell (1984, Study 3) found .38 between-subject agreement for the typicality of emotion terms.[3]

One might be willing to concede that different individuals use different representations for the same category but maintain that a given individual uses the same stable representation across situations. Consequently Barsalou et al. (1986) explored the extent to which a given individual produces the same graded structures for a category in different instances of the same context. To assess agreement, they correlated subjects' graded structure on one day with their graded structure in the same context a few weeks later. Across four experiments, they found that the average correlation was only around .8, indicating that a subject's graded structure in one session generally accounted for only about 64% of the variance in the other.

This low level of agreement was relatively unaffected by a variety of manipulations: Agreement was relatively unaffected by whether subjects took the self (.80), American (.79), housewife (.79), or redneck point of view (.78). Agreement was the same when subjects judged typicality (.80) versus exemplar goodness (.79). Subjects receiving the exemplars for each category in the same order across sessions (.85) showed no more stability than subjects receiving them in different orders (.84). Subjects judging 16 exemplars per category (.73) exhibited the same stability as subjects judging 8 exemplars per category (.74). Agreement was somewhat higher for subjects ranking exemplars (.78) than for subjects rating exemplars (.70). Agreement was relatively unaffected by category type, with common taxonomic categories only sometimes being slightly more stable than goal-derived categories. Similarly Fehr and Russell (1984, Study 3) found .55 within-subject agreement for the typicality of emotion terms.

Within-subject agreement was highly related to between-subject agreement, exhibiting an average correlation of around .75 across categories. The same factor(s) may be responsible for both between- and within-subject instability.

Graded structure also varies with context. Barsalou and Sewell (1984) found that subjects adopting different points of view generated very different graded structures for the same category. When American undergraduates judged typicality from the American and Chinese points of view, for example, they generated graded structures that were uncorrelated on the average across categories. Moreover, graded structures were inversely related for certain categories. Because between-subject agreement was comparable for the different points of view, these shifts in graded structure do not reflect random responding. Roth and Shoben (1983) similarly found that judging typicality and accessing exemplars in different linguistic contexts has a large impact on graded structure.

Property generation

One could argue that graded structure is a relatively indirect means of assessing category representations. Perhaps a more direct means is simply to have people describe category representations as they are thinking about them. Because people are reporting the contents of working memory, these accounts are likely to be fairly reliable (Ericsson & Simon, 1980, 1984).

Barsalou, Spindler, Sewell, Ballato, and Gendel (1987) used a variety of tasks to explore property generation. In one experiment, some subjects were asked to produce *average characteristics* of a category's exemplars, whereas other subjects were asked to produce *ideal characteristics* that a category's exemplars should have. Subjects in each condition were given examples of averages and ideals for two categories and asked not to generate the other kind of information. In another experiment, *prototype subjects* were asked to produce information that was typically true of a category and that did not have to be definitional, whereas *definition subjects* were asked to produce a strict dictionary definition for each category that did not contain nondefinitional information. Subjects in both experiments produced responses in a written form and were asked to spend a few minutes per category; they were not to spend a tremendous amount of time, or to provide only one or two properties per category. Whereas average and ideal subjects tended to produce lists of properties (e.g., *pretty, sings, feathers, builds nests,* and *catches worms* for *birds*), prototype and definition subjects tended to produce sentencelike strings of properties (e.g., *something/*that *people/use/*to *sit on/in a house* for *furniture;* slashes represent our division of the protocol into properties). In scoring subjects' protocols, we attempted to combine different surface forms of the same property as much as possible, which worked against observing instability. For example, we combined *transporting, form of transportation, carrying, hauling, getting, move, takes,* and *travel* into a single property for *vehicle*. Across experiments and conditions, subjects produced about five properties per category on the average, reminiscent of Miller's magic number minus two (Miller, 1956).

Variability across individuals. To assess agreement between subjects, Barsalou et al. (1987) computed the average overlap in properties between all possible pairs of subjects producing properties for a category. Overlap was measured with the *common element correlation,* namely, the number of properties common to two protocols divided by the geometric mean of the total properties in each (Bellezza, 1984a, 1984b, 1984c; Deese, 1965; McNemar, 1969). Across experiments, different subjects' protocols generally exhibited an overlap of around .32, indicating that only about one-third of a subject's description overlapped with another subject's description for the same category.

Only one variable had a relatively large impact on agreement. Subjects who produced definitions and prototypes (.44) showed much higher agreement than subjects who produced ideals and averages

(.20). Subjects producing definitions and prototypes may have generally reported information as it came to mind, whereas subjects producing averages and ideals may have had to perform more search and computation to produce properties (cf. Marbe's law; Woodworth, 1938; Woodworth & Schlosberg, 1960).

Otherwise this low level of agreement was relatively unaffected by a variety of manipulations: Agreement was only slightly higher for subjects taking their own point of view (.21) and the housewife point of view (.21) than for subjects taking the redneck point of view (.18). Subjects producing ideals (.22) showed more stability than subjects producing averages (.17). Ideals may be more stable because they are associated with relatively stable functional knowledge about categories, whereas averages may fluctuate with recently experienced exemplars. Stability may have been marginally higher for goal-derived (.22) than for common taxonomic categories (.18) because ideals represent goal-derived categories, whereas less stable averages also represent common taxonomic categories (Barsalou, 1985).

Subjects producing definitions (.44) showed no more agreement than subjects producing prototypes (.45). In addition, these two groups of subjects produced essentially the same properties overall and the same proportion of dictionary properties. On the basis of these null results, one could argue that no variable was manipulated. However, definition subjects took 1.41 sec longer on the average to generate a property than prototype subjects (9.40 vs. 7.99 sec per property). Even though definition subjects proceeded more carefully, they eventually retrieved the same information as prototype subjects. This pattern does not support the core-plus-identification view of categories, which proposes that category representations contain definitional cores and typicality-based identification procedures (Armstrong, Gleitman, & Gleitman, 1983; Osherson & Smith, 1981, 1982; Smith & Medin, 1981). According to this view, definitional cores, which reflect natural and logical invariants, should be more stable than identification procedures, which reflect personal experience. However, definition subjects did not show more stability or produce more definitional information than prototype subjects. Even though definition subjects were apparently more careful than prototype subjects, neither showed sensitivity to a distinction between definitional and nondefinitional information.

Agreement did not vary between well-defined concepts having necessary and sufficient conditions (e.g., *bachelor, mammal*), fuzzy concepts not having necessary and sufficient conditions (e.g., *game, furniture*), subordinates of the well-defined and fuzzy concepts (e.g., *dog, chair*), and concepts intermediate in definability between well-defined and fuzzy concepts (e.g., *window, dentist*). Nor did this factor interact with whether subjects produced definitions or prototypes.

Bellezza (1984b, 1984c) also observed the stability of property generation, as well as the stability of exemplar generation (1984a). Similar to our results, he found low levels of between-subject agreement for abstract categories (.18), superordinate categories (.20), basic-level categories (.28), and descriptions of famous people (.21).

Variability within individuals in the same context. To assess agreement within subjects, Barsalou et al. (1987) computed the overlap between a subject's protocol for a category on one day and his or her protocol in the same context a few weeks later. Across two experiments, they generally found an average overlap of around .55, indicating that only a little more than half a subject's protocol for a category in one session overlapped with his or her protocol in the other.

Similar to between-subject agreement, subjects producing definitions and prototypes (.67) were more stable than subjects producing ideals and averages (.43). Again this may have reflected a difference between subjects reporting information as it came to mind versus searching for – and possibly computing – less accessible types of information.

Otherwise this low level of agreement was relatively unaffected by a variety of manipulations: Agreement was unaffected by whether subjects took the self (.44), housewife (.45), or redneck point of view (.40). Agreement was the same when subjects produced ideals (.45) versus averages (.41) but was higher for goal-derived (.45) than for common taxonomic categories (.41) (only one of these identical differences was significant because the two tests varied in statistical power).

Within-subject agreement was the same for definition (.66) and prototype subjects (.67), offering further evidence against the core-plus-identification view. Only minor differences occurred among fuzzy (.64), subordinate (.65), intermediate (.69), and well-defined categories (.69). Bellezza (1984b, 1984c) observed comparable levels of agreement for abstract categories (.43), superordinate categories (.46), basic-level categories (.54), descriptions of famous people (.55), and descriptions of personal friends (.38).

Similar to graded structure, within-subject agreement was related to between-subject agreement, exhibiting average correlations of .3 for average and ideal subjects and .77 for prototype and definition subjects. Again the same factor(s) may be responsible for between- and within-subject instability.

Variability across contexts. Property generation also varies with context. Barsalou et al. (1987) computed the average overlap between all possible pairs of subjects *across* contexts and compared these values to the average overlap *within* contexts. Subjects taking different points of view (.16) agreed less than subjects taking the same point of view (.2). Subjects producing ideals versus averages (.15) agreed less than subjects producing the same kind of information (.2). The agreement that remains in these between-context comparisons suggests that certain core information is produced for a category regardless of context.

One might assume that subjects used the same representations for property generation and graded structure. However, when Barsalou et al. (1987) compared the relative stability of the same categories across these two tasks, they found no relationship. Because different categories were highly stable for each task, subjects must have represented the same category differently in each. Individual categories varied widely in stability, indicating that lack of variability was not responsible for no correlation. If categories had not varied, the correlations of between- and within-subject agreement within tasks would have not been as high as they were. Rips (this volume) similarly demonstrates that people use different information in different tasks.

Category membership

One could argue that instability in property generation simply reflects random sampling of information from invariant representations. Perhaps invariant representations manifest themselves only in more logical tasks, such as determining category membership or reasoning about categories (Armstrong et al., 1983; Osherson & Smith, 1981, 1982; Smith & Medin, 1981; but see Cherniak, 1984; Rips, 1975). If people have invariant representations but use them only in more logical tasks, then these tasks should demonstrate stability. If invariant representations are used in membership decisions, for example, then membership judgments should be relatively stable. However, McCloskey and Glucksberg (1978) found a pattern of instability similar to the one reported here: Different subjects showed substantial differences in how they assigned membership for a particular category; and given subjects frequently changed their minds about whether an entity was a category member in two sessions across a 1-month period. Similar to the representations used for graded structure and property generation, the representations used for category membership judgments are unstable.

Conclusion

Taken together, these findings illustrate substantial instability in category representations. Different people do not use the same representation for a particular category, and a given person does not represent a category the same way across contexts. Instead the representation of a given category varies substantially between and within individuals. This suggests that the invariant knowledge structures that many researchers attempt to identify through scaling, property listing, and linguistic analysis are analytic fictions. Instead of being actual representations that people sometimes use in a particular context, these theoretical constructs are averages or ideals of representations abstracted across a wide variety of people and contexts. Moreover the postulation and use of such constructs tend to obscure many important mechanisms and sources of information that underlie people's dynamic representational ability (also see Barsalou, 1987; Barsalou & Medin, 1986).

Sources of instability

What factors underlie this widespread instability in category representation? This section considers several possibilities.

Differences in knowledge

Instability between people could reflect differences in knowledge. Because different people acquire different knowledge for a category over their lifetime, they retrieve different knowledge when representing it. Differences in knowledge must certainly exist between members of different populations, between experts and novices, and even between particular individuals from the same population to some extent. Moreover these differences must certainly cause people to view categories differently on some occasions.

However this explanation does not appear to account for the instability in Barsalou et al.'s (1987) experiments. All the properties produced across subjects for a category seemed to be basic facts that would be known by all subjects. Although less than 20% of the subjects in one study produced *has a beak*, *builds nests*, or *lives in trees* for *bird*, all subjects must be familiar with these properties. Although subjects probably had idiosyncratic knowledge for the various categories, they apparently did not produce it. Instead, nearly all of the properties produced by subjects in these experiments were clearly facts and beliefs about the category known by all subjects. Some other mechanism appears responsible for the instability reviewed earlier.

Atypical exemplars

Instability both between and within individuals for graded structure could reflect uncertainty about the status of atypical exemplars. Because subjects lack knowledge for these exemplars, or are unsure about their category membership, they could frequently change their minds about these exemplars' typicality and thereby produce instability. According to this view, stability should increase monotonically with typicality.

Barsalou et al. (1986) assessed the stability of exemplars at various levels of typicality and found, across all experiments, that typical and atypical exemplars were equally stable and that both were more stable than moderately typical exemplars. Judgments for moderately typical exemplars were most likely to change across sessions within a given subject; and when judgments changed, judgments for moderately typical exemplars moved the farthest, relative to the average distance they could potentially move. Between subjects, variability was again highest for moderately typical exemplars. Consequently, atypical exemplars did not underlie the substantial instability we observed for graded structure. Judgments for exemplars at all levels of typicality frequently changed, with judgments for moderately typical exemplars changing the most.

This finding complicates unitary views of categorization that assume a single mechanism underlies typicality and category membership (e.g., Hampton, 1979; Zadeh, 1965). Because stability *increases* from moderate to low typical exemplars for typicality, whereas stability *decreases* from moderate to low typical exemplars for membership (McCloskey & Glucksberg, 1978), different mechanisms may underlie these two tasks to some extent.

Forgetting

Instability within individuals could reflect forgetting. On finding that subjects produced a smaller number of properties in Session 2 than in Session 1, Bellezza (1984c) suggested that subjects were trying to remember their Session 1 protocols but failed to remember all of them. Barsalou et al. (1987) also observed a decrease in the number of properties from Session 1 to Session 2.

Other findings argue against this interpretation. Bellezza (1984c) also found that between-subject agreement increased from Session 1 to Session 2, as did Barsalou et al. (1987). It is not clear how forgetting could improve agreement. An alternative interpretation is that subjects converge on core information across sessions. In Session 1, subjects may retrieve and report somewhat irrelevant information in the process of finding information they perceive as relevant. This initial experience may enable subjects to be more efficient in Session 2 by retrieving only relevant information. To the extent that relevant information is shared among subjects and irrelevant information is not, agreement should increase across sessions. In further support of this interpretation, Barsalou et al. (1987) also found that the proportion of dictionary properties retrieved for words increased from Session 1 to Session 2.

Barsalou et al. (1986) tested the forgetting hypothesis more directly. In one experiment, half the subjects received the exemplars for a category in the same order in both sessions, and half received them in different random orders. Almost any theory of memory would predict that receiving stimuli in the same order should provide higher retention of previous typicality judgments than receiving stimuli in different orders. Consequently, if forgetting underlies within-subject instability, more stability should be observed for subjects receiving the same order. However, order had no effect, with same-order subjects showing .85 agreement and different-order subjects showing .84 agreement.

Barsalou et al. (1986) provided one other test of the forgetting hypothesis. Half the subjects in another study judged 8 exemplars per category, and half judged 16. Again almost any theory of memory would predict that having to remember more judgments across sessions should increase forgetting. However, subjects receiving 16 exemplars (.73) were just as stable as subjects receiving 8 exemplars (.74).

As discussed in the next section Barsalou et al. (1986) also manipulated the delay between sessions from 1 hour to 4 weeks and observed a decline in stability. Notably the shape of this decline did not resemble standard forgetting functions (e.g., Bahrick, 1984; Bahrick, Bahrick, & Wittlinger, 1975; Ebbinghaus, 1885/1964; Rubin, 1982). Whereas standard forgetting functions show substantial change between 1 and 4 weeks, Barsalou, Sewell, and Ballato's function was asymptotic during this period. In general, forgetting does not appear to underlie instability.

Measurement error

Perhaps the least interesting explanation of instability is that it reflects measurement error, what Winer (1971, p. 283) defined as instability due "in part to the measuring device itself and in part to the conditions surrounding testing." But if measurement error were responsible for the low levels of stability observed in Barsalou et al. (1986), then we should always observe these low levels regardless of the items being ranked or rated. However, Galambos and Rips (1982, Experiment 1) report a result that disconfirms this prediction. Some of their subjects ranked script actions from most to least central, where the centrality of actions in a script is analogous to the typicality of exemplars in a category (Barsalou & Sewell, 1985). Other subjects ranked these *same* actions by temporal position, beginning with the action occurring first in the script and concluding with the action occurring last. Subjects ranking centrality exhibited between-subject agreement of .35, which is comparable to the between-subject agreement reported earlier for typicality.

In striking contrast, subjects ranking temporal position exhibited between-subject agreement of .89, indicating that the low agreement for centrality was not due to measurement error. Instead low agreement for centrality appears to reflect less stability in the information subjects retrieved to make those judgments. Furthermore it is highly plausible that Galambos and Rips (1982) would have also found higher stability *within* subjects for temporal position than for centrality if they had collected those data. Given the likely possibility that subjects would show nearly perfect between- and within-subject agreement for *some* dimensions of categories (e.g., weight), it follows that measurement error is not solely responsible for the instability of typicality judgments. If it were, then there should be no dimension for which subjects exhibit higher stability.

Mapping judgments onto response scales

Rather than reflecting variability in category representations, instability in graded structure could simply reflect uncertainty in mapping judgments onto response scales. When ranking exemplars, subjects may perceive two exemplars as tied in typicality but be forced to give one a higher ranking randomly. Between-subject instability could result because different subjects make different random responses to such ties. Within-subject instability could result because the same subject makes different random responses in different sessions. To test this, Barsalou et al. (1987) compared ranking of typicality to ratings of typicality. In contrast to rankings, ratings allow subjects to have ties because the same rating can be applied to more than one exemplar. As discussed earlier, however, between- and within-subject agreement were both significantly less for ratings than for rankings. Consequently the problem of exemplar discriminability does not appear to underlie instability.

Barsalou et al. (1987) provide further evidence that mapping judgments onto response scales does not underlie instability. If instability reflects subjects' difficulty in deciding which exemplar of a particular subset is more typical, then increasing the number of exemplars that subjects judge should aggravate this problem and thereby increase instability. As the number of exemplars increases, the number of ties between exemplars should increase thereby increasing the rate of random responding. As discussed earlier, however, both between- and within-subject stability were unaffected by whether subjects judged 8 or 16 exemplars per category. Moreover, number of exemplars did not interact with whether subjects were performing ratings or rankings. Again the problem of exemplar discriminability does not appear to underlie instability.

It should be noted that problems in mapping judgments onto response scales cannot explain instability in property generation, which does not involve a response scale. Moreover, patterns of instability were basically the same for property generation and graded structure (in terms of between-subject agreement, within-subject agreement, and contextual shift). If response scales were responsible for instability in graded structure, then it seems unlikely that we would observe such a similar pattern of instability in another task that does not involve a response scale.

Stochastic retrieval mechanisms

Instability for graded structure both between and within individuals could reflect random fluctuation in retrieval, or, more technically, stochastic retrieval mechanisms. Whenever an individual represents a category, every property has some probability of being retrieved, and a different random subset represents the category on each occasion.

One argument against this view is that it does not make much sense in terms of achieving everyday goals. If only a subset of information represents a category, then why would a mechanism have evolved that has a high probability of retrieving information that is irrelevant to current goals, as well as a high probability of not retrieving information that is relevant?

Barsalou et al. (1986) attempted to test the stochastic retrieval hypothesis directly by manipulating the delay between sessions from 1 hour to 4 weeks. If the stochastic retrieval hypothesis is correct, then within-subject agreement should not be affected by delay. Because properties are retrieved randomly, each session is an independent event, and sessions should not be related in any way. Consequently the delay that separates sessions should not affect the extent to which retrieved properties differ. However, within-subject agreement showed a large initial decrease from 1 hour to 1 week and then showed no change thereafter (.92 after 1 hour, .87 after one day, .81 after 1 week, .81 after 2 weeks, and .79 after 4 weeks). Contrary to the stochastic retrieval hypothesis, within-subject stability after a week's delay does not reflect random fluctuation. Other factors must be involved. One might suggest forgetting as such a factor, but this seems unlikely, as discussed in a previous section. A recency-based explanation is proposed shortly.

The .92 agreement in the 1-hour-delay condition indicates that the maximum amount of instability potentially reflecting stochastic retrieval is small. Moreover other mechanisms besides stochastic variability could underlie instability in this condition. For example, Session 1 processing could have changed category knowledge such that the knowledge underlying performance in Sessions 1 and 2 differed. This possibility receives further discussion later.

Deterministic retrieval mechanisms

Instead of reflecting random fluctuation, instability may reflect the systematic operation of basic retrieval mechanisms. Two such mechanisms – *accessibility* and *contextual cuing* – appear to provide a reasonable qualitative account of people's dynamic representational ability.

Accessibility provides a central source of instability. Even though most people in a population may have the same basic knowledge for a category (as discussed earlier), the accessibility of this information may vary widely between individuals. Because the highly accessible information for a category varies from individual to individual, different individuals retrieve different information when initially accessing it, even though they all share most of the information any one of them retrieves. People might eventually converge on the same basic information if allowed to produce properties long enough, although studies of precuing suggest that initially retrieved information would prevent convergence (Brown, 1968; Karchmer & Winograd, 1971). Accessibility may similarly underlie instability within individuals and between populations: Within individuals, everyday experience may constantly change the accessibility of category information and thereby produce instability. Between populations, patterns of accessibility may vary widely and thereby produce greater instability than found between individuals of the same population.

Contextual cuing makes category representations still more dynamic. Even though most people may have the same basic knowledge for a category, the contexts that different people experience have the potential to cue different information and thereby cause between-subject instability. Within an individual, experiencing a category in different contexts would similarly cue different information and thereby cause within-subject instability.

Stable knowledge use

Although accessibility and contextual cuing both produce instability, it is important to note that they can also produce stability under certain conditions. Consider the following examples. Imagine that a group of people all regularly use dial-in modems to access a computer via the same telephone number. Once everyone has memorized the number, they should show perfect between- and within-subject agreement in retrieving it, although occasional errors are a reminder of the potential for instability. Similarly imagine that an experimenter asks a group of people, "How many legs do dogs have?" We would again observe perfect between- and within-subject agreement for the information subjects retrieve.

Accessibility and contextual cuing provide a natural means of accounting for such stability. High levels of accessibility may sometimes produce high stability. Repeatedly retrieving particular information may cause it to become sufficiently accessible and integrated that it becomes retrieved as a static structure. Practicing a phone number, for example, should cause a relatively static structure to become well established in memory.

Contextual cuing can similarly produce high stability. Because highly specific cues focus on only a small amount of information in memory, they reduce variability in what is retrieved. *Dog*, for example, is not a specific cue because it is associated with a tremendous amount of information. Consequently a wide variety of information is retrieved that thereby produces instability. In contrast, *dog* conjoined with *number of legs* is so specific that it focuses on a single piece of information and results in perfect stability.

Much remains to be learned about how accessibility and contextual cuing simultaneously produce flexibility and stability. When are categories represented dynamically, and what purpose does this flexibility serve? When are category representations stable, and what purpose does this stability serve? Although Rey's (1983) claim that category representations are unstable appears true, so does Smith, Medin, and Rips's (1984) counterclaim that mechanisms exist for establishing stability.

A retrieval-based framework for dynamic knowledge representation

This section presents a more specific formulation of how accessibility and contextual cuing combine to produce instability (see Barsalou, 1987, for further discussion). According to this view, a person possesses a tremendous amount of loosely organized knowledge for a category in long-term memory. Much of this knowledge may be widely shared by a population, and its content may remain relatively stable over time within individuals. However, only a very small subset of an individual's total knowledge for a category is ever active on a given occasion to represent the category in working memory. Such subsets may contain many kinds of information, including abstracted properties, exemplars, fragments of exemplars, and fragments of intuitive theories. Although certain core information may occur in most subsets for a category, much of the information in a subset is either context-dependent or reflects recent experience. Because contexts and recent experience are rarely the same, the same subset of information for a category is rarely, if ever, activated as its representation. For this reason, instability, rather than invariance, better characterizes the representations of a category.

Following the terminology of Barsalou (1987), I use the term *concept* to refer *only* to temporarily constructed representations in working memory; *concept* will *never* refer to information in long-term memory. Instead, a concept is simply a particular individual's *conception* of a category on a particular occasion. And rather than being definitional – as they are often assumed to be – concepts simply provide an individual with useful expectations about a category based on long-term past experience, recent experience, and current context (Barsalou & Medin, 1986). This usage is similar to Kahneman and Miller's (1986) use of *norm*, which refers to standards constructed in working memory to evaluate events.

Viewing concepts as temporary constructs by no means implies that people do not have well-established knowledge. Instead this view *does* assume the presence of relatively stable knowledge in long-term memory. But rather than being a collection of invariant structures used over and over again across situations, category knowledge provides the material from which concepts in working memory are dynamically constructed.[4]

Types of information in concepts

This formulation proposes that three basic types of information provide concepts with both stability and flexibility: *context-independent information* constituting conceptual cores (CI information); *context-dependent information* activated by the current context (CD information); and *recent context-dependent information* activated in recent contexts (CD_{rec} information). These distinctions are *retrieval-based* in the sense that they classify information by its accessibility and cue specificity. In addition, they are somewhat orthogonal to content-based distinctions (e.g., whether a piece of information is an ideal, an average, an exemplar, or part of an intuitive theory).

Context-independent information. A number of studies have shown that certain information is automatically activated every time a concept is constructed for a category (Barsalou, 1982; Conrad, 1978; Greenspan, 1986; Whitney, McKay, & Kellas, 1985). When reading *skunk*, for example, *unpleasant smell* is activated automatically on all occasions independent of context and incorporated into the representation of *skunk*. The same appears true for *valuable* with respect to *diamond* and for *poisonous* with respect to *rattlesnake*. In terms of the retrieval mechanisms just discussed, CI information is high in accessibility and low in context specificity. As suggested by Barsalou (1982, p. 87), subsequent strategic processing may later inhibit this information if it is irrelevant in the current context (as for *sour* in *plastic lemon*).

Barsalou and Bower (1980) propose that information becomes CI after it has been incorporated into a concept on numerous occasions. Frequent incorporation of a property causes it to develop an automatized status with respect to the category such that its activation becomes obligatory every time the category is processed (cf. Schneider & Shiffrin, 1977; Shiffrin & Schneider, 1977). Barsalou and Bower further suggest that highly discriminative properties for a category, and properties that are functionally important, are likely to be processed frequently and thereby become CI. Medin (personal communication, March 1986) further suggests that properties become CI because they are central to an intuitive theory for a category and are therefore processed frequently. Because the CI information for a particular individual depends on his or her frequent experience with a category, the CI information for different individuals can vary widely, and the CI information for a particular individual can change over time.

The graded structure and property generation studies reviewed earlier corroborate the presence of CI information in concepts. Within an individual, concepts maintain a certain amount of stability over time, as measured by both graded structure and property generation. Concepts also possess a lesser amount of stability between different individuals in the same population. One interpretation of these stabilities is that they reflect the presence of CI information. Because the same CI information is incorporated into all of a person's concepts for a particular category, some stability is maintained across contexts. Because a lesser amount of CI information is shared by members of a population, some stability is maintained across individuals.

According to this view, a category's conceptual core contains CI information, namely, highly accessible information that is incorporated into all of an individual's category representations across contexts. However, most current theories view conceptual cores differently. Some propose that conceptual cores are definitional (e.g., Armstrong et al., 1983; Osherson & Smith, 1981, 1982; Smith & Medin, 1981). Others propose that conceptual cores contain intuitive theories and idealized cognitive models (e.g., Lakoff, 1987; Michalski, this volume; Miller and Johnson-Laird, 1976, pp. 280–301; Murphy & Medin, 1985; Nelson, 1974, 1978; Medin and Ortony, this volume, Rips, this volume). Whereas these latter views can be construed as stressing the importance of category competence, the CI-property view stresses performance, focusing on those properties most frequently central to category use.

CI information may often contain information from definitions and intuitive theories. However some information from definitions and intuitive theories may be relevant so rarely that it does not become CI. The chemical composition of water (H_2O), for example, may be relevant so rarely for *water* that it does not become CI, even though it is definitional. Moreover information that is neither definitional nor relevant to intuitive theories may become CI if processed frequently enough with a category. If someone frequently encounters brown dogs, for example, then *brown* may become CI for *dog*, even though it is neither definitional nor relevant to intuitive theories. Much remains to be learned about the relations among CI information, definitional information, and intuitive theories.

Context-dependent information. Contrary to CI information, other information becomes incorporated into concepts only because of its relevance in the current context. As proposed by Barsalou (1982), such information may become incorporated into a concept in two ways. First, CD information may be stored with knowledge about a category in long-term memory but be activated so rarely that its accessibility is far below the level necessary for context independence. Such information may be incorporated into a concept only when activated by highly associated cues in the current context. For example, *edible* may typically be inactive for *frog* and be incorporated into concepts only when cued by relevant contexts such as French restaurants. As suggested by Brooks (personal communication, December 1986), current contextual information may also retrieve category exemplars, both recent and from the distant past (Brooks, 1987; Jacoby & Brooks, 1984). The relatively inaccessible exemplars that underlie remindings may also fall within this class of CD information (cf. Ross, 1984, this volume; Schank, 1982).

Alternatively, CD information may not be stored in memory for a category but may instead by inferred. When reading about a zebra orienting to noises in the brush, for example, someone may infer *ears* for *zebra* by using a cognitive economy inference procedure: Because a *zebra* is a *mammal*, and because *mammals* have *ears*, *zebras* have *ears*. Michalski (this volume) similarly proposes that much of the information in category representations is inferred from base representations. These two formulations differ in that Michalski assumes that CD information is only inferred, whereas the view proposed here assumes that some CD information is also retrieved.

These accounts of CD information primarily concern focal context, namely, the specific tasks and information currently focal to a person's attention (e.g., reading about someone ordering frog legs at a restaurant). However, peripheral characteristics of a context may also activate CD information. Someone's current psychological state (e.g., euphoria), physical context (e.g., being in a cafe), recent mental activity (e.g., planning a vacation), and so forth, may also be sufficiently salient to act as retrieval cues and thereby select information about categories as they are processed.

A final source of CD information is the perception of exemplars. All the CD mechanisms mentioned so far involve *retrieving* or *computing* information in memory that becomes incorporated into a concept. If actual exemplars of the category are present, however, their *perceptual* characteristics may also become part of the CD information on that occasion.

Recent context-dependent information. As found in the graded structure and property generation studies described earlier, a given person shows substantial change in his or her concept for a category after a delay of a week or more, *even though experimental conditions remain constant.* In Barsalou et al. (1986), for example, within-subject agreement declined from .92 after an hour to .87 after a day to .8 after a week. Because the experimental contexts of the two sessions were the "same," these declines, along with instability after a week or more, probably do not reflect changes in CD information. Instead they appear to reflect another factor, CD_{rec} information.

Once CD information becomes activated for a category, it may temporarily remain at a high level of activation such that it acquires a *temporary* CI status. Within a short temporal window – perhaps a day or two – this information may be automatically incorporated into every concept constructed for the category, even when irrelevant. But beyond this window, CD_{rec} information loses its temporary CI status and once again becomes incorporated only if relevant to the current context (i.e., it returns to being CD). For example, if someone had frog legs at a French restaurant one evening, an encounter with a frog in the back yard the following day might bring the edibility of frogs to mind. But encountering a frog a week after consuming frog legs may no longer do so. Examples of such a recency effect have been reported in the social cognition literature, where subjects are more likely to use a trait during impression formation when it has been recently activated (e.g., Bargh, Bond, Lombardi, & Tota, 1986; Higgins & King, 1981; Wyer & Srull, 1986).

CD_{rec} information may also be created indirectly. Instead of being created by the construction of previous concepts for a category, it may also be created by the construction of concepts for *related* categories. A recent encounter with a vicious dog, for example, may temporarily elevate the activation level of *viciousness* in concepts for other animals. Evidence that events perturb more knowledge than directly applies has been reported in the frequency literature (e.g., Barsalou

& Ross, 1986; Leicht, 1968; Shaughnessy & Underwood, 1973). The current CD_{rec} information for a category may even reflect recent activity of the cognitive system *in general*. Such effects follow from theories in which every event is assumed to perturb more knowledge than directly applies, and perhaps all knowledge in memory (e.g., connectionist models; McClelland, Rumelhart, & the PDP Research Group, 1986; Rumelhart, McClelland, & the PDP Research Group, 1986). As stated by James in 1890:

> whilst we think, our brain changes, ... and its whole internal equilibrium shifts with every pulse of change. The precise nature of the shifting at a given moment is a product of many factors. ... But just as one of them certainly is the influence of outward objects on the sense-organs during the moment, so is another certainly the very special susceptibility in which the organ has been left at that moment by all it has gone through in the past. Every brain-state is partly determined by the nature of this entire past succession. Alter the latter in any part, and the brain-state must be somewhat different. ... It is out of the question, then, that any total brain-state should identically recur. Something like it may recur; but to suppose *it* to recur would be equivalent to the absurd admission that all the states that had intervened between its two appearances had been pure nonentities, and that the organ after their passage was exactly as it was before." [James, 1890/1950, p. 234]

The following example for *frog* shows how these three types of information account for the effect of delay on within-subject agreement for graded structure when context is held constant. Consider the 1-hour-delay condition. When a subject constructs a concept for *frog* during Session 1, CI information becomes automatically incorporated by virtue of its high accessibility (e.g., *green, hops*). CD_{rec} information that reflects recent processing also becomes incorporated automatically. *Edible*, for example, might be CD_{rec} if frog legs had been consumed recently. CD information activated by focal context becomes incorporated. If the subject's task is to classify exemplars into biological classes, for example, then focusing on *class* with respect to *frog* will activate *amphibian*, which might be CD for many subjects. Finally, CD information activated by peripheral context becomes incorporated. If the previous category judged were *insects*, for example, then the subliminal activation of *insects* that remained might activate *eats insects* for *frog*.

When the subject constructs another concept for *frog* an hour later in Session 2, the same CI information is incorporated as in Session 1 (*green, hops*). However, the CD_{rec} and CD information, although highly similar to their counterparts in Session 1, differ somewhat. First consider CD_{rec} information. The CD_{rec} information incorporated in Session 1 (*edible*) is also incorporated in Session 2, because both sessions are roughly within the same temporal window for the CD_{rec} information that accrued prior to Session 1. However, additional CD_{rec} information is also incorporated, namely, the CD information from Session 1 that was activated by peripheral context (*eats insects*). Consequently the CD_{rec} information is not identical in the two sessions.

CD information behaves similarly to CD_{rec} information, showing both constancy and change. Because experimental conditions were held constant in both sessions, the focal context should be the "same," and focusing on *class* should activate the same CD information (*amphibian*). In contrast, it is likely that peripheral context has changed such that new CD information is activated in Session 2. If the previous category judged were *musical instruments*, for example, then the subliminal activation of *musical instruments* that remained might activate the sound "rivet" for *frog*.

According to this account, the high stability within a subject over an hour reflects three sources of common information: CI information, CD_{rec} information that accrued *prior* to Session 1, and CD information activated by focal processing. The small amount of instability at this delay reflects two sources of unique information: CD_{rec} information in Session 2 that resulted from peripheral context in Session 1 and CD information resulting from a new peripheral context in Session 2.[5]

At longer delays, this account assumes that changes in CD_{rec} information are primarily responsible for instability. As delays become longer than the lifetime of CD_{rec} information, this information only serves to make concepts different, whereas within its lifetime it makes concepts similar. To the extent the CD_{rec} information active for Session 1 (*edible*) has become inaccessible and been replaced with new CD_{rec} information, the CD_{rec} information active for Session 2 will be different. Because within-subject stability stops decreasing after a week's delay, the lifetime of CD_{rec} information appears to be a week or less.

Different CD information activated by peripheral context may also play a role in decreasing stability. At very short delays, peripheral context may remain relatively constant and thereby cause stability, whereas it may differ at longer delays and thereby cause instability. Because a person's peripheral context changes so quickly, however, this factor may affect stability only at very short delays.

Factors affecting the volume of particular information types

Within an individual, the volume (amount) of CI information in his or her concepts for a category should not vary much across contexts. Because it takes much experience to establish and change this information, it should change slowly over time such that the same amount generally enters into all concepts for a category (although intense experience with a category, such as on-the-job training, may cause rapid change).

Between individuals, the volume of CI information in the concepts for a category may vary widely. Consider Figure 3.1(a) in which the width of a box represents the volume of information. As depicted there, someone who once owned a dog should have developed much more CI information about dogs than someone who never owned a dog (or who has but little experience with them). As is also depicted, this person has not had much recent experience with dogs and therefore has the same amount of CD_{rec} information as someone who never owned a dog (and who also has not had much recent experience with dogs).

Another variable that probably affects the volume of CI information is population. Because a certain population may make extensive use of a category, its members may generally develop a larger volume of CI information for the category than members of another population that makes less use of the category. For example, people from Michigan may have a larger volume of CI information for *snow plow* than people from Georgia, and even more so than people from New Guinea.

Contrary to CI information, the volume of CD_{rec} information in a person's concepts can change substantially from occasion to occasion. Consider the example in Figure 3.1(b). On the left is a person's concept prior to ever owning a dog. On the right is that person's concept after recently acquiring her first one. Although she has not had the dog long enough to increase the amount of CI information for *dog*, she has established a large amount of CD_{rec} information. Presuming that the dog is around for a long time, she will continue to have a large volume of CD_{rec} information that will be continually changing, at least somewhat. The volume of CD_{rec} information can vary widely both within and between individuals, depending on their recent experience.

Similar to CD_{rec} information, the volume of CD information in a person's concept can change substantially from occasion to occasion. Consider the example in Figure 3.1(c). On the left is a concept for

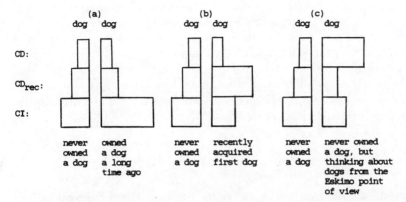

Figure 3.1. Examples of how (*a*) long-term, frequent experience affects the volume of CI information, (*b*) recent experience affects the volume of CD_{rec} information, and (*c*) current context affects the volume of CD information.

dog held by someone who has never owned a dog, who has not had much recent experience with dogs, and who is reading the word *dog* in no specified context. "No specified context" in this and later examples means reading a word or perceiving an exemplar in isolation (e.g., in the middle of an otherwise empty computer screen). In such situations, not much contextual information exists to activate CD information focally.

On the right of Figure 3.1(c) is the same person's concept after being asked to think about dogs from the Eskimo point of view. Because this person has previously acquired knowledge about the kinds of dogs that Eskimos have, about the roles these dogs play in Eskimo culture, and so forth, this information exists in his knowledge about dogs. However because he has not thought about this knowledge much in the past, and has not thought about it recently, Eskimo-related knowledge about dogs is not present in the CI and CD_{rec} information for the concept. When *Eskimo* is processed as the focal context, however, it cues this information by virtue of associative structure in memory. As a result, the total volume of CD information increases.

Intraconcept similarity

The first two sections demonstrated that concepts are unstable, and the next two presented a theoretical framework for viewing people's dynamic ability to represent categories. The final two sections explore implications of this framework for similarity.

Theories of similarity traditionally address the similarity of concepts for two different categories, what I will refer to as *intercategory similarity*. If category representations are unstable, however, then theories of similarity must consider another kind of similarity: the similarity between different concepts for the same category, what I will refer to as *intraconcept similarity*. Before discussing either intra- or intercategory similarity, it is first necessary to state several assumptions regarding similarity in general.[6]

Assumptions about similarity

Based on the analysis in previous sections, the similarity of two concepts depends on the amount of overlap between their CI, CD_{rec}, and CD information. For example, the two concepts juxtaposed along the vertical line on the left side of Figure 3.2(a) have less overlap for three kinds of information than the two concepts on the right (where overlap is represented by the amount of shaded area). Consequently the concepts on the left are less similar than those on the right.

However, the total volume of each kind of information must also be considered when assessing similarity. Although the two concepts on the left of Figure 3.2(b) have the same amount of overlap as the two concepts on the right, the total volume of the two concepts on the right is much greater. Following Tversky (1977), similarity is also a decreasing function of the amount of unique information in each concept, as well as the amount of information in common. Consequently the two concepts on the right are less similar than those on the left, even though their overlap is the same.

Also following Tversky (1977), various factors can cause subsets of information to be weighted differently. The relative weighting of common and unique information, for example, can vary across contexts. In addition, the relative weighting of CI, CD_{rec}, and CD information may also vary. For example, when people judge typicality from their own point of view, they may weight CD_{rec} information highly to maximize the contribution of their personal experience (assuming that similarity of exemplar and category concepts underlies typicality). In contrast, when taking the American point of view, people may weight this information closer to zero to minimize the contribution of personal experience. To simplify matters, nothing further will be said about weighting. How-

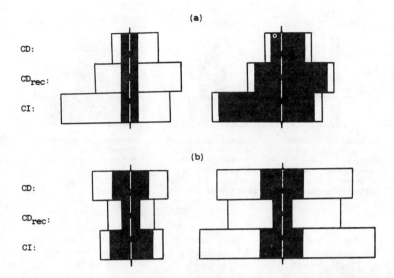

Figure 3.2. Examples of how (*a*) proportion of overlap and (*b*) total volume affect similarity. Two concepts are juxtaposed along the vertical line, with the shaded areas representing common information and the unshaded areas representing unique information.

ever it is certainly an important factor that a more complete analysis would have to consider.

Factors affecting intraconcept similarity

Cultural transmission of knowledge may largely involve establishing shared cores of CI information for categories within members of a population. For example, our culture may generally establish a core for *cow* that in part contains information about cows being a source of meat. Other cultures may transmit different cores for the same category. For example, the core in *cow* for citizens of India may contain information about cows *not* being a source of meat and about their religious significance.

As a baseline, then, intraconcept similarity should generally be lowest (although not necessarily) between individuals from different populations. As shown in Figure 3.3(a) there may generally not be much overlap *on the average* between two individuals from different populations with respect to CI, CD_{rec}, or CD information (e.g., as in Barsalou & Sewell, 1984; Schwanenflugel & Rey, 1986).

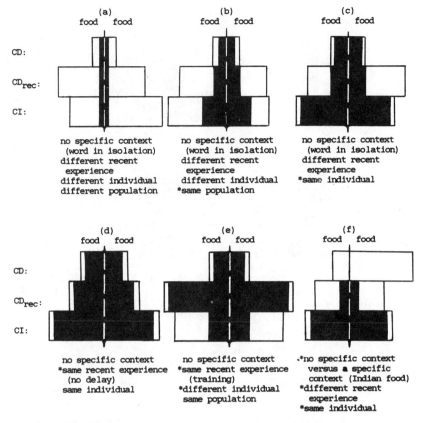

Figure 3.3. Examples of how population, individual, recent experience, and current context can affect intraconcept similarity. Two instances of the same concept are juxtaposed along the vertical line, with shaded areas representing common information and unshaded areas representing unique information. * indicates a change from the preceding example.

In contrast, two individuals from the same population may generally share more CI information by virtue of their shared cultural membership. As reviewed earlier, different individuals from the same population exhibit a low-to-moderate overlap in their concepts of the same category. The graded structures of different individuals generally correlate around .5 (accounting for 25% of the variance), and the properties produced by different individuals generally have an average overlap of around .32. Such agreement may reflect CI information shared by the population.

As suggested in Figure 3.3(b), this gain in CI overlap may often be accompanied by gains in CD_{rec} and CD information as well.

CD_{rec} overlap may increase because exemplars are more similar within populations, because actions performed on exemplars are more similar, and so forth. CD overlap may increase because the associative knowledge that underlies CD activation may be culturally bound, similar to CI knowledge. For example, people in the United States and the Soviet Union may have different stereotypes for Eskimos. Consequently, when thinking about dogs from the Eskimo point of view, these two populations may activate somewhat different CD information.

We turn now from populations to consider individuals. Because different people in a population often have different experiences with a category, they may develop different CI information to some extent. Consequently, instances of a concept constructed by the same person should be more similar than instances constructed by different people. As suggested by Figure 3.3(c), virtually the same CI information should be incorporated into a person's concepts for the same category across occasions. In support of this, we have generally found substantially higher agreement within subjects than between subjects, both for graded structure (.8 vs. .5) and for property generation (.55 vs. .32).

Again this gain in CI information may be accompanied by gains in CD_{rec} and CD information. CD_{rec} overlap may increase because exemplars are more similar within individuals, because actions performed on exemplars are more similar, and so forth. CD overlap may increase because the associative knowledge that underlies CD activation may be somewhat idiosyncratic.

Within the same individual, recent experience may increase intraconcept similarity in two ways. First, if a person constructs two concepts for the same category within the short lifetime of particular CD_{rec} information, then the presence of this information in both concepts should increase their similarity. When focal context also remains constant, intraconcept similarity may be quite high. As depicted in Figure 3.3(d), these may be the conditions under which intraconcept similarity is highest. As suggested by Barsalou (1987), such recency effects may facilitate goal-directed behavior by maintaining conceptual constancy while a particular goal is being achieved.

Second, recent experience may increase intraconcept similarity within the same individual across a long time period if similar events occurred prior to constructing instances of the same concept. For example, concepts constructed for *dog* on two occasions a year apart may be similar if the person was bitten by a dog just prior to both.

Similar recent experience may also increase intraconcept similarity between individuals. If two people were recently bitten by a dog, for example, then their concepts for *dog* should be more similar than if their recent experiences had differed. Analogously, if two people experience intense recent training with a concept, such as in a laboratory or on the job, then this should increase not only the proportion of CD_{rec} overlap but also the total volume of CD_{rec} overlap. As can be seen in Figure 3.3(e), this could substantially increase intraconcept similarity between individuals.

Context affects intraconcept similarity through the activation of CD information. To the extent contexts activate the same information, either within or between individuals, intraconcept similarity should increase. As shown in Figure 3.3(f), for example, reading a word in isolation may activate relatively little CD information, whereas reading a word in the context of a point of view may activate much CD information that is completely unrelated to the CD information in the other context. Conversely, constructing a concept from the same point of view on two occasions should result in a substantial amount of shared CD information, thereby causing a large increase in intraconcept similarity.

In summary, intraconcept similarity depends on the overlap of CI, CD_{rec}, and CD information. Population and individual subject factors may have large effects on the overlap of CI information and accompanying effects on the overlap of CD_{rec} and CD information. Recent experience is primarily responsible for the overlap of CD_{rec} information, which is maximized within individuals at short delays and between individuals who have had similar recent experiences. Current context is primarily responsible for the overlap of CD information. Depending on the composition of these factors, intraconcept similarity can range from extremely high to extremely low. Assuming invariant concepts for categories not only is unjustified but also obscures the presence of dynamic and important representational mechanisms. As discussed next, it also distorts interconcept similarity and obscures similar mechanisms there.

Implications for interconcept similarity

Theories of similarity generally address the similarity of concepts for two different categories and generally seem to assume that invariant concepts represent these categories (e.g., Krumhansl, 1978; Shepard, 1962a, 1962b; Tversky, 1977). But if the concepts representing a particular category are unstable, then it follows that the

similarity of two categories is also unstable. Contrary to an implication of traditional theories, the similarity of two categories is not
invariant.

Barsalou's (1982) Experiment 2 provides direct evidence that
the similarity of two categories varies across contexts. *Raccoon* and
snake, for example, were much less similar when judged in no explicit context than when judged in the context of *pets*. Because *pets*
activates similar CD information in *raccoon* and *snake*, their number of common properties increases, which thereby increases their
similarity. Barsalou (1982) also showed that this effect does *not* occur when a context is relevant to CI information. The similarity of
robin and *eagle*, for example, was the same in no explicit context
as in the context of *birds*. Because the common properties relevant
to *birds* are *context-independent*, they are active in the absence of the
birds context.

Moreover, interconcept similarity varies when context remains constant. Hutchinson and Lockhead (1977) obtained .55 between-subject
reliability and .73 within-subject reliability for subjects' judgments of
interconcept similarity (e.g., the similarity of *chicken* to *eagle*, of *plum*
to *robin*). These levels of agreement are reminiscent of those reported
earlier for graded structure and property generation, indicating that
concept instability also has a substantial effect on interconcept
similarity.

It should be noted that the *weighting of properties* typically provides
theories of similarity with potential for generating variability in interconcept similarity (e.g., as in Tversky's, 1977, diagnosticity principle). For example, by assuming that many properties in a concept
are weighted to zero in a particular context, and by assuming that the
properties weighted to zero can vary widely in different situations,
the content of concepts can *functionally* change across contexts. However, the actual content of the concept remains the same, unless a
further assumption is made that properties weighted to zero are not
part of the concept in that context. Generally speaking, most theorists
have not viewed weighting as a means of varying the content of concepts but instead have viewed it as a means of varying the effects of
an invariant set of properties.

Factors affecting interconcept similarity

All the factors that affect intraconcept similarity also affect interconcept similarity. As shown in Figure 3.4(a, b, c), the primary difference
between intra- and interconcept similarity is the average amount of

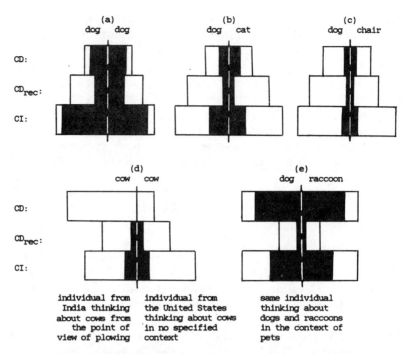

Figure 3.4. Examples of decreasing similarity among (*a*) instances of the same concept, (*b*) different but related concepts, and (*c*) unrelated concepts. Examples (*a*), (*b*), and (*c*) assume no specified context, different recent experience, and the same individual. Examples (*d*) and (*e*) demonstrate one way intraconcept similarity could be lower than interconcept similarity.

overlap: Intraconcept similarity should generally be higher than the interconcept similarity of two related concepts, which should generally be higher than the interconcept similarity of two unrelated concepts (these examples assume no specified context, different recent experience, and the same individual).

This ordering is not necessarily invariant, however, because the composition of concepts could be such that interconcept similarity in a particular situation is higher than intraconcept similarity. As shown in Figure 3.4(d), for example, someone from India thinking about *cow* from the point of view of *plowing* might have a fairly different concept than someone from the United States thinking about *cow* in no specified context. As shown in Figure 3.4(e), however, a single individual thinking about *dog* and *raccoon* from the point of view of *pets* might construct highly similar concepts for these different categories. Most important, the concepts for *dog* and *raccoon* may be more similar than the two concepts for *cow*, such that interconcept similarity is higher than intraconcept similarity. Dornbusch, Hastorf, Richardson, Muzzy, and Vreeland's (1965) classic study of interviewers' perceptions of campers demonstrates a similar effect in social cognition. They found that a given interviewer's personality assessments of two different campers were generally more similar than two interviewers' assessments of the same camper.

Figure 3.5 demonstrates how various factors influence interconcept similarity. These factors generally parallel those for intraconcept similarity in Figure 3.3. As a baseline, interconcept similarity should generally be lowest between concepts constructed by members of different populations. As shown in Figure 3.5(a, b), similarity should increase when constructed by members of the same population because of gains in CI overlap. Similar to intraconcept similarity, such gains may also be accompanied by gains in CD_{rec} and CD overlap. Interconcept similarity should generally increase further when concepts for two categories are constructed by the same individual as seen in Figure 3.5(c). Again, such gains may reflect gains in CI information, along with accompanying gains in CD_{rec} and CD information.

Similar recent experience with two categories, either within or between individuals, can further increase interconcept similarity. As shown in Figure 3.5(d), for example, someone who recently began work in a pet store may have had similar recent experiences with boas and dogs such that concepts constructed for these categories are similar at that point in time. As shown in Figure 3.5(e), once having worked in a pet store – but not recently – may also increase similarity, but in this case by increasing the overlap of CI information. Finally, interconcept similarity can be increased substantially by current context as in Figure 3.5(f). For example, if someone who has never worked in a pet store views *boa* and *dog* in the context of *pets*, the increase in CD overlap will increase interconcept similarity.

In summary, interconcept similarity, like intraconcept similarity, depends on the overlap of CI, CD_{rec}, and CD information. The primary difference between these two kinds of similarity may simply be that intraconcept similarity is generally higher than interconcept similarity, although not necessarily. Otherwise, intra- and interconcept similarity may both be produced by the same cognitive processes and reflect the same basic variables.

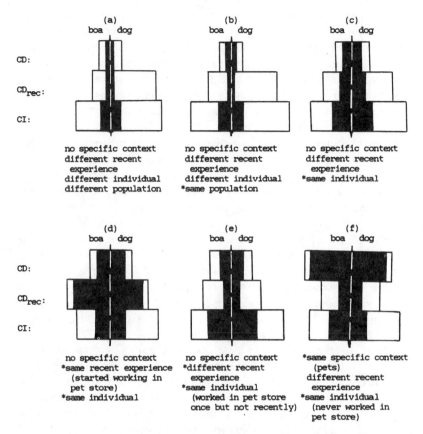

Figure 3.5. Examples of how population, individual, recent experience, and current context can affect interconcept similarity. Instances of two different concepts are juxtaposed along the vertical line, with shaded areas representing common information and unshaded areas representing unique information. * indicates a change from the preceding example.

Analogous to intraconcept similarity, population and individual subject factors may have large effects on the overlap of CI information and accompanying effects on the overlap of CD_{rec} and CD information. Again recent experience is responsible for the overlap of CD_{rec} information, and current context is responsible for the overlap of CD information. Depending on the composition of these factors, the similarity of concepts for two categories can vary widely. Assuming invariant concepts and static similarity relations between categories obscures the operation of important factors affecting interconcept similarity.

What do averages of scaling data represent?

Averaging data across subjects and across trials within the same subject is standard practice in empirical studies of human knowledge. But given the substantial instability of concepts, what do these averages represent? According to the analysis here, the answer depends on what is averaged. Consider averaging the typicality judgments of different subjects in the "same" context. As shown in the left two panels of Figure 3.6(a), the concepts constructed for an exemplar by different subjects overlap on CI information shared by the population, have no CD_{rec} overlap, and overlap on CD information shared by the population. Assume for simplicity that the effects of nonoverlapping information on typicality are uncorrelated (i.e., nonoverlapping CI effects are uncorrelated, all CD_{rec} effects are uncorrelated, and nonoverlapping CD effects are uncorrelated). Then typicality averaged across subjects should reflect only overlapping information between subjects, as shown in the right panel of Figure 3.6(a). In other words, averaging across subjects nets the effects of population CI information for the exemplar plus population CD information. All other information has no effect.

Next consider averaging multiple typicality judgments made by the same subject in the "same" context at two times more than a week apart. As shown in the left two panels of Figure 3.6(b), concepts constructed for the same exemplar should have a complete CI overlap, no CD_{rec} overlap, and a partial CD overlap. Again assume for simplicity that the effects of nonoverlapping information on typicality are uncorrelated (i.e., all CD_{rec} effects are uncorrelated, and nonoverlapping CD effects are uncorrelated). Then typicality, as averaged across sessions, should reflect only overlapping information, as shown in the right panel of Figure 3.6(b). In other words, averaging across trials nets the effects of the individual's CI information for the exemplar, plus the individual's CD information that is affected only by focal context. All other components have no effect.

Averaging across subjects and contexts obscures the effects of certain sources of information in concepts. What remain are the effects of information common to the particular concepts observed. There may be certain situations in which we would like to know this information, and averaging may be a good way to determine it. To the extent we assume that this information represents a person's concept in a particular situation, however, we are misinterpreting data. If we wish to identify actual concepts constructed by an individual, and the

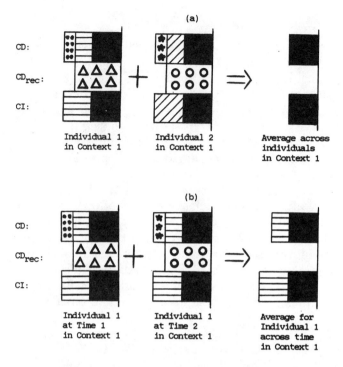

Figure 3.6. Examples of how (*a*) averaging across individuals, and (*b*) averaging across contexts within an individual obscures certain sources of information in concepts. Shaded areas represent population cores. Lined areas represent idiosyncratic, individual cores. Areas containing figures represent the contribution of recency and nonfocal context.

relations between them, we cannot do so by averaging across individuals or contexts. Instead we must assess concepts in specific individuals in specific contexts.

Two other points should be noted. First, averaging does not necessarily identify CI cores. As suggested in Figure 3.6, averaging may net not only CI information occurring across individuals and contexts but also CD information occurring across contexts. Moreover, if subjects have had similar recent experience with a category, such as laboratory training, then averaging may also net CD_{rec} information across individuals. The point is that using averaging to identify CI cores may be difficult, and care should be taken to cancel out all other sources of information. Second, averaging may not yield accurate estimates of information occurring across contexts or individuals when the effects of nonoverlapping information *are* correlated. Under these conditions, it is impossible to know what averages mean without knowing the nature of the correlations.

Specific applications

When the inputs to scaling procedures such as multidimensional scaling and hierarchical clustering procedures are data averaged across subjects and contexts, only information common to the particular concepts observed enters into scaling solutions. Nonoverlapping information between individuals and contexts will not have an effect, to the extent the effects of this information are uncorrelated. Although these procedures may be valuable for identifying common information across individuals and contexts, they do not provide complete information about any individual's concepts in any particular context.

Another scaling procedure, INDSCAL, does exhibit sensitivity to the concepts of particular subjects by identifying weightings that individuals place on dimensions. When the inputs to this procedure are averages across contexts, however, the basis of solutions will only be information common to the individual's concepts across contexts. Nonoverlapping information unique to specific contexts will not be captured, to the extent its effects are uncorrelated. In contrast, when the inputs are an individual's nonaveraged data from specific contexts, the solution will reflect all the information in concepts constructed during the experiment. Because of changes that can occur in CD_{rec} and CD information, however, care should be taken in generalizing these results to other contexts for that subject.

In comparing group versus individual points of view, Barsalou and Sewell (1984) found that the average graded structures constructed by undergraduates taking the faculty point of view were *identical* to the average graded structures constructed by faculty taking their own point of view. Sewell (1985), however, found that specific individuals were far from perfect at constructing graded structures from the point of view of a close friend. How could the average graded structure of faculty and undergraduates taking the faculty point of view be identical when the graded structures of close friends were highly divergent? One possible account concerns the effects of averaging. Averaging across subjects may eliminate the effects of all information not common to the population. Consequently, if information common to one population is the same as information common to the other, then the effects of this information on average graded structures should be identical, because all nonoverlapping information cancels out. In contrast, when comparing the nonaveraged concepts of individuals, idiosyncratic information is not canceled out, and differences between individuals are observed. The apparent identity of population averages is therefore misleading: A concept held by a member of one population is *not* identical to a concept held by a member of the other – in fact, there is probably substantial non-overlapping information. The illusion of identity exists only because averaging eliminated the nonoverlapping information.

In Barsalou, Sewell, and Ballato (work in progress), subjects taking their own point of view generated average graded structures for common taxonomic categories that were identical to those of subjects taking the American point of view. However, subjects taking their own point of view showed lower between-subject agreement, suggesting that these subjects' judgments were more idiosyncratic. Again the equivalence of average graded structures reflects nonoverlapping information being canceled by averaging. Even though the self condition had more nonoverlapping information than the American condition, this difference was not captured by average graded structures.

Conclusion

Categories are not represented by invariant concepts. Different individuals do not represent a category in the same way, and a given individual does not represent a category in the same way across contexts. Instead there is tremendous variability in the concepts that represent a category. This variability engenders the consideration of intraconcept similarity, namely, how instances of the same concept are related. Intraconcept similarity depends on (a) whether concepts are constructed by members of the same or different populations, (b) whether concepts are constructed by the same or different individuals, (c) recent experiences with the category, and (d) current context. Because concepts for the same category are not invariant, neither is intercategory similarity. The similarity of the concepts for two categories can vary widely as a function of the same factors that determine intraconcept similarity. Accurate assessments of how an individual in a given context perceives the similarity of two concepts cannot be based on data averaged across either individuals or contexts. Averaging tends to obscure important sources of information in concepts and to leave only sources that are constant across the concepts observed. Though obtaining such information may be of value for certain purposes, it should not be construed as completely representing a person's concept in a particular context. As James (1890/1950, p. 236) states:

No doubt it is often *convenient* to formulate the mental facts in an atomistic sort of way, and to treat the higher states of consciousness as if they were all built out of unchanging simple ideas. It is convenient often to treat curves as if they were composed of small straight lines, and electricity and nerve-force as if they were fluids. But in the one case as in the other we must never forget that we are talking symbolically, and that there is nothing in nature to answer to our words.

NOTES

I am grateful to Lee Brooks, J. Wesley Hutchinson, Douglas Medin, Andrew Ortony, Jayna Spindler, and especially Stella Vosniadou for helpful comments on previous drafts of this chapter. I am also grateful to Jayna Spindler, Daniel Sewell, Susan Ballato, and Elaine Gendel for their contributions to the research described herein, and to Ulric Neisser for pointing out that William James had much to say about instability. Work on this chapter was supported by Grant IST–8308984 to the author from the National Science Foundation. Correspondence and reprint requests should be sent to Lawrence W. Barsalou, School of Psychology, Georgia Institute of Technology, Atlanta, GA 30332.

1 For examples of relevant literature, see Armstrong, Gleitman, and Gleitman (1983), Katz (1972), Osherson and Smith (1981, 1982), on definitions; see Hampton (1979), Rosch and Mervis (1975), on prototypes; see Brooks (1978), Hintzman (1986), Jacoby and Brooks (1984), Medin and Schaffer (1978), on exemplars; see Minsky (1975), Rumelhart and Ortony (1977), on frames and schemata; see Schank and Abelson (1977), on scripts; see Gentner and Stevens (1983), Johnson-Laird (1983), on mental models.
2 Although people make extensive use of stereotypes such as *American, housewife*, and *redneck*, and even though such stereotypes may lead to accurate inferences on some occasions, they often lead to inaccurate inferences and offer a narrow and prejudiced view of the world. Our use of stereotypes is not meant to condone their use. Instead we have chosen to study stereotypes because of the extensive role they play in cognition (Fiske & Taylor, 1984).
3 Rosch (1975) and Armstrong et al. (1983) report that between-subject agreement is .9 and higher. As discussed by Barsalou (1987) and Barsalou, Sewell, and Ballato (1987), these values do not actually represent between-subject agreement but instead represent the stability of *average* typicality judgments. Because the reliability of averages increases monotonically with the number of subjects in a sample, a .9 level of agreement can be obtained with a modest number of subjects, even though between-subject agreement may actually be quite low.
4 It is important to note that retrieval has been central to previous theories of knowledge. Quillian (1968), Collins and Loftus (1975), and McCloskey

and Glucksberg (1979), for example, all assume *continuous retrieval* of category information during classification and question answering; that is, information is retrieved until a sufficient amount is available to make a response. Moreover the first two of these theories, through intersecting search, have some capability of handling context effects (as a conjunction of probes). Exemplar models are also oriented toward the importance of retrieval in representation and have much potential for explaining instability (e.g., Brooks, 1978, 1987; Hintzman, 1986; Jacoby & Brooks, 1984; Medin & Schaffer, 1978). In general, however, none of these theories has yet addressed issues associated with between-subject instability, within-subject instability, and contextual shift.

5 CD_{rec} information at Session 2 that resulted from peripheral context in Session 1 (*eats insects*) need not necessarily be a source of instability. Because this information was also present during Session 1 as CD information, it could increase stability rather than decrease it. This depends on the extent to which *memory* of CD information from Session 2 is the same as its initial activation in Session 1.

6 Previous theories have discussed the similarity of a concept to itself, which could be construed as a kind of intraconcept similarity (e.g., Krumhansl, 1978; Tversky, 1977). Because this previous work has addressed a stimulus' overall confusability with other stimuli, however, rather than how instances of the same category are related, it has addressed a very different kind of intraconcept similarity than the kind addressed here.

REFERENCES

Anderson, R. C., & Ortony, A. (1975). On putting apples into bottles: A problem of polysemy. *Cognitive Psychology, 7,* 167–180.

Anderson, R. C., Pichert, J. W., Goetz, E. T., Schallert, D. L., Stevens, K. V., & Trollip, S. R. (1976). Instantiation of general terms. *Journal of Verbal Learning and Verbal Behavior, 15,* 667–679.

Armstrong, S. L., Gleitman, L. R., & Gleitman, H. (1983). What some concepts might not be. *Cognition, 13,* 263–308.

Bahrick, H. P. (1984). Semantic memory in permastore: Fifty years of memory for Spanish learned in school. *Journal of Experimental Psychology: General, 113,* 1–37.

Bahrick, H. P., Bahrick, P. O., & Wittlinger, R. P. (1975). Fifty years of memories for names and faces: A cross-sectional approach. *Journal of Experimental Psychology: General, 104,* 54–75.

Barclay, J. R., Bransford, J. D., Franks, J. J., McCarrell, N. S., & Nitsch, K. (1974). Comprehension and semantic flexibility. *Journal of Verbal Learning and Verbal Behavior, 13,* 471–481.

Bargh, J. A., Bond, R. N., Lombardi, W. J., & Tota, M. E. (1986). The additive nature of chronic and temporary sources of construct accessibility. *Journal of Personality and Social Psychology, 50,* 869–878.

Barsalou, L. W. (1982). Context-independent and context-dependent information in concepts. *Memory & Cognition, 10,* 82–93.

Barsalou, L. W. (1983). Ad hoc categories. *Memory & Cognition, 11,* 211–227.

Barsalou, L. W. (1985). Ideals, central tendency, and frequency of instantiation as determinants of graded structure in categories. *Journal of Experimental Psychology: Learning, Memory, and Cognition, 11*, 629–654.

Barsalou, L. W. (1987). The instability of graded structure: Implications for the nature of concepts. In U. Neisser (Ed.), *Concepts and conceptual development: Ecological and intellectual factors in categorization* (pp. 101–140). Cambridge: Cambridge University Press.

Barsalou, L. W., & Bower, G. H. (1980, September). A priori determinants of a concept's highly accessible information. Paper presented at the meeting of the American Psychological Association, Montreal.

Barsalou, L. W., & Medin, D. L. (1986). Concepts: Static definitions or context-dependent representations? *Cahiers de Psychologie Cognitive, 6*, 187–202.

Barsalou, L. W., & Ross, B. H. (1986). The roles of automatic and strategic processing in sensitivity to superordinate and property frequency. *Journal of Experimental Psychology: Learning, Memory, and Cognition, 11.* 116–134.

Barsalou, L. W., & Sewell, D. R. (1984). *Constructing representations of categories from different points of view* (Emory Cognition Project Rep. No. 2). Atlanta: Emory University.

Barsalou, L. W., & Sewell, D. R. (1985). Contrasting the representation of scripts and categories. *Journal of Memory and Language, 24*, 646–665.

Barsalou, L. W., Sewell, D. R., & Ballato, S. M. (1986). *Assessing the stability of category representations with graded structure.* Unpublished manuscript.

Barsalou, L. W., Spindler, J. L., Sewell, D. R., Ballato, S. M., & Gendel, E. M. (1987). *Assessing the instability of category representations with property generation.* Unpublished manuscript.

Barsalou, L. W., Usher, J. A., & Sewell, D. R. (1985). *Schema-based planning of events.* Paper presented at the meeting of the Psychonomic Society, Boston.

Bellezza, F. S. (1984a). Reliability of retrieval from semantic memory: Common categories. *Bulletin of the Psychonomic Society, 22*, 324–326.

Bellezza, F. S. (1984b). Reliability of retrieval from semantic memory: Information about people. *Bulletin of the Psychonomic Society, 22*, 511–513.

Bellezza, F. S. (1984c). Reliability of retrieval from semantic memory: Noun meanings. *Bulletin of the Psychonomic Society, 22*, 377–380.

Brooks. L. R. (1978). Nonanalytic concept formation and memory for instances. In E. Rosch & B. B. Lloyd (Eds.), *Cognition and categorization* (pp. 169–211). Hillsdale, NJ: Erlbaum.

Brooks. L. R. (1987). Decentralized control of categorization: The role of prior processing episodes. In U. Neisser (Ed.), *Concepts and conceptual development: Ecological and intellectual factors in categorization* (pp. 141–174). Cambridge: Cambridge University Press.

Brown, J. (1968). Reciprocal facilitation and impairment of free recall. *Psychonomic Science, 10*, 41–42.

Buss, D. M., & Craik, K. H. (1983). The act–frequency approach to personality. *Psychological Review, 90*, 105–126.

Buss, D. M., & Craik, K. H. (1985). Why *not* measure that trait? Alternative criteria for identifying important dispositions. *Journal of Personality and Social Psychology, 48*, 934–946.

Cherniak, C. (1984). Prototypicality and deductive reasoning. *Journal of Verbal Learning and Verbal Behavior, 23*, 625–642.

Collins, A., & Loftus, E. F. (1975). A spreading-activation theory of semantic processing. *Psychological Review, 82*, 407–428.

Conrad, C. (1978). Some factors involved in the recognition of words. In J. W. Cotton & R. L. Klatzky (Eds.), *Semantic factors in cognition.* Hillsdale, NJ: Erlbaum.

Deese, J. (1965). *The structure of associations in language and thought.* Baltimore: Johns Hopkins University Press.

Dornbusch, S. M., Hastorf, A. H., Richardson, S. A., Muzzy, R. E., Vreeland, R. S. (1965). The perceiver and the perceived: Their relative influence on the categories of interpersonal cognition. *Journal of Personality and Social Psychology, 1*, 434–440.

Ebbinghaus, H. E. (1964). *Memory, a contribution to experimental psychology.* (H. A. Ruger & C. E. Bussenius, Trans.). New York: Dover. (Original work published 1885.)

Epstein, S. (1979). The stability of behavior: 1. On predicting most of the people much of the time. *Journal of Personality and Social Psychology, 37*, 1097–1126.

Ericsson, K. A., & Simon, H. A. (1980). Verbal reports as data. *Psychological Review, 87*, 215–251.

✓ Ericsson, K. A., & Simon, H. A. (1984). *Protocol analysis: Verbal reports as data,* Cambridge, MA: MIT Press.

Fehr, B., & Russell J. A. (1984). Concept of emotion viewed from a prototype perspective. *Journal of Experimental Psychology: General, 113*, 464–486.

✓ Fiske, S. T., & Taylor, S. E. (1984). *Social cognition.* Reading, MA: Addison-Wesley.

Galambos, J. A., & Rips, L. J. (1982). Memory for routines. *Journal of Verbal Learning and Verbal Behavior, 21*, 260–281.

Geis, M. F., & Winograd, E. (1975). Semantic encoding and judgments of background and situational frequency of homographs. *Journal of Experimental Psychology: Human Learning and Memory, 104*, 385–392.

✓ Gentner, D., & Stevens, A. L. (Eds.) (1983). *Mental models.* Hillsdale, NJ: Erlbaum.

Greenspan, S. L. (1986). Semantic flexibility and referential specificity of concrete nouns. *Journal of Memory and Language, 25*, 539–557.

Halff, H. M., Ortony, A., & Anderson, R. C. (1976). A context-sensitive representation of word meanings. *Memory & Cognition, 4*, 378–373.

Hampton, J. A. (1979). Polymorphous concepts in semantic memory. *Journal of Verbal Learning and Verbal Behavior, 18*, 441–461.

Higgins, E. T., & King, G. (1981). Accessibility of social constructs: Information processing consequences of individual and contextual variability. In N. Cantor & J. F. Kihlstrom (Eds.), *Personality, cognition, and social interaction* (pp. 69–120). Hillsdale, NJ: Erlbaum.

Hintzman, D. L. (1986). "Schema abstraction" in a multiple-trace memory model. *Psychological Review, 93*, 411–428.

Hutchinson, J. W., & Lockhead, G. R. (1977). Similarity as distance: A structural principle for semantic memory. *Journal of Experimental Psychology: Human Learning and Memory, 3*, 660–678.

Jacoby, L. L. & Brooks, L. R. (1984). Nonanalytic cognition: Memory, perception, and concept learning. In G. H. Bower (Ed.), *The psychology of learning and motivation: Advances in research and theory* (Vol. 18, pp. 1–47). New York: Academic Press.

James, W. (1950). *The principles of psychology* (Vol. 1). New York: Dover. (Original work published 1890.)

✓ Johnson-Laird, P. N. (1983). *Mental models: Towards a cognitive science of language, inference, and consciousness.* Cambridge, MA: Harvard University Press.

Kahneman, D., & Miller, D. T. (1986). Norm theory: Comparing reality to its alternatives. *Psychological Review, 93,* 136–153.

Karchmer, M. A. & Winograd, E. (1971). Effects of studying a subset of familiar items on recall of the remaining items: The John Brown effect. *Psychonomic Science, 25,* 224–225.

Katz, J. J. (1972). *Semantic theory.* New York: Harper & Row.

Krumhansl, C. L. (1978). Concerning the applicability of geometric models to similarity data: The interrelationship between similarity and spatial density. *Psychological Review, 85,* 445–463.

✓ Lakoff, G. (1987). *Women, fire, and dangerous things: What categories tell us about the nature of thought.* Chicago: University of Chicago Press.

Leicht, K. L. (1968). Recall and judged frequency of implicitly occurring words. *Journal of Verbal Learning and Verbal Behavior, 7,* 918–923.

Loftus, E. F. & Loftus, G. R. (1980). On the permanence of stored information in the human brain. *American Psychologist, 35,* 409–420.

✓ McClelland, J. L., Rumelhart, D. E., & the PDP Research Group (1986). *Parallel distributed processing: Explorations in the microstructure of cognition:* Vol. 2: *Psychological and biological models.* Cambridge, MA: MIT Press (Bradford Books).

McCloskey, M., & Glucksberg, S. (1978). Natural categories: Well-defined or fuzzy sets? *Memory & Cognition, 6,* 462–472.

McCloskey, M., & Glucksberg, S. (1979). Decision processes in verifying category membership statements; Implications for models of semantic memory. *Cognitive Psychology, 11,* 1–37.

McNemar, A. (1969). *Psychological statistics* (4th ed.). New York: Wiley.

Medin, D. L., & Schaffer, M. M. (1978). Context theory of classification learning. *Psychological Review, 85,* 207–238.

Miller, G. A. (1956). The magical number seven, plus or minus two: Some limits on our capacity for processing information. *Psychological Review, 63,* 81–97.

Miller, G. A., & Johnson-Laird, P. N. (1976). *Language and perception.* Cambridge, MA: Harvard University Press.

Minsky, M. L. (1975). A framework for representing knowledge. In P. H. Winston (Ed.,), *The psychology of computer vision* (pp. 211–277). New York: McGraw-Hill.

Mischel, W. (1968). *Personality & assessment* (pp. 1–72). New York: Wiley.

Mischel, W. (1983). Alternatives in the pursuit of the predictability and consistency of persons: Stable data that yield unstable interpretations. *Journal of Personality, 51,* 578–604.

Mischel, W., & Peake, P. K. (1982). Beyond deja vu in the search for cross-situational consistency. *Psychological Review, 89,* 730–755.

Murphy, G. L., & Medin, D. L. (1985). The role of theories in conceptual coherence. *Psychological Review, 92,* 289–316.

Nelson, K. (1974). Concept, word, and sentence: Interrelations in acquisition and development. *Psychological Review, 81*, 267–285.

Nelson, K. (1978). Explorations in the development of a functional semantic system. In W. Collins (Ed.), *Child psychology* (Vol. 12). Hillsdale, NJ: Erlbaum.

Osherson, D. N. & Smith, E. E. (1981). On the adequacy of prototype theory as a theory of concepts. *Cognition, 9*, 35–58.

Osherson, D. N. & Smith, E. E. (1982). Gradedness and conceptual combination. *Cognition, 12*, 299–318.

Quillian, M. R. (1968). Semantic memory. In M. L. Minsky (Ed.), *Semantic information processing* (pp. 227–270). Cambridge, MA: MIT Press.

Rey, G. (1983). Concepts and stereotypes. *Cognition, 15*, 237–262.

Rips, L. J. (1975). Inductive judgments about natural categories. *Journal of Verbal Learning and Verbal Behavior, 14*, 665–681.

Rips, L. J., & Turnbull, W. (1980). How big is big? Relative and absolute properties in memory. *Cognition, 8*, 145–174.

Rosch, E. H. (1975). Cognitive representations of semantic categories. *Journal of Experimental Psychology: General, 104*, 192–233.

Rosch, E. H., & Mervis, C. B. (1975). Family resemblances: Studies in the internal structure of categories. *Cognitive Psychology, 7*, 573–605.

Ross, B. H. (1984). Remindings and their effects in learning a cognitive skill. *Cognitive Psychology, 16*, 371–416.

Roth, E. M., & Shoben, E. J. (1983). The effect of context on the structure of categories. *Cognitive Psychology, 15*, 346–378.

Rubin, D. C. (1982). On the retention function for autobiographical memory. *Journal of Verbal Learning and Verbal Behavior, 21*, 21–38.

Rumelhart, D. E., McClelland, J. L., & the PDP Research Group (1986). *Parallel distributed processing: Explorations in the microstructure of cognition: Vol. 1. Foundations.* Cambridge, MA: MIT Press (Bradford Books).

Rumelhart, D. E. & Ortony, A. (1977). The representation of knowledge in memory. In R. C. Anderson, R. J. Spiro, & W. E. Montague (Eds.), *Schooling and the acquisition of knowledge.* Hillsdale, NJ: Erlbaum.

Schank, R. C. (1982). *Dynamic memory.* Cambridge: Cambridge University Press.

Schank, R. C., & Abelson, R. P. (1977). *Scripts, plans, goals, and understanding: An inquiry into human knowledge structures.* Hillsdale, NJ: Erlbaum.

Schneider, W., & Shiffrin, R. M. (1977). Controlled and automatic information processing: 1. Detection, search and attention. *Psychological Review, 84*, 1–66.

Schwanenflugel, P. J., & Rey, M. (1986). The relationship between category typicality and concept familiarity: Evidence from Spanish and English speaking monolinguals. *Memory & Cognition, 14*, 150–163.

Sewell, D. R. (1985). *Constructing the points of view of specific individuals.* Unpublished doctoral dissertation, Emory University, Atlanta.

Shaughnessy, J. J., & Underwood, B. J. (1973). The retention of frequency information for categorized lists. *Journal of Verbal Learning and Verbal Behavior, 12*, 99–107.

Shepard, R. N. (1962a). The analysis of proximities: Multi-dimensional scaling with an unknown distance function (Pt. 1). *Psychometrika, 27*, 125–140.

Shepard, R. N. (1962b). The analysis of proximities: Multi-dimensional scaling with an unknown distance function (Pt. 2). *Psychometrika, 27,* 219–246.

Shiffrin, R. M., & Schneider, W. (1977). Controlled and automatic information processing: 2. Perceptual learning, automatic attending, and a general theory. *Psychological Review, 84,* 127–190.

Smith, E. E., & Medin, D. L. (1981). *Categories and concepts.* Cambridge, MA: Harvard University Press.

Smith, E. E., Medin, D. L., & Rips, L. J. (1984). A psychological approach to concepts: Comments on Rey's "Concepts and stereotypes." *Cognition, 17,* 265–274.

Smith, E. E., Shoben, E. J., & Rips, L. J. (1974). Structure and process in semantic memory: A featural model for semantic decisions. *Psychological Review, 81,* 214–241.

Tabossi, P. (1988). Effects of context on the immediate interpretation of unambiguous nouns. *Journal of Experimental Psychology: Learning, Memory, and Cognition, 14,* 153–162.

Tabossi, P., & Johnson-Laird, P. N. (1980). Linguistic context and the priming of semantic information. *Quarterly Journal of Experimental Psychology, 32,* 595–603.

Thompson, D. M., & Tulving, E. (1970). Associative encoding and retrieval: Weak and strong cues. *Journal of Experimental Psychology, 86,* 255–262.

Tulving, E., & Thompson, D. M. (1973). Encoding specificity and retrieval processes in episodic memory. *Psychological Review, 80,* 352–373.

Tversky, A. (1977). Features of similarity. *Psychological Review, 84,* 327–352.

Whitney, P., McKay, T., & Kellas, G. (1985). Semantic activation of noun concepts in context. *Journal of Experimental Psychology: Learning, Memory and Cognition, 11,* 126–135.

Winer, B. J. (1971). *Statistical principles in experimental design.* New York: McGraw-Hill.

Woodworth, R. S. (1938). *Experimental psychology.* New York: Holt.

Woodworth, R. S., & Schlosberg, H. (1960). *Experimental psychology* (rev. ed.). New York: Holt.

Wyer, R. S., & Srull, T. K. (1986). Human cognition in its social context. *Psychological Review, 93,* 322–359.

Zadeh, L. A. (1965). Fuzzy sets. *Information and Control, 8,* 338–353.

4

Two-tiered concept meaning, inferential matching, and conceptual cohesiveness

RYSZARD S. MICHALSKI

Introduction

Suppose we asked someone how to get to some place in the city we were visiting and received needed instructions in response. Clearly, we would say that this person *knew* the answer, no matter whether the person knew the place personally or just had to figure out its location on the basis of general knowledge of the city, that is, by conducting inference. We would say this, of course, only if the answer were given to us in a reasonable amount of time.

The above example illustrates a general principle: One knows what one remembers, or what one can infer from what one remembers within a certain time constraint. Thus our knowledge can be viewed as a combination of two components, memorized knowledge and inferential extension, that is, knowledge that can be created from recorded knowledge by conducting inference within a certain time limit.

The main thesis of this chapter is that individual concepts – elementary components of our knowledge – parallel such a two-tiered nature of knowledge. We hypothesize that processes of assigning meaning to individual concepts recognized in a stream of information, or of retrieving them from memory to express an intended meaning are intrinsically inferential and involve, on a smaller scale, the same types of inference – deductive, analogical, and inductive – as processes of applying and constructing knowledge in general. This hypothesis reflects an intuition that the meaning of most concepts cannot, in principle, be defined in a crisp and context-independent fashion.

Specifically, the meaning of most concepts cannot be completely defined by some necessary or sufficient features, by a prototype, or by a set of representative exemplars. Rather, the meaning of a concept is a dynamic structure built each time anew, in the course of an interaction between some initial base meaning and the interpreter's background knowledge in the given context of discourse.

122

This view leads us to the proposition that the meaning we assign to a concept in any given situation is a result of an interplay between two parts: the *base concept representation* (BCR), and the *inferential concept interpretation* (ICI). The base concept representation is an explicit structure residing in memory that records both specific facts about the concept and general characteristics of it. The specific facts may include representative examples, exceptions, and counterexamples. The general characteristics are teacher-defined, or inferred by induction from examples or by analogy. They include typical, easily definable, and possibly context-independent assertions about the concept. These characteristics tend to capture the principle, the ideal or intention behind a given concept. If this principle changes to reflect a deeper knowledge about the concept involved, the BCR is redefined. To see this, consider, for example, the changes of our understanding of concepts such as *whale* (from fish to mammal) or *atom* (from the smallest indivisible particle to the contemporary notion of a dual wave–matter form).

The inferential concept interpretation is a process of assigning meaning to a concept using the BCR and the context of discourse. This process involves the interpreter's relevant background knowledge and inference methods and transformations that allow one to recognize, extend, or modify the concept meaning according to the context. These methods are associated with the concept or its generalizations, and, together with relevant background knowledge, constitute the second tier in concept representation.

The main goal of this chapter is to sketch ideas and underlying principles for constructing an adequate cognitive model of human concepts. It is not to define such a model precisely or to present specific algorithms. It is also hoped that the proposed ideas will suggest better computational methods for representing, using, and learning concepts in artificial intelligence systems.

Inference allows us to remember less and know more

This section will attempt to show that the two-tiered representation of concept meaning outlined above can be justified on the basis of cognitive economy – that is, economy of mental resources, memory and processing power – and that it reflects some general aspects of the organization of human memory. For a discussion of issues concerning cognitive economy see Lenat, Hayes-Roth, and Klahr (1979).

Let us start by assuming that the primary function of our knowledge is to interpret the present and predict the future. When one is exposed to any sensory inputs, one needs knowledge to interpret them. The more knowledge and the stronger the inferential capabilities (i.e., roughly the number of production and inference rules) one possesses, the greater the amount of information one can derive from a given input.

Interpreting observations in the context of the available knowledge makes it possible to derive more information from the input than is presented on the surface. It also allows one to build expectations about the results of any action and to predict and/or influence future events. The latter is possible because events and objects in our world are highly interrelated. If our world consisted of totally unrelated random events, one following the other, our knowledge of the past would be of no use for predicting the future, and this would obviate the need to store any knowledge. Moreoever, this, in turn, would presumably obviate the need for having intelligence, as the primary function of intelligence is to construct and use knowledge.

On the other hand, if our world were an eternal repetition of exactly the same scenes and events, knowledge once acquired would be applicable forever, and the need for its extension and generalization would cease. No wonder that in old, slow-changing traditional societies the elderly enjoyed such high status. The slower the rate of change in an environment, the higher the predictive value of past specific knowledge and the lower the need to extend and generalize knowledge. This suggests a hypothesis that the degree to which our innate subconscious capabilities for generalizing any input information corresponds to the rates of change in our environment. Thus, in a world that was evolving and changing at a different rate, our innate capabilities for generalization would presumably be different.

From the myriad sensory inputs and deluge of information received, we select and store only a minuscule fraction. This selection is done by a goal-dependent filtering of the inputs. The fraction actually stored contains a spectrum of structures representing different levels of abstraction from reality and different beliefs in their correctness. This spectrum spans the low-level, highly believed facts and observations, through partial plausible abstractions and heuristics, to high-level and highly hypothetical abstractions. The highest belief usually is assigned to our own personal sensory experiences, and the lowest belief to vague abstractions made by people whom we do not especially trust. These various assertions, together with a degree of belief in them, are automatically memorized when they are received or generated by inference. They then can be forgotten but not consciously erased.

The filtering of input information is done by conducting inferences – deductive, analogical, and inductive – that engage the input information and the goals and the knowledge of the person. The idea that a person's knowledge is involved in the processes of interpreting inputs is, of course, not new. An interesting illustration of it is presented, for example, by Anderson and Ortony (1975). They conducted experiments showing that the comprehension of a sentence depends heavily on the person's knowledge of the world and his or her analysis of the context.

Our ability to make inferences seems to come from a naturally endowed mechanism that is automatically activated in response to any input of information. One may ask why this is so. As our memory and information-processing powers are limited, it seems natural that the mind should tend to minimize the amount of information stored and maximize the use of that which is already stored. Consequently, one may hypothesize that the inferential processes that transfer any input information to stored knowledge are affected by three factors:

1. what is important to one's goals
2. what knowledge will be maximally predictive
3. what knowledge will allow one to infer the maximum amount of other knowledge.

The first factor reflects the known phenomenon that facts considered very important tend to be remembered before other facts. The second factor is significant because the predictive power of knowledge enables us to develop expectations about the future, and thus to prevent or avoid undesirable courses of actions, and to achieve goals. The third factor relates to cognitive economy: If we can infer B from A without much cognitive effort, then it is enough just to remember A. The second and third factors have interesting consequences. They suggest a memory organization that is primarily oriented toward storing analogies and generalizations, but facilitates the process of efficiently performing deduction on the knowledge stored.

These three factors explain the critical role of analogical and inductive inference in the process of transforming information received from the environment to knowledge actually memorized. This is so because it is analogical inference that transfers knowledge from known objects or problem solutions to new but related objects or problems. And it is inductive inference that produces generalizations and causal explanations of given facts (from which one can deduce original facts and predict new ones). Strict deductive inference and various forms of plausible inference (plausible deductive, analogical,

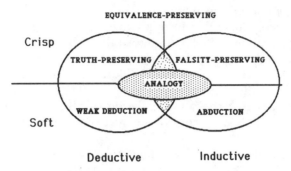

Figure 4.1. Types of inference.

and inductive) are means for extending/deriving more knowledge from our base knowledge, though such derived knowledge may be of lesser certainty.

The relationship between different types of inference is shown in Figure 4.1. The types of inference are divided according to two dimensions: (a) mode of inference: deductive versus inductive; and (b) strength of inference: crisp versus plausible. "Crisp" deductive inference is the truth-preserving inference studied in formal logic. "Soft" deductive inference uses approximate rules of deductive inference and produces probable rather than strict consequences of given premises. This type of inference is implemented, for example, in various expert systems that generate advice together with an estimate of its certainty.

Inductive inference produces hypotheses (or explanations) that crisply or softly imply original facts (premises). This means that original facts are deductive consequences of the hypotheses. Crisp inductive inference is a falsity-preserving inference. For example, hypothesizing that all professors at a particular university are bright on the basis that all professors of the Computer Science Department at this university are bright is a falsity-preserving inductive inference. (If the initial premise is true, the conclusion can be true or false; but if the premise is false, the hypothesis must be false also. Conversely, if the hypothesis is true, then the premise clearly must be true also.) Soft inductive inference produces hypotheses that only plausibly imply the original facts. For example, seeing smoke, one may hypothesize that there is a fire somewhere. It is a soft inductive inference, because there could be smoke without a fire.

Analogical inference is placed in the middle because it can be viewed as inductive and deductive inference combined (Michalski, 1987). The process of noticing analogy and creating an analogical mapping between two systems is intrinsically inductive; the process of deriving inferences about the analog using the mapping is deductive. This view, derived by the author through purely theoretical speculations, seems to be confirmed by the experimental findings of Gentner and Landers (1985) and Gentner (this volume). In order to explain difficulties people have in noticing analogies, they decomposed analogical reasoning into three parts, which they call "access," "structure-mapping," and "inferential power." They found that access and structure-mapping are governed by different rules than inferential power. Access is facilitated by literal similarity or mere appearance, and structure-mapping is governed by similarity of higher-order relations. These are inductive processes, as they produce a structure that unifies the base and the target systems. Inferential power corresponds to deduction.

The view of analogy as induction and deduction combined explains why it is more difficult for people to notice analogy than to use it once it is observed. This is so because inductive inference, being an underconstrained problem, typically consumes significantly more cognitive power than deductive inference, which is a well-constrained problem.

Figure 4.2 illustrates levels of knowledge derived from the base knowledge by conducting various types of inference (the "trumpet" model). The higher the type of inference, the more conclusions can be generated, but the certainty of conclusions decreases. A core theory and a discussion of various aspects of human plausible inference can be found in Collins and Michalski (1986).

Let us now return to the discussion of the third factor influencing inferential processes, namely, what knowledge allows us to infer the maximum amount of other knowledge. This issue, obviously, has special significance for achieving cognitive economy. The need for cognitive economy implies that it is useful for individual words (concepts) to carry more than one meaning, when considered without any context and without inferential extension of their meaning. By allowing that the meaning of words can be context-dependent and inferentially extensible, one can greatly expand the number of meanings that can be conveyed by individual words. This context dependence, however, cannot be unlimited, again because of cognitive economy. To be economical, context dependence should be employed only when the context can be identified with little mental effort. Inferential extensions

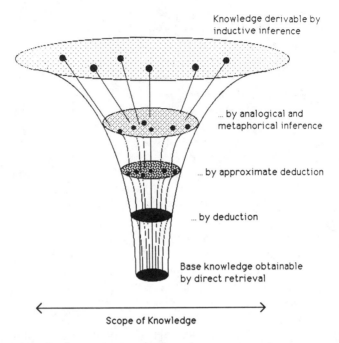

Knowledge derivable by
inductive inference

... by analogical and
metaphorical inference

... by approximate deduction

... by deduction

Base knowledge obtainable
by direct retrieval

Scope of Knowledge

Figure 4.2. A "trumpet" model of inferential knowledge extension. Shading represents decreasing strength of belief in inferentially derived knowledge.

also have natural limits, which are dictated by the mental power available, and the decreasing confidence in conclusions as the levels of inference increase.

Concept meaning is distributed between representation and interpretation

Concepts are mental structures representing classes of entities united by some principle. Such a principle might be a common use or goal, the same origin or behavior, or just similar perceptual characteristics. In order to use concepts, one must possess efficient methods for recognizing them in streams of sensory signals or in mental processing. To do so, one needs to have appropriate mental representations of concepts.

The traditional work on concept representation assumes that the whole meaning of a concept resides in a single stored structure, for example, a semantic network, a frame, or a graph, that captures all relevant properties of the concept (e.g., Collins & Quillian, 1972;

Minsky, 1975; Sowa, 1984). The process of recognizing a concept involves simple matching between the stored representation and perceived facts. Such matching may include comparing attribute values or nodes of corresponding networks, but has not been assumed to involve any complex inferential processes.

In contrast, our view is that such a matching may involve a significant amount of deductive, analogical, or inductive inference and that this inference takes into consideration the context of discourse and the person's background knowledge. Therefore, we postulate a two-tiered representation of concept meaning, which draws a distinction between the base concept representation (BCR) and the inferential concept interpretation (ICI). The BCR is a stored-knowledge structure associated with the concept. It specifies the most common, typical properties of the concept and the principle unifying different instances of it. It may also include representative examples, counter-examples, exceptions, and other known facts about the concept.

The ICI uses methods, relevant background knowledge, and rules of inference for interpreting the BCR according to various contexts. The methods incorporate metaknowledge about the concept, that is, which properties of the concept are crucial and which are not in a given context, what transformations are allowed on the BCR, and how these properties or transformations can vary among instances of the concept. These methods contain procedures for matching the BCR with observations. In the case of physical objects, the methods include permissible physical transformations (i.e., transformations that do not remove an object from the given class, for example, the transformations of a chair that do not remove it from the class of chairs).

Figure 4.3 illustrates the two-tiered concept meaning. The rectangular area denotes the scope of a concept as defined by the base concept representation. The irregularly shaped area depicts the changes in the concept meaning due to the inferential concept interpretation. For example, the rectangular area may represent all animals sharing typical physical characteristics of fish, and the irregularly shaped area may represent animals that can be considered fish in various contexts.

It is easy to see that to recognize an object – that is, to assign it to a concept – one may need to match only a small portion of properties observed in the object with properties stated in the base representation. The properties that need to be matched depend on the context in which the recognition process occurs.

For example, one may recognize a given person just by some of this person's facial features, silhouette, voice, handwriting, medical

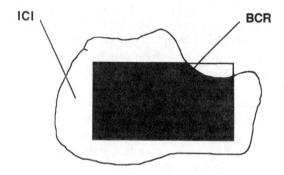

BCR - the scope of the concept defined by the Base
Concept Representation

ICI - the scope of the concept as derived by Inferential
Concept Interpretation for a given context and
background knowledge

Figure 4.3. An illustration of two-tiered concept representation.

record, fingerprints, any combination of these, or by a host of other characteristics. Thus, if the concept recognition process were based on a direct match of a fixed number of features of the target concept with properties of an observed object, then one would need to store representations for all these possibilities. Such a method would be hopelessly memory-taxing and inefficient. It is practical only in simple cases, such as those considered in many current expert systems.

In the proposed theory, the process of relating the base representation of a concept to observations is done by inferential concept interpretation. This process "matches" the base concept representation with observations by conducting inference involving the contextual information (e.g., What are other candidate concepts?) and relevant background knowledge. This inference determines what features are needed or sufficient to be matched in order to recognize a concept among a context-dependent set of candidates, and what kind of match is required. Thus the degree of match between a concept representation (CR) and an observed entity (OE) is not just a function of CR and OE, as traditionally assumed, but rather a four-argument function, which also includes a parameter, CX, for context, and BK, for background knowledge:

Degree of match (CR, OE) = f(CR, OE, CX, BK)

The context is computed dynamically in the process of using or recognizing concepts. Thus the proposed view requires an efficient method for representing and using contexts for any given concept. A simple introspection of our mental processes appears to confirm this: We seem to have little difficulty in determining and maintaining the context in any discourse.

There is no unique way of distributing the concept meaning between BCR and ICI. We expect that the actual distribution of the concept meaning between these two parts represents a desired trade-off between the economy of concept representation and the economy of inferential concept interpretation. Thus, learning a concept involves acquiring not only the base concept representation but also the methods for inferential concept interpretation.

Let us illustrate the proposed approach by a few examples. Consider the concept of *fish*. Typical and general characteristics of fish are that they have a certain elongated shape, a tail, live in water, and swim. These and other typical physical properties of fish, as well as representative examples, would be stored in the BCR. Suppose someone finds an animal that matches many characteristics of fish but does not swim. Suppose that this animal appears to be sick. The ICI would involve background knowledge that sick animals may not be able to move and that swimming is a form of moving. By deductive reasoning from these facts one concludes that lack of ability to swim should not be taken as negative evidence for the animal being a fish. On the contrary, the fact that the animal does not swim might even add to the confidence that it is a fish, once the animal was recognized as being sick.

Suppose that we learned the concept of *fish* by reading a general description and seeing a few examples. The BCR consists of this general description and the memorized examples. Suppose that we visit a zoo and see an animal defined as *fish* that is of a shape never seen in the examples or stated in the general description – say, a horselike shape. We may add this example to our BCR without necessarily modifying our general notion of *fish*. If we see another horse-shaped fish, we may recall that example and recognize the new instance as a fish without evoking the general notion of *fish*. This explains why we postulate that the BCR is not just a representation of the general, typical, or essential meaning of a concept but may also include examples of a concept.

The rules used in the above reasoning about sick fish would not be stored as the base concept representation for *fish*. They would be a part of the methods for inferential concept interpretation. These methods would be associated with the general concept of *animal*, rather than with the concept of *fish*, because they apply to all animals. Thus we postulate that the methods for inferentially interpreting a concept can be inherited from those applicable to a more general concept.

As another example, consider the concept of *sugar maple*. Our prototypical image of a sugar maple is that it is a tree with three- to-five-lobed leaves that have V-shaped clefts. Some of us may also remember that the teeth on the leaves are coarser than those of the red maple, that slender twigs turn brown, and that the buds are brown and sharp-pointed. Being a tree, a sugar maple has, of course, a trunk, roots, and branches.

Suppose now that while strolling on a nice winter day someone tells us that a particular tree is a sugar maple. Simple introspection tells us that the fact that the tree does not have leaves would not strike us as a contradiction of our knowledge about sugar maples. This is surprising, because, clearly, the presence of leaves of a particular type is deeply embedded in our typical image of a maple tree. The two-tiered theory of concept representation explains this phenomenon simply: The inferential concept interpretation associated with the general concept of *tree* evokes a rule; "In winter deciduous trees lose leaves." By deduction based on the subset relationship between a tree and a maple tree, the rule would be applied to the latter. The result of this inference would override the stored standard information about maple trees, and the inconsistency would be resolved.

Suppose further that when reading a book on artificial intelligence we encounter a drawing of an acyclic graph structure of points and straight lines connecting them, which the author calls a tree. Again, calling such a structure a tree does not evoke in us any strong objection, because we can see in it some abstracted features of a tree. Here, the matching process involves inductive generalization of the base concept representation. Once such a generalized notion of a tree is learned in the context of mathematical concepts, it will be used in this context.

These examples clearly show that the process of relating observations with concept representations is much more than matching features and determining a numerical score characterizing the match, as done in various mechanized decision processes, for example, expert systems.

It should be noted that the distribution of the concept meaning between the representation and interpretation parts is not fixed but can be done in many ways. Each way represents a trade-off between the amount of memory for concept storage and computational complexity of concept use. At one extreme, all the meaning can be expressed by the representation. In this case the representation explicitly defines all properties of a concept, including any concept variations, exceptions, and irregularities. It states directly the meaning of the concept in every possible context. It stores all known examples of the concept. This results in a very complex and memory-taxing concept representation. The concept interpretation process would, however, be relatively simple. It would involve a straightforward matching of the properties of the unknown object with information in the concept description.

At the other extreme, the concept is explicitly represented only by the most simple description characterizing its idealized form. In this case, the process of matching a concept description with observations might be significantly more complex.

As far as memory representation of concepts is concerned, we assume that their base concept representations are stored as a collection of assertions and facts. These collections are organized into *part* or *type* hierarchies with inheritance properties (e.g., Collins & Michalski, 1986). The methods used by inferential concept interpretation are also arranged into hierarchies. For example, as already indicated, the rule that a sick fish may not swim is stored not with the ICI methods associated with the concept of *fish* but rather with the concept of *animal*.

As mentioned earlier, the process of inferential concept interpretation may involve performing not just truth-preserving deductive inference on the base concept interpretation but also various forms of plausible inference. In particular, it may create an inductive generalization of the base concept representation, draw analogies, run mental simulations, or envision consequences of some acts or features. The background knowledge needed for inferential interpretation includes information about methods for relating concept representations to observations, about which properties are important and which are not in various contexts, and about typicality of features, statistical distribution of properties and concept occurrences, and so on. An inferential interpreter may produce a yes/no answer or a score representing the degree to which the base representation matches given observations. Extending the meaning of a single concept by conducting inference corresponds on a small scale to extending any knowledge by inference.

When an unknown entity is matched against a base concept representation, it may satisfy it directly or it may satisfy some of its in-

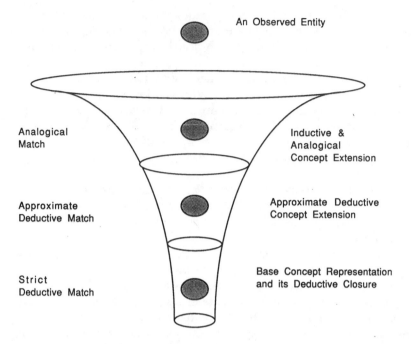

An Observed Entity

Analogical
Match

Inductive &
Analogical
Concept Extension

Approximate
Deductive Match

Approximate Deductive
Concept Extension

Strict
Deductive Match

Base Concept Representation
and its Deductive Closure

Figure 4.4. Types of inferential concept matching.

ferential extensions. The type of inference performed to match the description of the entity with the base concept representation determines the type of match (Figure 4.4). If the description of an entity matches the BCR precisely – satisfies it directly or satisfies its specialization (falls into its deductive extension) – then we have a *strict match*; if it satisfies an approximate deductive extension, then we have an *approximate match*; if it matches an analogical or inductive extension – satisfies a generalization that unifies the BCR with the description of the entity – then we have an *analogical* or, generally, an inferential match.[1]

As mentioned earlier, when we are recognizing an entity in the context of a finite set of candidate entities, usually only a small subset of its properties will need to match the properties in the base representation of candidate concepts. This set is defined by a *discriminant concept description* (Michalski, 1983). Such a description can be determined by conducting inductive inference on the base representation of the candidate concepts. A method for an efficient recognition of concepts in the context of candidate concepts, called *dynamic recognition,* is described in Michalski (1988).

The process of inferential concept interpretation can be viewed as a vehicle for extending the base concept meaning into a large space of variations by the use of context, rules of inference, and general knowledge. This process is an important means for achieving flexibility of concepts and thus leads to cognitive economy. Later, in the section describing experimental results, we present an example of a very simple inferential interpretation of a logic-style base concept representation.

Some other views on concept representation

There seems to be universal agreement that human concepts, except for special cases occurring predominantly in science (concepts such as a prime number, a triangle, a vertebrate, etc.), are structures with flexible and imprecise boundaries. I call such concepts *flexible*. They allow a varying degree of match between them and observed instances and have context-dependent meaning. Flexible boundaries make it possible to "fit" the meaning of a concept to changing situations and to avoid precision when it is not needed or not possible. The varying degree of match reflects the varying representativeness of a concept by different instances. According to the theory presented, this is accomplished by applying inferential concept matching, which takes into consideration the context and background knowledge of the interpreter.

Instances of a concept are rarely homogeneous. Among instances of a concept people usually distinguish a "typical instance," a "nontypical instance," or, generally, they rank instances according to their typicality. By using context, the meaning of almost any concept can be expanded in directions that cannot be predicted in advance. An illustration of this is given by Hofstadter (1985, chap. 24), who shows how a seemingly well-defined concept, such as *First Lady*, can express a great variety of meanings depending on the context. For example, it might include the husband of Margaret Thatcher.

Despite various efforts, the issue of how to represent concepts in such a rich and context-dependent sense is not resolved. Smith and Medin (1981) distinguish among three approaches: the *classical view*, the *probabilistic view*, and the *exemplar view*. The classical view assumes that concepts are representable by features that are singly necessary and jointly sufficient to define a concept. This view seems to apply only to very simple cases. The probabilistic view represents concepts as weighted, additive combinations of features. It postulates that concepts should correspond to linearly separable subareas in a feature space. Experiments indicate, however, that this view is also not adequate (Smith & Medin, 1981; Wattenmaker, Dewey, Murphy, & Medin, 1986). The exemplar view represents concepts by one or more typical exemplars rather than by generalized descriptions. Although it is easy to demonstrate that we do store and use concept exemplars for some particular purposes, it seems clear that we also create and use abstract concept representations. For important ideas on concept representation and organization from the computational viewpoint, see papers by Minsky (1980), Sowa (1984), and Lenat, Prakash, and Shepherd (1986).

The notion of typicality can be captured by a measure called *family resemblance* (Rosch & Mervis, 1975). This measure represents a combination of frequencies in which different features occur in different subsets of a superordinate concept, such as *furniture, vehicle*, and so on. The individual subsets are represented by typical members. Nontypical members are viewed as corruptions of the typical, differing from them in various small aspects, as children differ from their parents (e.g., Rosch & Mervis, 1975; Wittgenstein, 1953). The idea of family resemblance is somewhat related to the two-tiered representation, except that the BCR is a much more general concept than a prototype, and the ICI represents a significantly greater set of transformations than "corruptions" of a prototype.

Another approach uses the notion of a *fuzzy set* as a formal model of imprecise concepts (Zadeh, 1976). Members of such a set are characterized by a graded set-membership function rather than by the in/out function employed in the classical notion of a set. This set-membership function is defined by people describing the concept and thus is subjective. This approach allows one to express explicitly the varying degree of membership of entities in a concept, as perceived by people, which can be useful for various applications. It does not explain, however, what are the computational processes that determine the set-membership functions. Neither is it concerned with developing adequate computational mechanisms for expressing, handling, and reasoning about the context-dependence and background-knowledge dependence of the concept meaning.

The idea of two-tiered representation attributes the graded concept membership to the flexibility of inferential concept interpretation. Thus, instead of explicitly storing the membership function, one obtains an equivalent result as a by-product of the method of interpreting the base concept representation. This method also handles the context and background-knowledge dependence, via a store of rules and allowable concept transformations.

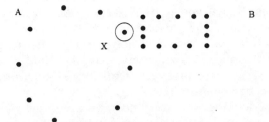

Figure 4.5. An illustration of conceptual cohesiveness. Object *X* has higher conceptual cohesiveness with concept *A* than with concept *B* though it is "closer" to *B*.

The idea of two-tiered representation first appeared in a simple form in the experiments conducted by Michalski and Chilausky (1980) on inductive knowledge acquisition for expert systems. In these experiments, two-valued logic-based diagnostic decision rules were created by induction from examples. When these rules were applied to diagnosing new cases, however, they were interpreted not by the standard two-valued logic evaluation scheme but by various many-valued logic evaluation schemes. For example, logical disjunction was interpreted either as the maximum function or as the probabilistic sum. Logical conjunction was interpreted as the minimum function, the average, or the probabilistic product. The experiments showed that such modifications of rule interpretations can lead to an improvement of the rule performance on new cases.

A more advanced inferential matching was proposed in the method of conceptual clustering described by Michalski and Stepp (1983). The method utilized the idea of *conceptual cohesiveness*. Suppose that an observed object does not match any concept description precisely. There are, however, several concepts that are candidates for an imprecise or, generally, an inferential match. The proposed solution is to generalize each concept minimally, so that it includes the object under consideration. The resulting generalized concepts are then evaluated from the viewpoint of conceptual cohesiveness. This criterion tries to minimize the degree of generalization necessary to include the new object and to maximize the simplicity of the description of the generalized concept. The concept that receives the highest score is viewed as the right "home" for the object. The concept of conceptual cohesiveness is illustrated in Figure 4.5.

Closely related to our ideas is the work by Murphy and Medin (1985) and by Barsalou and Medin (1986). Computational techniques for using knowledge for interpreting observations via *deductive* inference are presented in the work by DeJong (1986), DeJong and Mooney (1986), and Mitchell, Keller, and Kedar-Cabelli (1986). A computational framework for applying *plausible* inference for interpreting observations (specialization, generalization, and similarity-based transformations) is described by Collins and Michalski (1986). Various issues involved in creating mental representations of concepts are described by Collins and Gentner (1987).

The next section describes an experimental study investigating a simple form of two-tiered concept representation in the context of learning decision rules from examples in the area of medicine.

The two-tiered representation can reduce memory needed: an experiment

This section describes the results of an experiment investigating a simple form of two-tiered representation of four different types of lymphography. In the experiment, the base concept representation, called a *cover*, is in the form of a disjunction of conjunctive statements, called *complexes*. Interpreting a complex as the condition part of a rule, CONDITION → CONCEPT NAME, a cover can be viewed simply as a set of rules with the same right-hand side.

The complexes are conjunctions of relational assertions, called *selectors*. Each selector characterizes one aspect of the concept. It states a value or a set of values that an attribute may take on for the entities representing the concept. Here are two examples of selectors:

> [blood type = A or B] (*Read*: The blood type is A or B.)
> [Diastolic blood pressure = 65...90] (*Read*: The diastolic blood pressure is between 65 and 90.)

Thus selectors relate an attribute to one or more of the attribute's possible values. A selector is *satisfied* by an entity if the selector's attribute applied to this entity takes on one of the values stated in the selector. Each complex (a conjunction of selectors) in the base concept representation (cover) is associated with a pair of weights, t and u, representing, respectively, the *total* number of known cases that it covers and the number of cases that it covers alone (*uniquely*) among other complexes associated with this concept. For example, suppose that the complex:

> [blood pressure = 140/90] & [blood type = A or O]: 60, 55

is one of the complexes characterizing patients with some disease. The weights $t = 60$ and $u = 55$ mean that the blood pressure 140/90 and

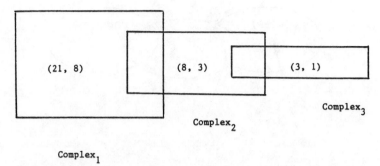

Figure 4.6. An ordered disjunctive concept representation. The numbers in parentheses denote the *t* weight and *u* weight, respectively.

the blood type A or O occurred in a total of 60 patients with this disease, and in 55 patients it occurred uniquely (i.e., these patients did not have properties satisfying other complexes associated with this disease). Statements with high *t* weights may be viewed as characterizing typical cases of a concept, and statements with low *t* weights and *u* weights can be viewed as characterizing rare, exceptional cases, or errors.

In the experiment, initial covers for the diseases were determined by applying the inductive learning program AQ15 to a set of known cases of diseases (Hong, Mozetic, & Michalski, 1986; Michalski, Mozetic, Hong, & Lavrac, 1986). Complexes in each cover were ordered according to decreasing values of *t* weights, as shown in Figure 4.6. (If two complexes had the same *t* weight, then they were ordered by decreasing values of *u* weights). Thus, the first complex in each cover is likely to characterize the most typical properties of the concept, the next complex less typical properties, and so on.

As mentioned earlier, a cover serves here the role of the base concept representation. The diagnosis of a case is determined by matching each cover with the case, and finding the cover with the highest match. The way the cover is matched against a disease case is determined by the inferential concept interpretation (see the discussion of flexible matching below).

To determine the most desirable distribution of the concept meaning between the BCR and ICI, the so-called TRUNC method was applied.

First, the initial covers for each disease obtained from AQ15 were used to diagnose a set of new disease cases, and the performance score was calculated. Next, each such cover was reduced by removing from it the "lightest" complex (i.e., the complex with the smallest *t* weight).

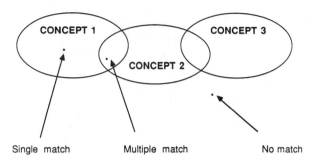

Figure 4.7. Three possible outcomes of matching an event with the base concept representation of different concepts.

The so-truncated cover was then used to diagnose the same new cases, and the performance score was calculated again. The above process was repeated until the truncated cover of each disease had only one complex (termed the *best complex*). Each such iteration represents a different split between the BCR and the ICI. Thus this experiment enabled us to compare the performance of concept descriptions for different distribution between BCR and ICI.

The diagnosis of any new disease case was determined by a simple inferential matching, called *flexible matching*, of the case with the set of covers representing different diseases (here, types of lymphography). This matching treated covers not as logical expressions that are either satisfied or not satisfied by a given case but as descriptions with flexible context-dependent boundaries. The confidence in the diagnosis was defined by the maximum degree of match found between the given case and a cover. Thus the diagnostic decision is determined in the context of all diagnoses under consideration.

The computation of the degree of match distinguished among three possible outcomes of matching an event (here, a disease case) with a set of covers: *single match* – only one cover is strictly matched (i.e., the case completely satisfies only one cover); *no match* – the case satisfies no cover; and *multiple match* – the case satisfies several covers. These three possible outcomes are illustrated in Figure 4.7.

When there is a single match, the diagnosis is defined by the cover satisfied. When there is no match or a multiple match, the degree of (approximate) match is computed for each cover. This computation takes into consideration the strength of conditions represented by individual selectors[2] and t weights of complexes (the t weights are treated as estimates of prior probabilities). The evidence provided by

Table 4.1. *Experimental results*

Domain	Cover reduction	Complexity		Accuracy 1st choice (percentage)	Human experts	Random choice
		# Sel	# Cpx			
	none	37	12	81		
Lymphography	unique >1	34	10	80	60/85%	25%
	best cpx	10	4	82	(estimate)	

individual complexes in a cover is summed as probabilities. Specifically, the degree of match is computed according to these rules:

- The degree of match (DM) between an event and a selector is 1 when the selector is satisfied; otherwise, it is the inverse of the strength of the selector.
- The DM between an event and a complex is the product of DMs of individual selectors times the relative t weight of the complex (the ratio of the t weight to the total number of past events).
- The DM between an event and a cover is the probabilistic sum[3] of DMs for complexes in the cover.

The choice of this particular interpretation was experimental. Technical details on the matching function are described by Michalski et al. (1986). A selection of results is shown in Table 4.1, which presents results for three cases of cover reduction:

- "no" (no cover reduction), when the BCR included all complexes that were needed to represent all known cases of the given disease, that is, the *complete* description
- "unique > 1," when the cover included only complexes with a u weight greater than 1
- "best cpx," when the BCR was reduced to the single complex with the highest t weight (the "heaviest")

The system's performance was evaluated by counting the percentage of the correct diagnoses, defined as the diagnosis that receives the highest degree of match and that is considered correct by an expert (see Table 4.1, "Accuracy 1st choice"). For comparison, the table columns "Human experts" and "Random choice" show the estimated performance of human experts (general practitioner/specialist) and the performance representing random choice.

As shown in Table 4.1, the best performance (82%) was obtained, surprisingly, when the BCR consisted of only *one conjunctive statement* ("best cpx") per concept. This representation was also, of course, the simplest, as it required approximately one-fourth the memory of the complete description.

These results show that by using a very simple concept representation (here, a single conjunction) and only a somewhat more complex concept interpretation (as compared to the one that would strictly match the complete concept description) one may significantly reduce the amount of storage required, without affecting the performance accuracy of the concept description. Further details and more results from this experiment are described in Michalski et al. (1986).

This research is at an early stage, and further work is required, both theoretical and experimental. There is, in particular, a need to determine whether similar results can be obtained in other domains of application. Among interesting topics for further research are development and experimentation with more advanced methods for inferential matching and base concept representations, new techniques for representing contexts, and algorithms for learning two-tiered concept representations. For representing physical objects, one needs to develop methods for defining and/or learning permissible transformations of the base concept representations of these objects (e.g., transformations of a typical table that will not change it to some other object). The latter topic is of special importance for understanding sensory perception.

Conclusion

The two-tiered concept representation postulates that the total concept meaning is distributed between a base concept representation and an inferential concept interpretation. The BCR covers the typical, easily explainable concept meaning and may contain a store of examples and/or known facts about the concept. The ICI is a vehicle for using concepts flexibly and for adapting their meanings to different contexts. The inferential interpretation involves contextual information and relevant background knowledge. It may require all types of inference, from truth-preserving deductive inference through approximate deductive and analogical inference to falsity-preserving inductive inference. When dealing with physical objects, the interpretation may involve various transformations of the BCR (e.g., a prototype or a set of prototypes).

Experiments testing some of the ideas on a simple medical example showed that distributing concept meaning more toward inferential concept interpretation than toward the base concept representation (as compared with storing the complete BCR) was highly advantageous, leading to a significant reduction in the size of memory needed for storing concept descriptions while preserving the diagnostic performance.

NOTES

The author thanks Doug Medin, Andrew Ortony, Gail Thornburg, and Maria Zemankova for comments and useful criticisms of the earlier versions of this chapter. Remarks of Intelligent Systems Group members P. Haddawy, L. Iwanska, B. Katz, and H. Ko were also helpful.

This work was supported in part by the National Science Foundation under Grant DCR 84–06801, in part by the Defense Advanced Research Projects Agency under grants N00014–85–K–0875 and N00014–87–K–0874 administered by the Office of Naval Research, and in part by the Office of Naval Research under grants N00014–88–K–0226 and N00014–88–K–0397.

1 The above-mentioned analogical match is not to be confused with the analogical mapping discussed in the structure-mapping theory of analogy by Gentner (1983; this volume). The analogical match is related to what Gentner and Landers (1985) call "analogical access." It involves finding semantic correspondences between attributes and relations of the entity to be recognized and the base knowledge representation.
2 The strength of a selector $\{A = R\}$, where R is a set of values of A, is defined as the ratio of the number of all possible values of attribute A over the number of values in R.
3 The probabilistic sum is defined as $p_1 + p_2 - (p_1 \times p_2)$.

REFERENCES

Anderson, R. C., & Ortony, A. (1975). On putting apples into bottles: A problem of polysemy. *Cognitive Psychology, 7,* 167–180.
Barsalou, L. W., & Medin, D. L. (1986). Concepts: Static definitions or concept-dependent representations. *Cahiers de Psychologie Cognitive, 6,* 187–202.
Collins, A., & Gentner, D. (1987). How people construct mental models. In D. Holland & N. Quinn (Eds.), *Cultural models in language and thought,* (pp. 243–265). Cambridge: Cambridge University Press.
Collins, A. M., & Quillian, M. R. (1972). Experiments on semantic memory and language comprehension. In L. W. Gregg (Ed.), *Cognition learning and memory* (pp. 117–137). New York: Wiley.
Collins, A., & Michalski, R. S. (1986). *Logic of plausible inference.* Reports of the Intelligent Systems Group, no. ISG 85–17, Urbana-Champaign: University of Illinois, Department of Computer Science. An extended version appears in *Cognitive Science, 13* (1989).
DeJong, G. (1986). An approach to learning from observation. In R. S. Michalski, J. G. Carbonell, & T. M. Mitchell (Eds.), *Machine learning: An artificial intelligence approach,* (Vol. 2, pp. 571–590). Los Altos, CA: Morgan Kaufmann.

DeJong, G., & Mooney, R., (1986). Explanation-based learning: An alternative view. *Machine Learning, 1*, 145–176.

Gentner, D. (1983). Structure-mapping: A theoretical framework for analogy. *Cognitive Science, 7*, 155–170.

Gentner, D., & Landers, R. (1985, November). Analogical reminding: A good match is hard to find. *Proceedings of the International Conference on Systems, Man, and Cybernetics*, Tucson, AZ.

✓ Hofstadter, D. R. (1985). *Metamagical themas: Questing for the essence of mind and pattern*. New York: Basic Books.

Hong, J., Mozetic, I., & Michalski, R. S. (1986). *AQ15: Incremental learning of attribute-based descriptions from examples, the method, and user's guide*. Intelligent Systems Group Rep. no. ISG86–5. Urbana-Champaign: University of Illinois, Department of Computer Science.

Lenat, D. B., Hayes-Roth, F., & Klahr, P. (1979). Cognitive economy in artificial intelligence systems. *Proceedings of International Joint Conference on Artificial Intelligence, 6*, Tokyo.

Lenat, D., Prakash, M., & Shepherd, M. (1986). CYC: Using common sense knowledge to overcome brittleness and knowledge acquisition bottlenecks. *AI Magazine, 6*, 65–85.

Michalski, R. S. (1983). Theory and methodology of inductive learning. In R. S. Michalski, J. G. Carbonell, & T. M. Mitchell (Eds.), *Machine learning: An artificial intelligence approach* (pp. 83–130). Los Altos, CA: Kaufmann.

Michalski, R. S. (1987). Concept learning. In S. C. Shapiro (Ed.), *Encyclopedia of artificial intelligence* (pp. 185–194). New York: Wiley.

Michalski, R. S. (1988). *Dynamic recognition: An outline of the theory*. Report of Machine Learning and Inference Laboratory. Fairfax: George Mason University, Department of Computer Science.

Michalski, R. S., & Chilausky, R. L. (1980). Learning by being told and learning from examples: An experimental comparison of two methods of knowledge acquisition in the context of developing an expert system for soybean disease diagnosis. *International Journal of Policy Analysis and Information Systems, 4*, 125–161.

Michalski, R. S., Mozetic, I., Hong, J., & Lavrac, N. (1986). The multi-purpose incremental learning system AQ15 and its testing application to three medical domains. *Proceedings of the American Association for Artificial Intelligence Conference*, Philadelphia.

Michalski, R. S., & Stepp, R. E. (1983). Learning from observation: Conceptual clustering. In R. S. Michalski, J. G. Carbonell, & T. M. Mitchell (Eds.), *Machine learning: An artificial intelligence approach* (pp. 331–363). Los Altos: CA: Kaufmann.

Minsky, M. (1975). A framework for representing knowledge. In P. H. Winston (Ed.), *The psychology of computer vision* (pp. 211–277). New York: McGraw-Hill.

Minsky, M. (1980). K-lines: A theory of memory. *Cognitive Science, 4*, 117–133.

Mitchell, T. M., Keller, R. M., & Kedar-Cabelli, S. T. (1986). Explanation-based generalization: A unifying view. *Machine Learning, 1*, 47–80.

Murphy, G. L., & Medin, D. L. (1985). The role of theories in conceptual coherence. *Psychological Review, 92*, 289–316.

Rosch, E. H. & Mervis, C. B. (1975). Family resemblances: Studies in the internal structure of categories. *Cognitive Psychology, 7*, 573–605.

✓ Smith, E. E., & Medin, D. L. (1981). *Categories and concepts.* Cambridge, MA: Harvard University Press.

Sowa, J. F. (1984). *Conceptual structures: Information processing in mind and machine.* Reading, MA: Addison-Wesley.

Wattenmaker, W. D., Dewey, G. I., Murphy, T. D., & Medin, D. L. (1986). Linear separability and concept learning: Context, relational properties, and concept naturalness. *Cognitive Psychology, 18,* 158–194.

✓ Wittgenstein, L. (1953). *Philosophical Investigations.* New York: MacMillian.

Zadeh, L. A. (1976). A fuzzy-algorithmic approach to the definition of complex or imprecise concepts. *International Journal of Man-Machine Studies, 8,* 249–291.

5

From global similarities to kinds of similarities: the construction of dimensions in development

LINDA B. SMITH

is similar to functions as little more than a blank to be filled ...
Goodman, 1972, p. 445

Introduction

We compare objects to each other in a variety of ways. We experience our world in terms of a complex system of distinct kinds of perceptual similarities. We judge objects to be similar or different. We also judge objects to be similar and different in part – to be, for example, similar in color and different in size. We categorize objects by their attributes and in so doing judge them to be similar; for example, we categorize objects as red, as blue, as big, as small. We compare objects in terms of their direction of difference – judging, for example, one object to be smaller than another. This variety of kinds of judgments clearly indicates that perceptual similarity is not one thing but is of many interrelated kinds. In brief, we seem to possess a complex system of perceptual relations, a complex system of kinds of similarity. The concern of this chapter is with the development of a system of knowledge about such relations.

The evidence suggests that an understanding of perceptual relations develops quite slowly during the preschool years. Indeed, working out a system of perceptual dimensions, a system of *kinds* of similarities, may be one of the major intellectual achievements of early childhood. The evidence for an emerging dimensional competence is widespread – and includes developments in Piagetian conservation tasks (e.g., Piaget, 1929), in seriation and transitive inference tasks, in classification tasks (e.g., Inhelder & Piaget, 1958, 1964), in transposition learning (e.g., Keunne, 1946) and discriminative learning tasks (e.g., Kendler, 1979). The relative lateness of children's acquisition of dimensional adjectives also suggests the slow emergence of a system of knowledge about perceptual relations (e.g., Blewitt, 1982;

146

Johnston, 1985). However, despite all the empirical work and the clear importance of relational concepts, there is no unified framework for thinking about their structure and about how they develop.

My purpose is to present a preliminary theoretical framework. Briefly, I propose that early in development we understand the similarities between objects in terms of two dimensionally nonspecific relations: global resemblances and global magnitude. Distinct kinds of relations of sameness (overall similarity, identity, part identity and dimensions) and distinct kinds of relations of magnitude (global polarity, greater-than, less-than, and dimensionally specific directions of difference) are hypothesized to emerge in a structured way from the more global beginnings. The basic developmental notion is one of differentiation, from global syncretic classes of perceptual resemblance and magnitude to dimensionally specific kinds of sameness and magnitude. However, prior to an analysis of relational concepts and hypotheses about their development, we need to consider a preliminary issue concerning wholes and parts and relevant levels of analyses.

A preliminary issue: wholes and their parts

Some of you, upon hearing that I propose a trend from holistic similarity (and magnitude) relations to dimensional ones, may have frowned; such a proposal is sure to be wrong. What I want to do first is to convince you that it may be the wrong answer to some questions (perhaps the question you are interested in), yet still be the right one to the question of how a knowledge system about perceptual relations develops.

My proposal may seem wrong on logical grounds. The idea that dimensions emerge from dimensionless similarity has been said to be logically flawed. Carnap (1928/1967) in his system known as the Aufbau attempted to develop a logical system of relations from the primitives of unitary indivisible objects, similarity, and the usual operations of logic. He failed. The principal source of his failure, at least according to his fellow philosopher Goodman (1951), was the use of similarity. The problem with similarity, says Goodman, is that it requires for its explanation just what it purports, in Carnap's system, to explain. One cannot get *red* from the likeness between *A* and *B* and *round* from the likeness between *B* and *C* unless, as Goodman has shown, there is some specification of distinct kinds of likeness to begin with. The problem with similarity is that it has no meaning unless one specifies the kind of similarity. My proposal, then, would seem to fail like Carnap's. How can one get dimensions from global similarity if similarity gains its meaning from dimensions?

A proposal that the relational knowledge system begins with dimensionless relations may seem not just logically wrong but computationally wrong as well. A classic controversy asked whether whole objects were built from elementary features and attributes or whether, somehow, objects were perceived as unitary wholes, and attributes and features secondarily derived from the wholes. Current evidence (and, as we noted, logic) favors the former view – that whole objects are built up from the prior processing of attributes and features. Treisman and Gelade's (1980) findings of illusory conjunctions strongly suggest this view. The finding is that adults, when shown a red square and blue circle, sometimes (under certain circumstances) perceive a red circle and a blue square. This finding, that the parts sometimes get put together wrongly, strongly suggests the construction of whole objects from their constituent attributes. Studies of infant perception (e.g., Cohen & Younger, 1983) also suggest that the features and attributes of objects may be processed prior to the representation of the whole object. In the habituation paradigm, at least, infants appear to represent and discriminate objects on the basis of individual features (e.g., *red*) at an earlier age than they represent and discriminate on the basis of joint features that form the object as a whole (e.g., *red* and *square*). Models of the perceived similarity of one object to another (e.g., Nosofsky, 1984; Tversky, 1977) also support a components-to-whole view of the perception of multidimensional objects. In virtually all such models, similarity is some function of the *combination of the constituent dimensional* similarities (or differences). It is difficult to imagine how it could be otherwise. My proposal, then, would seem to fly in the face of what we know about the processing and comparison of multidimensional objects. If the wholes are built from the parts, how can holistic relations be developmentally prior to relations between parts?

Global similarity may make no sense as a logical primitive and may have no meaning without dimensions. Global, whole-object relations may well be secondary to the prior processing of features and attributes. Nonetheless, I suggest that dimensionally nonspecific relations are experientially and developmentally prior in an emerging relational knowledge system. As Susan Carey (1982) has argued, what is logically and/or computationally primitive need not be developmentally early. My specific suggestion is that represented whole objects are built from the prior analyses of separate features and dimensions and that global similarities and differences are calculated from the constituent dimensions. However, it is the whole object and whole-object relations that are given first to experience. The constituent dimensional differences and similarities are rather inaccessible, not immediately experienced, and, more important for the present proposal, not conceptually simple (see Smith, 1989, for more on the processing of dimensions and objects).

This proposal – that what is prior and simple at one level of analysis is secondary and complex at another – is neither paradoxical nor without precedent. The constituent steps to perception are often not accessible to thought and seem particularly not accessible for children. Thus phonemelike segments seem to be the constituents of words in the perception and production of speech; but it is the word that is experientially primary, and phonemelike segments of words seem inaccessible to children (and adults) without training (i.e., without learning to read; e.g., Gattuso, Smith, & Treiman, 1986; Morais, Cary, Alegria, & Bertelson, 1979). As another example, infants categorically discriminate colors much like adults, but preschool children have considerable difficulty learning color terms (Bornstein, 1985). Again, what is simple in perception seems not so simple in conception. As a final example, even as adults we do not *understand*, that is, we do not have represented in our knowledge system (at least I don't) the geometry that underlies our perception of biological motion. So, in the present case, similarity may have no meaning without dimensions, and perceived similarity may have no psychological reality except as some combination of dimensional kinds of similarity; nonetheless, at the level of experience and understanding, dimensionless similarity and difference may be prior to dimensional kinds of similarity and difference.

Further, changes in the *understanding* of kinds of perceptual similarity and difference seem to be a major force in intellectual growth in the preschool years. There are real and measurable developmental changes in the perception of objects during this period (e.g., Smith & Kemler, 1978), but these seem not to be the principal limiting factors in children's performances in many cognitive tasks – particularly such tasks as conservation, seriation, classification, and language acquisition (see Smith & Evans, 1989). The major constraint on children's uses of similarity in many tasks appears to be, instead, in their conceptual organization of their experiences, in what they *know* about kinds of perceptual similarity. That is the issue to which I now turn.

An analysis of relational concepts

My proposal for the development of a system of knowledge about perceptual relations consists primarily of an analysis of kinds of relations, and hypotheses as to their order of development. In this section, I present my analysis, which is a listing of the concepts I propose to be distinct parts of the relational knowledge system. These are given in Figures 5.1 through 5.4. This listing is meant as a framework and introduction. It is not exhaustive. Further, the hypothesized concepts are listed in the figures so as to illustrate the structure of the concepts and do not represent any notions about the developmental progression. To begin, I propose that there are two basic kinds of relations: relations of sameness and relations of magnitude.

Sameness relations

Object-specific sameness relations. Relations of sameness can be partitioned into two kinds: concrete relations between objects and abstract *kinds* of relations. Listed in Figure 5.1 are five concrete relations of sameness that may exist between objects and by which categories of objects may be formed. Illustrated below each listing are examples of pairs of objects that instantiate the relation. Given first is the relation of *resemblances*; that is, an all-encompassing relation that includes the other relations of sameness and is, therefore, similarity at its most "undisciplined" – unconstrained and unspecified. The next two relations of sameness, *overall similarity* and *identity*, are better behaved. These are whole-object relations that take into account all of an object's characteristics at once; no particular parts or attributes are emphasized. So a brown shoe and a black boot would be holistically similar; a brown shoe and a brown wagon would not. The two holistic relations, identity and overall similarity, differ in degree of similarity. Identity concerns objects that are not discriminably (or significantly) different. Whole object identity is, for example, the relation that exists between two dinner plates in a matched set of china. Overall similarity includes identity but is broader and is the relation between objects that are (perhaps) discriminably different but also highly similar overall. Overall similarity is the sort of relation that presumably exists between distinct members of the same basic category – between, for example, two chairs or two dogs. The last two sameness relations, *part similarity* and *part identity*, concern the constituent parts of objects; one aspect or attribute is emphasized in the comparison. Part similarity and part identity, like whole-object identity and overall similarity, differ in degree of sameness. A red ball and a pink thread are part-similar; a red ball and a red thread are part-identical.

These sameness relations are interrelated in several ways. First, identity and overall similarity are undifferentiated relations between

1. Resemblances (part-similarity) --- sets of objects that are "alike"

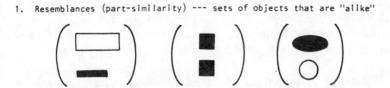

2. Overall similarity --- sets of objects similar overall

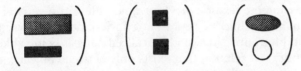

3. Identity --- equivalence sets of identical objects

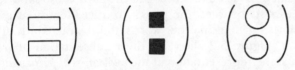

4. Part-similarity --- sets of objects similar in part

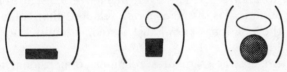

5. Part-identity --- sets of objects identical in part or sharing a common attribute

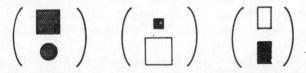

Figure 5.1. List of concrete sameness relations. Pairs of objects instantiating each relation are given as examples only. These relations are not mutually exclusive, and more than one relation may exist between a given pair of objects. Thus a given pair of objects may be an example of more than one relation.

whole objects whereas part identity and part similarity are relations between the constituent attributes of objects. Second, identity is an equivalence relation whereas overall similarity, part-similarity, and part identity are not (being neither transitive nor symmetric). Further, there are intricate inclusion relations between the extensions of these relations, as illustrated in Figure 5.5. All identity sets are both overall-similarity sets *and* part-identity sets. However, not all sets that are both overall-similarity sets and part-identity sets are identity sets. Further, all identity sets, overall-similarity sets, and part-identity sets are part-similar, and part similarity and resemblance are coextensive.

Kinds of sameness relations. Figure 5.2 lists abstract kinds of sameness relations. These are relations on relations – relations that organize the concrete samenesses that are listed in Figure 5.1. For example, the concrete relation of whole-object identity given in Figure 5.1 might enable a child to represent two identical yellow cups as being alike and to represent two identical red pens as being alike. But concrete identity is a relation that exists only between objects; and so the child, by concrete identity alone, could not represent the fact that the kind of alikeness that exists between the cups is the same kind of alikeness that exists between the pens. Abstract identity as given in Figure 5.2 allows for that. In other words, the abstract kinds of samenesses given in Figure 5.2 allow for the representation of *relations*, rather than just the representation of the *relatedness of particular objects*. There is possible an abstract relation of sameness for each object relation listed in Figure 5.1. However, in Figure 5.2, I list only the two abstract counterparts of the concrete relations that I think most important in the relational knowledge system: identity and overall similarity.

The next two abstract sameness relations, dimensional identity and dimensional similarity, do not have direct counterparts in Figure 5.1. Rather, they stem from the further organization of part identities and/or part similarities into dimensional kinds. So, not only are part-identity relations as a class distinct from overall similarity and (absolute) identity, but part identities, unlike global similarities and absolute identities, can be further differentiated into kinds according to the particular part. For example, two blue objects are part-identical; two red objects are part-identical; two square objects are part-identical. But the particular parts involved in the first two cases are of the same kind and are different in kind from the part involved in the third case. Two blue objects are not just part-identical; they are the same color, just as are two red objects. This representation of kind of part results in the two new sameness relations: dimensional identity and dimensional similarity. It is this organization of part identities and part similarities by qualitative kinds that constitutes a *psychological* dimension in the knowledge system. To understand particular dimensional identities and particular dimensional similarities is to understand that partic-

1. Abstract identity --- sets of equivalence sets organized by identity

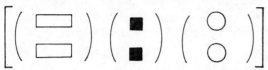

2. Abstract overall similarity --- sets of sets organized by overall similarity

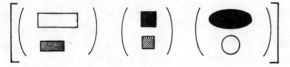

3. Dimensions

    a. Dimensional identity --- sets of equivalence sets organized by kind of part-identity

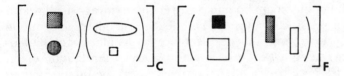

    b. Dimensional similarity --- sets of sets organized by kind of part-similarity

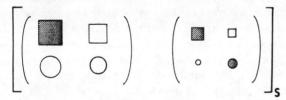

Figure 5.2. List of abstract kinds of sameness relations. These are relations on relations; the critical relation is the *kind* of relation that exists between pairs of particulars. In the illustration, brackets group together pairs of objects that are related in the same abstract kind of way.

ular dimensions exist. The specification of the *kind* of part identity also affords more logically powerful classes. Dimensional identity, like whole-object identity (but unlike part identity), is an equivalence relation: reflexive, symmetric, and transitive.

Relations of magnitude

The sameness relations illustrated in Figures 5.1 and 5.2 concern an understanding of the relations that exist between objects varying on both nominal and ordinal dimensions. Figures 5.3 and 5.4 list the further special relations of *difference* between objects varying on dimensions of magnitude. Figure 5.3 lists relations of global or dimensionally undifferentiated magnitude. Just as I suggest that there are dimensionally nonspecific relations of sameness, I suggest that there are dimensionally nonspecific relations of magnitude.

Global magnitude. The first holistic relation of magnitude given in Figure 5.3 is that of *global polarity*. Global polarity is the categorical contrast that exists between objects (or events) that are on the one hand relatively intense (across all dimensions) and on the other hand not intense (across all dimensions). For example, a large, warm object and a small, hot object are both intense relative to a very small, warm object and a small, cold object.[1] The next set of global magnitude relations concerns directions of difference across all varying dimensions of magnitude. *Global greater-than* concerns the iteration of directional difference between pairs of objects and the understanding that greater than is inherently relative and applies across the full range of magnitudes. So if A is more intense than B, B may be more intense than some other object, C; further, A may be very intense overall but still less intense than some other, even more intense object. The inverse relation of *global less-than* is listed separately from *global greater-than*, since it is in principle possible (and I think likely for children) that opposing directions of difference are initially understood separately; *greater-than* may be understood without *less-than* being understood, or both may be represented without an understanding of their necessary connection (i.e., $A > B$ if $B < A$).

The distinction between global polarity and global directions of difference is meant to capture the distinction between our categorical uses of magnitude (polarity) and our comparative uses (directions). We often partition objects into polar categories according to their position on the judged continuum – categorizing several different objects as the big ones or the high ones, as hot, as cold.

1. Overall polarity --- categorical contrast between sets of objects in magnitude across all dimensions

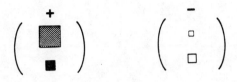

2. Directions of difference --- ordering of objects according to relative magnitude across all varying dimensions

   a. Greater than

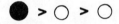

   b. Less than

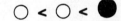

   c. Opposing directions

$$X > Y \quad \text{iff} \quad Y < X$$

Figure 5.3. List of relations of global magnitude.

Our comparative use of magnitude relations, in contrast, centers on the directional difference between objects *regardless of their absolute positions on the continuum*. So, given two categorically large objects, we may judge one to be smaller than the other. Any level of magnitude may be judged greater than some and less than others. These two uses of magnitude have often been contrasted in discussions of dimensionally specific magnitudes (e.g., Clark, 1970; Nelson & Benedict, 1974), and there is considerable evidence to suggest that categorical uses are developmentally prior to comparative ones. I suggest that, just as the distinction between categorical and comparative concepts of magnitude is useful for thinking about quantitative dimensions, so may such a distinction be useful for thinking about global notions of magnitude.

1. Polarity --- contrastive differences between values on a single dimension

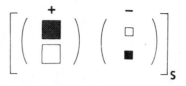

2. Dimensions of difference --- ordering of values on a single dimension according to relative magnitude

    a. Greater than

$$\left[\left(\begin{array}{c}\square\\\blacksquare\end{array}\right)\overset{>}{}_{s}\left(\begin{array}{c}\boxtimes\\\square\end{array}\right)\overset{>}{}_{s}\left(\begin{array}{c}\square\\\blacksquare\end{array}\right)\right]_{s}$$

    b. Less than

$$\left[\left(\begin{array}{c}\square\\\blacksquare\end{array}\right)\overset{<}{}_{s}\left(\begin{array}{c}\boxtimes\\\square\end{array}\right)\overset{<}{}_{s}\left(\begin{array}{c}\square\\\blacksquare\end{array}\right)\right]_{s}$$

    c. Opposing directions

$$X \gtrless_s Y \quad \text{iff} \quad Y \lessgtr_s X$$

    d. Transitivity

$$\text{if } X \gtrless_s Y \text{ and } Y \gtrless_s Z, \text{ then } X \gtrless_s Z$$

Figure 5.4. List of dimensional relation of magnitude.

Dimensionally specific magnitude. Figure 5.4 lists dimensional magnitude relations. The first four listed relations, *polarity, greater-than, less-than,* and the necessary connection between *greater-than* and *less-than,* are the dimensionally specific analogs to the global relations of magnitude. Given these relations, objects are not just represented as intense or not intense, or more intense than some object and less intense than others. Rather, objects are represented as intense in particular ways – as big and little, as bigger than some object and littler than another, as loud and quiet, as louder than some event and quieter than another. Such a dimensionally specific representation of magnitude results in a new power in magnitude relations that has no global counterpart. The dimensionalization of directions of difference means a *unique linear* ordering of values by their magnitude on the dimension. A complete understanding of dimensional relations of magnitude should include an understanding of this unique linear ordering; that is, an understanding of betweenness, that if $A > B$ and $B < C$, then B is between A and C, and an understanding of transitivity, that if $A > B$ and $B > C$, then $A > C$. Global relations of magnitude do not have these properties that afford such powerful inferences, since objects are not necessarily ordered linearly by global magnitude relations.[2] Quantitative relations *on a dimension* are therefore inferentially more powerful than global magnitude relations.

Significance of the analysis

To this point, all I have provided is an analysis, truly just a list, of potential relational concepts. The value of this list is that it emphasizes the complexity of our concepts about perceptual relations and their connection to each other. The potential interdependencies among the concepts, both logically and in development, may prove quite intricate. For example, identity, dimensional identity, overall similarity, and part similarity are all relations by which categories may be formed, but identity and dimensional identity provide for a specific kind of category: the equivalence class. Global polarity and directions of difference are the ordinal counterparts of the holistic relations of sameness. Of potential importance is the fact that there would seem to be two routes to the understanding of dimensions, through sameness relations and through magnitude relations. Dimensions may be understood by organizing part identities (or attributes) according to qualitative kind. Quantitative dimensions may also be understood as *linear* orderings of attributes by opposing directions of difference. These are highly interrelated specifications of a dimension. One can get a linear ordering of attributes only if they are of the same kind (see Goodman, 1951, for proof). A dimension exists, that is, attributes are organized by qualitative kind, if the attributes can be linearly ordered by the relations of greater-than and less-than. Further, interdefining opposing directions of difference requires the organization of directions of difference by dimensional kind, an organization isomorphic to the organization of attributes by kind. If A is bigger than B, B is necessarily smaller than A, but A is not necessarily quieter.

Ultimately, what one would like, of course, is a complete specification of the *psychological* structure of these concepts and their inter-
relationships in development. Unfortunately, we are not close to such
an understanding. The reason is lack of relevant evidence, and the
lack of evidence stems directly from the lack of a framework such as
the one provided here. The lack of a guiding framework is obvious
in existing empirical data. There is confusion in the literature as to
just what aspects of knowledge some performance by children indicates. For example, some investigators have assumed that the ability
to sort reds in one pile and blues in another indicates an understanding of the dimension of color (e.g., Aschkenasy & Odom, 1982; Fischer
& Roberts, 1980). However, the present analysis suggests that sorts
by part identity (or part similarity) could occur within an understanding of dimensions. A child could know that two red objects are alike
and two blue objects are alike and two square objects are alike, without
knowing that the likeness between two blue objects is of the same
qualitative kind as that between two red objects. A second example
of the weakness of current evidence and conclusions from that evidence concerns children's understanding of quantitative dimensions
and their performance in (certain) seriation and transitive inference
tasks (e.g., Bryant & Trabasso, 1971). In such tasks, objects usually
vary on one dimension (e.g., size), and thus we have no way of knowing
whether children order objects by dimensionally nonspecific directions of difference (e.g., *more*) or by dimensionally specific ones (e.g.,
bigger). We cannot know what children know unless we dissect the
structure of potential knowledge.

The current literature also fails in its lack of comparisons between
emerging concepts. There is no unified "relational knowledge" literature. Rather, separate studies, and indeed separate groups of investigators, examine children's use of sameness relations in
classification and their use of magnitude relations in seriating objects
and making transitive inferences. There are few hypotheses and little
information about interdependencies among aspects of the relational
knowledge system. The value of the present listing of potential relational concepts is that it provides a way of organizing the currently
disjointed evidence and points to some of the questions that ought to
be asked about just what children know about the structure of perceptual relations.

Hypotheses and evidence

The general claim that I want to make is that the emergence of relational concepts proceeds from dimensionless relations to dimen-

sionally specific ones – that there is a *dimensionalization* of the knowledge system. There is considerable evidence for such a trend in general terms. Children's early word acquisitions suggest such a trend. Among the first words acquired by children are the names for basic categories – categories such as *dog* and *chair*, which seem well organized by overall similarities. Words that refer to superordinate categories (e.g., *animal*) are not well organized by global similarity, and the words that refer to dimensional relations themselves (e.g., *red* or *tall*) appear to be understood relatively late (see Anglin, 1977; MacNamara, 1982; Rescorla, 1980). The evidence from classification tasks also suggests such a trend. School-age children consistently assign objects to groups by single dimensions, categorizing reds versus blues, bigs versus littles. Children under age 5 do not (e.g., Bruner, Olver, & Greenfield, 1966; Inhelder & Piaget, 1964; Vygotsky, 1962); instead they consistently classify objects by their similarity overall, preferring, for example, to group a red ellipse with an orange circle rather than a red ellipse with a blue ellipse (Kemler, 1983; Shepp, Burns, & McDonough, 1980; Smith, 1985). Evidence from discriminative learning tasks and transposition tasks also corroborate the trend: In such tasks, older children learn rules about component attributes, dimensions, and dimensional directions of difference, whereas preschool children tend to learn rules about whole objects (Kendler, 1979; Keunne, 1946; Tighe & Tighe, 1978). Thus the evidence concerning children's *use* of relations suggests that early in development holistic ones dominate. But the question I would like to turn to now is not quite answered by these data. The relevant question is what, in detail, do children know about relations of sameness and of magnitude. What follows is some evidence and much speculation concerning the answer to this question.

Relations of sameness

Identities, part identities, and dimensions. I will begin where I think there is some strong evidence suggesting that, initially, part identities are not organized into dimensional kinds. In this study (Smith, 1984), I employed an imitation task. Children aged 2, 3, and 4 watched while first one experimenter and then a second experimenter selected objects by a particular rule. The question was whether the children would imitate the rule in their selections. The three types of rules examined were identity, part identity, and dimension rules as shown in Table 5.1. On identity trials, the first experimenter might select two large yellow cups, and the second experimenter might select two small red houses. The child would show an understanding of

Table 5.1. *Sets for imitation task (from Smith, 1984)*

	Identity	Part identity	Dimension
E₁	lg yellow cup	lg red dog	lg red ball
	lg yellow cup	sm red dog	sm red ball
	sm blue car	sm blue dog	sm yellow ball
E₂	sm red house	med red dog	med blue ball
	sm red house	lg red dog	lg blue ball
	med brown dog	lg green dog	lg red ball
Child	sm purple boot	sm red dog	sm yellow ball
	sm purple boot	med red dog	med yellow ball
	med green table	med yellow dog	med red ball

abstract identity if he or she selected from the possible available objects two objects that were identical to each other (in the example in Table 5.1, the child should select the two purple boots). The relation, here, is an abstract one; there is no common property or similarity between the choices of the two experimenters and the correct choice by the child; what is common is the kind of relation. Nonetheless, even the 2-year-olds imitated identity choices with ease, showing the ability to represent this relation.[3] These choices do appear to be imitations by identity; 2-year-olds did not select identical objects in a control condition in which the experimenters did not choose by identity.

On part-identity trials, the experimenters selected objects that shared the same part identity but were different on other dimensions (e.g., each would select red objects, or each would select 8-inch tall objects). At issue here is imitation by a concrete property (e.g., redness) possessed by all objects selected by the experimenters and existing between correct choices for the child. Thus one might think this a simpler task than that concerning abstract identity. However, the critical relation concerns parts, not whole objects, and only half the 2-year-olds (but all the 3- and 4-year-olds) succeeded in this task. Particular part identities, such as *red*, then, are not clearly represented by all the youngest children. Finally, on dimension trials, the rule governing the experimenters' choices was sameness on a particular dimension. For example, if the dimension were color, the first experimenter might select two red objects and the second experimenter might select two blue objects. A correct choice by the child might consist of selecting two yellow objects. At issue is *dimensional kind* of part identity and not a concrete property. In this task, none of the 2-year-olds, some of the 3-year-olds, and all the 4-year-olds imitated by dimensional kind of sameness. The errors on these trials were particularly telling. Children virtually always chose objects that were part identical, but the youngest children did not preserve the dimensional kind of part identity. So, if the experimenters chose by same color, the 2-year-olds were equally likely to choose two objects that were same in color or same in size. Apparently, 2-year-olds can represent and infer rules about (abstract) whole-object identity, and many can represent and infer rules about part identities, but they do not have part identities organized into dimensional kinds. Dimensions appear not to be given but to emerge with development.

Concrete relations versus abstract kinds of relations. In the imitation study, 2-year-olds successfully imitated choices by abstract identity. They clearly represented the relation between two identical cups as being the same as between two identical houses. Are abstract kinds of relations, albeit perhaps only holistic ones, represented as such from the beginning? Maybe, but I think not. The best evidence for the representation of a kind of relation would be for the child to demonstrate knowledge of some *rule* based on that relation. Merely using the relation is insufficient. To clarify this point, consider an example. Assume that a child judges object A to be like object A' and to be different from object B – as might be done in a habituation paradigm, if after habituation of some response to A the infant demonstrated dishabituation given B but not A'. Now assume that the child judges (in some similar manner) object B to be like object B' but to be different from object C. The child has judged the identity (or overall similarity) relation across two distinct item sets. But all this means is that the child "has" a relation *same as A* and a relation *same as B*. There is nothing in such judgments to indicate an understanding that the judgment made between A and A' is the same kind as that between B and B'. The kind of evidence that *demands* explanation in terms of an abstract relation of sameness is rule use.

Children show evidence of forming these sorts of rules at the end of the second year. Evidence for rules about kinds of relations, as opposed to particular things, can be found in children's understanding of the distinction between proper and class nouns in article use ("a Dax" implies the existence of more than one of this kind of thing; see, e.g., MacNamara, 1982) and in the rule-based use of the plural (e.g., dog/dogs, foot/foots; see, e.g., Bowerman, 1982). I think additional evidence from a variety of other tasks – object banging (Forman, 1982), iterative naming, and classification (Sugarman, 1983) – also points to the child's clear use of rules based on abstract sameness

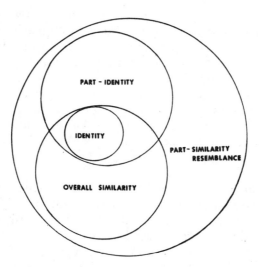

Figure 5.5. Inclusion relations of the various sameness relations.

relations by the end of the second year. Interestingly, I could find no unambiguous evidence for abstract relations prior to 20 months of age. So abstract relations (again, though, perhaps only global ones) may emerge very early in development and begin to organize the infinite number of distinct perceptible similarities between specific objects.

Resemblance, similarity, and identity. Figure 5.5 shows the overlapping extensions of the various relations of sameness. Early in development, these relations may not be differentiated from each other; such differentiation may require the organization as abstract kinds. So, very early, there may only be resemblances – a myriad of possible concrete relations noticeable by the child. We know that certainly by 1 year of age children represent and notice overall similarities, and it may be that strong similarity across all (or many) object characteristics is particularly salient. However, quite young children also notice weaker resemblances or part similarities. Bowerman (1982) and MacNamara (1982) both report generalizations in noun use by their own children, between the ages of 15 and 20 months, that clearly suggest attention to partial similarities or resemblances. For example, Bowerman's daughter called the following items *moon*: grapefruit, hangnail, lemon section, ball of spinach. These uses may be metaphorical; the child may be saying "The grapefruit is like a moon." Indeed, MacNamara's son explicitly used the phrase *like a*. He said,

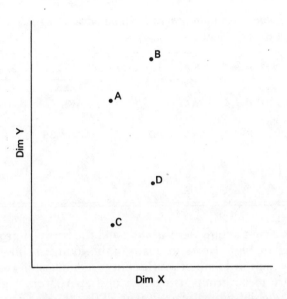

Figure 5.6. The coordinates in multidimensional space of the four unique stimulus objects used in an experiment by Smith and Evans.

for example, that searchlights were "like a helicopter." It may be that all varieties of similarity are available from the beginning. However, they may not be represented distinctly; and as a class of relations, such various resemblances are complexive and syncretic. Specific kinds of similarities may gain differential status only with development. In this emergence of kinds of similarities, *degree* of overall similarity may take precedence; this is the relation that governs earliest object category acquisitions. So, at this first step toward differentiated relations, all that may be represented is degree of overall similarity; objects may be very similar overall or not very similar.

The subsequent step in the differentiation of relations of sameness may be the according of special status to a particular degree of overall similarity – that of identity. Identity may not be a special relation at first, it may only come to be represented as such. Paul Evans and I have collected some suggestive evidence on this issue from 2-, 3-, and 4-year-olds in a classification task. As illustrated in Figure 5.6 and Table 5.2, the children were sometimes given Similarity sets that could be partitioned into two groups such that all objects within a group were *similar* (but not identical) and the between-group *dissimilarity* was high. All children readily classified these sets in this way. All the children also easily classified the Identity and Similarity sets, the sets

Table 5.2. *Exact stimulus items given to children on particular trials and proportion of correct classifications*

	SIM vs. DIM	SIM + IDENTITY	IDENTITY vs. SIM
Objects to be classified	ABCD	AADD	AABB
"Correct" classification	AB vs. CD	AA vs. DD	AA vs. BB
Age			
2 years	.65	.88	.26
3 years	.70	.93	.67
4 years	.70	.97	.90

in which objects within a group were *identical* and the between-group *dissimilarity* was, again, high. However, many of the youngest children refused to classify the third kind of set (Identity vs. Similarity). Here, *identical* objects are to be grouped together and apart from highly *similar* objects. The children maintained that all the objects went together. These refusals to classify probably do not reflect an inability to discriminate between similar objects; all children who participated discriminated successfully between all pairs of objects in a prior oddity task. What I suggest is that, for the youngest children, whole-object identity is just a strong form of overall similarity and not a special kind of sameness. If this is true, and if the children were attempting to classify by overall similarity, then all objects in this third set do properly belong together.

The specialness of identity for older children is particularly well illustrated in a second classification task. In this task, 3-, 4-, and 5-year-old children were first given the four unique objects illustrated in the top panel of Figure 5.7. All children classified these objects in the same way – large objects versus small ones. Subsequent to this classification, these same objects were "mixed up" *and* a new object was added, and the children were asked to reclassify. As illustrated in the bottom panel of Figure 5.7, the new object was identical to one of the already present objects. The new object did not change the classifications by the 3-year-olds. They still partitioned the objects into the large ones versus small ones. The older children, however, changed their classification. They now grouped the two identical objects together and did not include any other objects in that group. Most of the children classified the objects into three groups by relative size (large, small, and the two identical smallest objects). However,

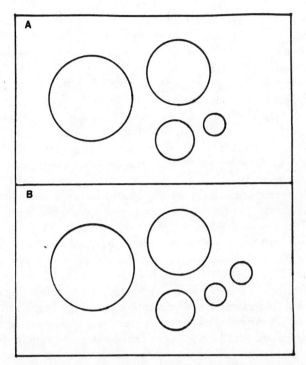

Figure 5.7. Two sets of objects (A and B) varying in size and given, separately, to children to classify. Set B differs from Set A only in the addition of one object that is identical to one already present object.

several children used the identity relation throughout their classification; they classified the two identical objects together and then classified each of the remaining, unique, objects singly.

   The finding that identity emerges as a special relation with development is intriguing. The value of identity is its logical power. As an equivalence relation, identity is both transitive and symmetric; these are valuable properties that similarity relations do not possess. The power of identity as an equivalence relation may even help the emergence of the second equivalence relation, dimensional identity, by providing the motivation for attending to part identities and organizing them by dimensional kind.

Relations of magnitude

   Global relations. Just as young children show a proclivity for categorizing objects by holistic similarity, so they may tend to compare objects in terms of contrasts in holistic magnitude. I suggest that children represent magnitude relations at a very early age, but those relations are initially dimensionally nonspecific. There is considerable suggestive evidence. Results from cross-modal transfer studies are certainly consistent with this possibility (see, e.g., Gibson & Spelke, 1983). The errors that children make in acquiring dimensional terms are also suggestive. For example, 3- and 4-year-olds have been reported to confuse *high* with *tall*, *low* with *short*, *big* with *bright*, *small* with *dim*, and *big* with *many* (Carey, 1978; Ehri, 1976; Gitterman & Johnston, 1983; Maratsos, 1974). These confusions make sense if the child has general notions of moreness and lessness that are not linked to specific dimensions.

Children's free classifications of objects also suggest a sensitivity to dimensionally nonspecific relations of magnitude. In one study (Smith, 1985), I gave children objects varying in size and saturation to put into groups. The 3- and 4-year-olds spontaneously formed contrasting groups of large, vividly colored objects versus small, pale objects more than twice as often as they formed contrasting groups of large, pale objects versus small, vivid ones. Apparently, objects that were intense in both size and color were perceived as being alike and being very different from objects that were not intense in both size and color. For these children *moreness* and *lessness* across both dimensions, but not *moreness* and *lessness* on a specific dimension, mattered. Interestingly, older children and adults do not spontaneously categorize by joint magnitude on saturation and size. However, in a forced-choice task they show some knowledge that *big* is like *vivid*, and *small* like *pale* (Smith, Sera, & McCord, 1986). Thus global magnitude relations may become less salient with age in certain tasks, but they are apparently not lost altogether.

Young children not only categorize objects by global polarity but also seriate objects by global directions of difference. While collecting data in tasks directed to other questions, we have repeatedly observed children trying to seriate objects on two dimensions of magnitude at once. The behavior of one child, a 3½-year-old, illustrates the phenomenon. The child was given three objects, a 2-inch saturated green circle, a 1½-inch saturated green circle and a 1½-inch desaturated circle as shown in Figure 5.8. As many children seem to do spontaneously, this child labeled the objects as "Daddy," "Mommy," and "Baby." In the first set (Set A in Figure 5.8) "Daddy" and "Mommy" differed appropriately in size; "Mommy" and "Baby" were the same size, but the object labeled "Mommy" was more intense in color than the one labeled "Baby." This child's labelings, then, are consistent

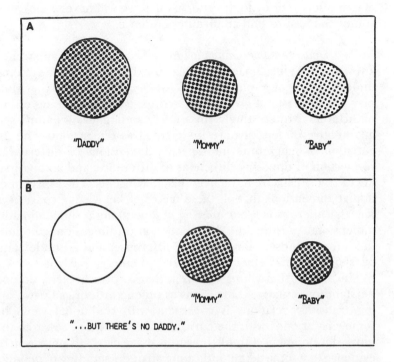

Figure 5.8. Schematic illustrations of two sets of three objects and their labeling by a child. The objects varied in size and saturation (of green color). Degree of saturation is indicated by density of pattern.

with an ordering of the objects by their global magnitude. On another trial (Set B in Figure 5.8), this same child was given a 2-inch desaturated circle, a 1½-inch medium-saturation circle, and a 1-inch desaturated circle. The child immediately moved the second and third objects together and said "Mommy and Baby." He then picked up the remaining object, put it down, and said, "There's no Daddy." This rejected object was a perfectly appropriate "Daddy" by size, but across both dimensions it was, perhaps, less intense than the other two.

What we may be seeing here is an early dimensionally undifferentiated notion of directions of difference. This possibility contrasts with the traditional evidence in both the cognitive (e.g., Inhelder & Piaget, 1964) and language literature (e.g., Ehri, 1976; Layton & Stick, 1979; Nelson & Benedict, 1974) that seriation and an understanding of comparative relations are late emerging. Perhaps only dimensionally differentiated understandings are late. At any rate, these global seriations by a 3-year-old suggest that if polar notions of global magnitude are prior to directional ones, we will have to look to quite young children to find confirming evidence.

Understanding quantitative dimensions. Children's apparent early knowledge of global magnitude may not, however, include a complete understanding of *greater-than* and *less-than*, in the sense that children may not understand *greater-than* and *less-than* as opposing directions of difference. Interestingly, this understanding may wait until specific quantitative dimensions are understood as dimensions. The differentiation of magnitude into specific dimensions of difference, the connection of opposing directions of difference, and an understanding of transitivity are intimately related concepts. The aspect of quantitative dimensions that all these pieces of knowledge concern is the fact that there is *only one ordering of items* along a single quantitative dimension. And thus the differentiation of dimensions, the interdefinition of opposing directions of difference, and an understanding of transitivity may emerge together and emerge fairly late.

This notion that young children, that is, preschoolers, do not understand quantitative dimensions as unique orderings by two opposing transitive relations is consistent with traditional views but is somewhat at odds with the current "can do" bias of research in cognitive development. I think, however, that a closer examination of the evidence that some take as indicating an understanding of quantitative dimensions by young children will reveal that children have bits and pieces of ideas about more and less and some dimensions but nothing like a full understanding.

Consider preschool children's "successes" in transitive inference tasks as shown in the elegant series of experiments begun by Bryant and Trabasso (1971). In the experiments, children were required to memorize pairs of premises, for example, "The red one is taller than the blue one," "The blue one is taller than the yellow one," "The yellow one is taller than the green one." After the premises were well learned, the children were asked to make inferences, for example, about the relation between the red one and the green one. Even 3-year-olds made the appropriate inferences. Further, the pattern of performance suggests that the children represented the premise information by mentally constructing an ordered list of individual objects, that is, by seriating the objects in their mind. Clearly, the mental machinery is such that quantitative dimensions can be represented. However, children's success in this task requires some very precise conditions. For example, the premise statements must be learned in both directions for each pair (e.g., "The red one is taller than the blue one" *and* "The blue one is shorter than the red one"; Trabasso & Riley, 1975). Apparently, young children do not spontaneously realize that if one object is taller than a second, then the second object is necessarily shorter than the first. Further, young children succeed only when the premises are limited to adjacent pairs and cannot include *both* adjacent and nonadjacent pairs. More specifically, Halford (1984) found that children often did not seriate the items correctly given the following premises about colored sticks: "Red is longer than blue," "Blue is longer than green," *and* "Red is longer than green." The children appear to have wanted to form a series where "longer" meant something like *next-to-on-the-right* and "shorter" meant *next-to-on-the-left*. So young children may make what look like transitive inferences, but, apparently, they do not understand the necessary connection between opposing directions or the uniqueness of the ordering of values. Further, there is nothing in any of these transitive inference results to suggest that children understand dimensional magnitude relations as opposed to global ones. I wonder, if children were told "*A* is bigger than *B*," "*B* is louder than *C*," and "*C* is heavier than *D*," would they infer that *A* is bigger/louder/heavier than *D*?

Young children's incomplete and fragmented understandings of quantitative relations are also evident in their use of the dimensional adjectives. In one study, we (Ratterman & Smith, 1985) examined children's use of *high* and *low* in contrastive and comparative form. On some trials 3- and 4-year-old children were shown two objects at 5 feet and 6 feet aboveground; all children labeled the two objects as "high." When asked which of the two "high" objects was higher, the children maintained correctly that the one at 6 feet was. When asked which was lower, the children maintained that *neither* was. Analogously, on other trials the children were shown objects at 1 foot and 2 feet from the ground. They labeled these objects as "low" and maintained that the object at 1 foot was lower but that *neither* was higher. These children apparently do not realize that *higher* and *lower* refer to opposite directions of difference. Rather, they appear to have the two comparative forms organized as separate directions of difference that apply within distinct categories; an object can be *higher* than the other only if it is not *low*, and an object can be *lower* than the other only if it is not *high*. These young children's uses of *higher* and *lower* are rather like our mature use of comparatives to refer to differences on (some) nonquantitative dimensions. We can judge, for example, which of two red objects is redder, but we cannot judge which of two red objects is greener. In sum, a complete understanding of dimensions of magnitude includes the integration and interconnection of various relations and may therefore emerge fairly late in complete form, despite many clear beginnings of pieces of knowledge in young children.

Putting it together: the relational knowledge system

So far, what I have done is consider in somewhat piecemeal fashion existing evidence as it relates to my list of potential relational concepts. What I will do now is try to put it all together into a coherent system. Figure 5.9 shows my attempt – a diagram of a portion of our knowledge about perceptual relations. I do not view this diagram as anything more than illustrative. It is certainly not complete; and it may be wrong in many details. Nevertheless, I hope it serves to summarize and clarify my proposal.

In the figure, earlier concepts are represented at the top. Arrows indicate structural connections between earlier and later concepts, that is, later concepts that include or reorganize pieces of earlier concepts. At this point, it is important to recognize that, when I say *earlier* and *later*, I mean earlier and later in emerging, not earlier and later in existence. Later concepts do *not replace* earlier ones. Rather, I think both the immature and mature systems, for example, represent global similarities and magnitudes; however, mature individuals also represent and use more differentiated levels. Notice also that this is not a componential system. Pieces are not acquired and added up to form some other piece. Rather, the notion is that relational knowledge is structured and that what develops is that structure. Development consists of the organization and reorganization of relations of sameness and magnitude.

Figure 5.9 illustrates the basic proposal that we begin with global notions of resemblance and magnitude by representing them at the top. Resemblances become differentiated into overall similarities, identities, and part identities. Early relations of magnitude consist of polarity and directions of difference. A dimension exists when the part identities are organized by dimensional kind; an ordinal dimension exists when there are opposing directions of difference that are logically linked. I indicate in the figure the emergence from part identities of two possible classes of dimension: color and extent. The dimension of color exists for the child when the child represents, for example, *red* and *blue* as attributes of one kind. The ordinal dimension of overall size exists for the child when the child represents *big* and *little* as attributes of a distinct kind *and* knows that *bigger* and *littler* are opposing directions of difference.

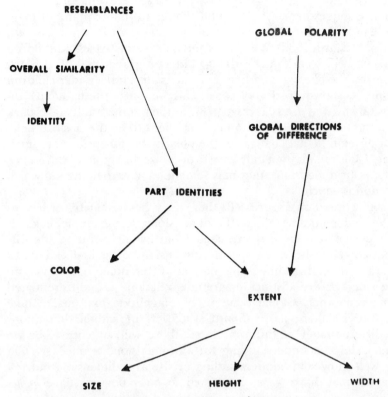

Figure 5.9. A schematic illustration of a possible portion of the relational knowledge system.

Interestingly, it is perhaps at the emergence of dimensions, when part identities become organized by kind and when opposing directions of magnitude become interdefined, that relations of sameness become integrated with relations of magnitude. The initial union between relations of sameness and relations of magnitude may not come easily to the child, and there may be mistakes. Children may sometimes try to map magnitude relations onto dimensions where they do not belong. As one possible example of such an attempt, Park, Tsukagoshi, and Landau (1985) report that preschool children organize colors into the polarized categories of *warm-light* and *cool-dark*. Warm-light colors are red, orange, and yellow, and cool-dark colors are green, blue, and purple. Park et al. found that both children learning English and children learning Japanese confused the warm-light color names with each other (e.g., *red* with *yellow*) and the cool-dark color names with each other (e.g., *green* with *purple*). We also have some preliminary evidence suggesting developmental change in the mapping of magnitude onto the dimension of (surface) darkness (or lightness) (Smith, Sera, & McCord, 1986). We have found that 2- and 3-year-old children consistently link dark gray with big, and light gray with little. So dark seems intense like big, and light not intense like little. Older children and adults, however, do not consistently organize the light/dark dimension this way (see Marks, 1978). Rather, some adults take dark to be the positive pole, and others take light to be the positive pole. Such developmental changes in the polarity of dimensions are intriguing. Children may not only have to organize directions of difference into specific dimensions; they may sometimes have to figure out which direction is which.

As illustrated in Figure 5.9, there may be systematic orderings of the understanding of specific dimensions. For example, color as a dimension may be differentiated from extent, prior to the differentiation of the three specific dimensions of spatial extent. In general, qualitative dimensions may be differentiated from magnitude ones before distinct magnitude relations are differentiated from each other. Global relations of magnitude may make some dimensions cohere more (Smith, 1985). If individual dimensions are differentiated at different rates, there will, of course, be no unitary shifts in understanding for all dimensions at once. A child may well show some understanding of size as a dimension, but not distance; may have *bigger* connected to *littler* but not have *higher* linked to *lower*. Individual dimensions and categories of dimension (e.g., extent or space) may have to be worked out individually. With development there may be a continuous process of organizing and reorganizing resemblances into kinds. Indeed, there may be no true end state; we may keep differentiating and dimensionalizing experience and relations even in adulthood, though presumably at a much slower rate.

Language and thought

One final but cogent issue concerns the interaction between emerging relational concepts and emerging relational language. To this point I have used evidence about relational language acquisition and conceptual development equally – as if they were the same thing. I am aware that this is a gross simplification. The nature of conceptual development must constrain language acquisition. At the same time, the acquisition of language may have a major impact on – even alter

– conceptual growth. Language may point the child to regularities and dimensions that he or she otherwise might not notice, or it may help the child to notice some regularities earlier than otherwise. For example, it seems possible that language helps the child discover the color dimension. Adults regularly ask young children, "What color is it?" And long before young children correctly name individual colors, they know the *class* of possible answers and reply "red," "blue," or "green," and not, for example, "big." They know the possible answers, not necessarily because of any latent knowledge of the dimension but because adults permit only certain labels as answers (Carey, 1978; Cruse, 1977). This class of allowable labels may point the child to the relevant dimension. If language does help organize the relational knowledge system, there may be cross-language differences; colors, for example, may be polarized within the conceptual systems as well as the language system of the mature speakers of some language (Berlin & Kay, 1969). The structure of language may also sometimes obscure the structure of relations and be a roadblock to overcome. For example, English-speaking children's tendency at one point in development to use *big* to mean *tall* may reflect solely the nature of usage of these terms in English and may actually slow the ultimate division of extent into three kinds (see, on this issue, Gathercole, 1982; Maratsos, 1974). The interaction of emerging language and emerging concepts in this domain is sure to be complicated but is clearly central to understanding the development of a relational knowledge system and how we judge a thing to be like another.

Conclusion: relations, similarity, and analogy

Before concluding, I consider the place of this work in the larger context of similarity and analogy. The present chapter with its focus on emerging concepts *about* perceptual similarity seems far afield from the more usual worry about the role of similarity in complex concepts. Such seemingly elementary ideas as *red*, *bigger*, and *same color* seem not to be the same stuff at all as concepts such as *feminist bank teller* (Smith & Osherson, this volume), *minting of coins* (Rips, this volume), and *floating basketball* (Barsalou, this volume). Nonetheless, there may be some useful contacts to be made. At the very least, the issues raised in this chapter about concepts of similarity suggest that there is no such thing as "pure similarity" (Rips, this volume). Just in terms of what objects *look like*, there are a variety of kinds of similarity – a structured system of kinds of relatedness. Surely, such complex ideas as *coins* and *pizzas* also contain many kinds of similarity. Instead of arguing about whether "similarity" is good or bad as an explanatory construct, we should, as admonished by Goodman in the epigraph to this chapter, fill in the blanks that similarity stands for.

As we fill in those blanks, we may find more specific relations between emerging concepts about perceptual similarities and the role of distinct kinds of similarities in structuring complex concepts. One intriguing possibility concerns the emerging specialness of identity. The specialness of identity may form the basis of people's beliefs in "essences" – the belief that all instances of some concept (say, *cow*) are absolutely identical in some way (e.g., DNA structure) even if that way is not specifiable (see Medin & Ortony, this volume; Murphy & Medin, 1985). Such beliefs appear to emerge with development (see Keil & Batterman, 1984). Children's early concepts of such things as islands, for example, seem to be structured initially by undifferentiated resemblances (e.g., usually near water, often having palm trees, sandy, etc.) but become structured by criterial particulars (land surrounded by water). This shift from complexive similarity to specified kinds of identities in the structure of complex concepts may depend on the earlier differentiation of perceptual identity relations as a special class of similarity. There may be other dependencies between emerging concepts about relations and the structuring of more complex ideas. I wonder, for example, if the structural properties (e.g., transitivity) of quantitative relations might first be induced from perception – say, from the structure of the size dimension – and then transported to more abstract domains.

In conclusion, there seem to be considerable complexity and growth in basic concepts of perceptual similarity and difference. Early in development there is similarity and difference, without, at the conceptual level, specification of the dimensional kind of similarity and difference. With development, the relational knowledge system becomes dimensionalized and highly organized into distinct and interrelated kinds of similarity and difference. Understanding the structure and development of these seemingly basic perceptual relations would seem to be a good place to begin specifying exactly what psychological similarity is.

NOTES

This paper was supported by Public Health Service grants K04–HD–589 and RO1–HD–19499. I thank Rob Nosofsky for his comments on an earlier version of this paper.

1 I assume that global magnitude is some monotonically increasing function of combined dimensional magnitudes, just as overall similarity is some monotonically increasingly function of the combined dimensional similarities (see Smith, 1985).

2 It is *possible* that there could be a unique linear ordering of objects by global magnitude – if there were absolute correspondences (see Marks, 1978) in magnitude across dimensions. I think that unlikely for the total class of dimensions that I am considering as dimensions of magnitude. It is also possible that a unique linear ordering by global magnitude could result from the combined intensities across all varying dimensions *if there were no variation in the weightings applied to the dimensions*, an assumption I also think unwarranted (see Tversky, 1977).

3 Although we call this relation *identity* because the objects are identical, given the inclusion relations between the various sameness relations, the young child might well have succeeded by the relation of overall similarity and not by an identity relation distinct from overall similarity.

REFERENCES

Anglin, J. M. (1977). *Word, object, and conceptual development.* New York: Norton.

Aschkenasy, J. R., & Odom, R. D. (1982). Classification and perceptual development: Exploring issues about integrality and differential sensitivity. *Journal of Experimental Child Psychology, 34*, 435–448.

Berlin, B. D., & Kay, P. (1969). *Basic color terms, their universality and evolution.* Berkeley: University of California Press.

Blewitt, P. (1982). Word meaning acquisition in young children: A review of theory and research. In W. Reese (Ed.), *Advances in Child Development and Behavior* (Vol. 17, pp. 139–195). New York: Harcourt Brace Jovanovich.

Bornstein, M. H. (1985). Colour-name versus shape-name learning in young children. *Journal of Child Language, 12*, 387–393.

Bowerman, M. (1982). Reorganizational processes in lexical and syntactic development. In E. Wanner & L. R. Gleitman (Eds.), *Language acquisition: The state of the art* (pp. 319–346). Cambridge: Cambridge University Press.

Bruner, J. S., Olver, R. R., & Greenfield, P. M. (1966). *Studies in cognitive growth.* New York: Wiley.

Bryant, P. E., & Trabasso, T. R. (1971). Transitive inferences and memory in young children. *Nature, 232*, 456–458.

Carey, S. (1978). The child as a word learner. In M. Halle, J. Bresnan, & G. Miller (Eds.), *Linguistic theory and psychological reality* (pp. 264–293). Cambridge, MA: MIT Press.

Carey, S. (1982). Semantic development: The state of the art. E. Wanner & L. R. Gleitman (Eds.), *Language acquisition: The state of the art* (pp. 347–389). Cambridge: Cambridge University Press.

Carnap, R. (1967). *The logical structure of the world and pseudoproblems in philosophy.* Berkeley: University of California Press. (Original work published 1928.)

Clark, H. H. (1970). The primitive nature of children's relational concepts.

In J. R. Hayes (Ed.), *Cognition and the development of language* (pp. 269–278). New York: Wiley.

Cohen, L. B., & Younger, B. A. (1983). Perceptual categorization in the infant. In G. K. Scholnick (Ed.), *New trends in conceptual representation: Challenge to Piaget's theory* (pp. 197–220). Hillsdale, NJ: Erlbaum.

Cruse, D. A. (1977). A note on the learning of colour names. *Journal of Child Language, 4*, 305–311.

Ehri, L. (1976). Comprehension and production of adjectives and seriation. *Journal of Child Language, 3*, 369–384.

Fischer, K. W. (1980). A theory of cognitive development: The control and construction of hierarchies of skills. *Psychological Review, 87*, 477–531.

Fischer, K. W., & Roberts, R. J. (1980). *A developmental sequence of classification skills in preschool children.* Unpublished manuscript, University of Denver.

Forman, G. E. (1982). A search for the origin of equivalence concepts through a microanalysis of block play. In G. E. Forman (Ed.), *Action and thought: From sensorimotor schemes to symbolic actions* (pp. 97–134). New York: Academic Press.

Gathercole, V. A. (1982). Decrements in children's responses to "big" and "tall": A reconsideration of the potential cognitive and semantic cues. *Journal of Experimental Child Psychology, 34*, 156–173.

Gattuso, B., Smith, L. B., & Treiman, R. (1986). *Classification by dimensions: A comparison of the auditory and visual modalities.* Unpublished manuscript, Indiana University.

✓ Gibson, E. J., & Spelke, E. S. (1983). The development of perception. In J. H. Flavell & E. M. Markman (Eds.), *Handbook of child psychology* (4th ed.): Vol. 3. *Cognitive development* (pp. 1–76). New York: Wiley.

Gitterman, D., & Johnston, J. R. (1983). Talking about comparisons: A study of young children's comparative adjective usage. *Journal of Child Language, 10*, 605–621.

Goodman, N. (1951). *The structure of appearance.* Cambridge, MA: Harvard University Press.

Goodman, N. (1972). *Problems and projects.* Indianapolis: Bobbs-Merrill.

Halford, G. S. (1984). Can young children integrate premises in transitivity and serial order tasks? *Cognitive Psychology, 16*, 65–93.

✓ Inhelder, B., & Piaget, J. (1958). *The growth of logical thinking from childhood to adolescence.* New York: Basic Books.

✓ Inhelder, B., & Piaget, J. (1964). *The early growth of logic in the child.* New York: Norton.

Johnston, J. R. (1985). Cognitive prerequisites: Cross linguistic study of language acquisition. In D. Slobin (Ed.), *Universals of language acquisition*: Vol. 2. *Theoretical issues* (pp. 961–1004). Hillsdale, NJ: Erlbaum.

Keil, F. C., & Batterman, N. A. (1984). A characteristic-to-defining shift in the development of word meaning. *Journal of Verbal Learning and Verbal Behavior, 23*, 221–236.

Kemler, D. G. (1983). Exploring and reexploring issues of integrality, perceptual sensitivity, and dimensional salience. *Journal of Experimental Child Psychology, 36*, 365–379.

Kendler, T. S. (1979). Cross-sectional research, longitudinal theory, and discriminative transfer ontogeny. *Human Development, 22*, 235–254.

Keunne, M. R. (1946). Experimental investigation of the relation of language to transposition. *Journal of Experimental Psychology, 6*, 471–490.

Layton, T. L., & Stick, S. L. (1979). Comprehension and production of comparatives and superlatives. *Journal of Child Language, 6*, 511–527.

✓ MacNamara, J. (1982). *Names for things: A study of human learning.* Cambridge, MA: MIT Press

Maratsos, M. P. (1974). When is the high thing the big one? *Developmental Psychology, 10*, 367–375.

Marks, L. E. (1978). *The unity of the senses.* New York: Academic Press.

Morais, J., Cary, L., Alegria, J., & Bertelson, P. (1979). Does awareness of speech as a sequence of phones arise spontaneously? *Cognition, 7*, 323–331.

Murphy, G. L., & Medin, D. L. (1985). The role of theories in conceptual coherence. *Psychological Review, 92*, 289–316.

Nelson, K., & Benedict, H. (1974). The comprehension of relative, absolute, and contrastive adjectives by young children. *Journal of Psycholinguistic Research, 3*, 333–342.

Nosofsky, R. M. (1984). Choice, similarity, and the context theory of classification. *Journal of Experimental Psychology: Learning, Memory, and Cognition, 10*, 104–114.

Park, S., Tsukagoshi, K., & Landau, B. (1985). *Young children's mis-naming of colors.* Paper presented at the biennial meeting of the Society for Research in Child Development, Toronto.

✓ Piaget, J. (1929). *The child's conception of the world.* New York: Harcourt, Brace.

Ratterman, M. J., & Smith, L. B. (1985). *Children's categorical use of "high" and "low."* Paper presented at the biennial meeting of the Society for Research in Child Development, Toronto.

Rescorla, L. A. (1980). Overextension in early language development. *Journal of Child Language, 7*, 321–335.

Shepp, B. E., Burns, B., & McDonough, D. (1980). The relation of stimulus structure to perceptual and cognitive development: Further tests of a separability hypothesis. In F. Wilkening, J. Becker, & T. Trabasso (Eds.), *The information integration by children* (pp. 113–146). Hillsdale, NJ: Erlbaum.

Smith, L. B. (1984). Young children's understanding of attributes and dimensions: A comparison of conceptual and linguistic measures. *Child Development, 55*, 363–380.

Smith, L. B. (1985). Young children's attention to global magnitude: Evidence from classification tasks. *Journal of Experimental Child Psychology, 39*, 472–491.

Smith, L. B. (1989). A model of perceptual classification in children and adults. *Psychological Review, 96*, 125–144.

Smith, L. B., & Evans, P. (1989). Similarity, identity, and dimensions: Perceptual classification in children and adults. In B. E. Shepp & S. Ballesteros (Eds.), *Object perception: Structure and process.* Hillsdale, NJ: Erlbaum.

Smith, L. B., & Kemler, D. G. (1978). Levels of experienced dimensionality in children and adults. *Cognitive Psychology, 10*, 502–532.

Smith, L. B., Sera, M., & McCord, C. (1986, November). *Developmental changes in the organization of relations of magnitude.* Paper presented at the meeting of the Psychonomic Society, New Orleans.

Sugarman, S. (1983). *Children's early thought.* Cambridge: Cambridge University Press.

Tighe, T. J., & Tighe, L. S. (1978). A perceptual view of conceptual development. In R. D. Walk & H. L. Pick (Eds.), *Perception and experience* (pp. 387–416). New York: Plenum Press.

Trabasso, T., & Riley, C. A. (1975). The construction and use of representations involving linear order. In R. L. Solso (Ed.), *Information processing and cognition: The Loyola Symposium* (pp. 381–410). Hillsdale, NJ: Erlbaum.

Treisman, A. M., & Gelade, G. (1980). A feature-integration theory of attention. *Cognitive Psychology, 12,* 97–136.

Tversky, A. (1977). Features of similarity. *Psychological Review, 85,* 327–352.

✔ Vygotsky, L. S. (1962). *Thought and language.* Cambridge, MA: MIT Press.

6

Psychological essentialism

DOUGLAS MEDIN and ANDREW ORTONY

> What is common to them all? – Don't say: "There *must* be something
> common, or they would not be called 'games' " – but *look and see*
> whether there is anything common to all. – For if you look at them
> you will not see something that is common to *all*, but similarities,
> relationships, and a whole series of them at that. To repeat: don't
> think, but look!
>
> Wittgenstein, *Philosophical Investigations*

Wittgenstein's admonition "don't think, but look" has had the important effect of stimulating psychologists to reconsider their common
practice of equating concept formation with the learning of simple
definitional rules. In the early 1970s, psychologists like Eleanor Rosch
(e.g., Rosch, 1973), responding to the difficulty of identifying necessary and sufficient conditions for membership of all kinds of categories, proposed alternative models of category representation based
on clusters of correlated features related to the categories only prob-
abilistically. Without denying the importance and impact of this
changed view of concepts (reviewed, e.g., by Smith & Medin, 1981),
we think that in certain respects the "don't think, but look" advice
may have been taken too literally. There are problems with equating
concepts with undifferentiated clusters of properties and with aban-
doning the idea that category membership may depend on intrinsically important, even if relatively inaccessible, features. For example,
on the basis of readily accessible properties that can be *seen*, people
presumably will not judge whales to be very similar to other mammals.
However, if they *think* about the fact that whales are mammals not
fish, they will probably acknowledge that with respect to some important, although less accessible property or properties whales *are*
similar to other mammals. This observation suggests that restricting
oneself to relatively accessible properties may make it difficult to account for the perceived similarity of whales to other mammals. If one

179

cannot appeal to "hidden" properties, it is difficult to explain the fact that people might recognize such similarities. Thus there might be a price to pay for looking rather than thinking.

The question of how best to conceptualize possible forms of similarity is intimately related to the question of how to conceptualize the nature of the "stuff" to which judgments of similarity are applied. Similarity judgments are always made about presented or represented entities. Because even presented entities are perceived and interpreted in terms of an existing set of concepts, there is a sense in which similarity judgments are always made with respect to *representations* of entities (rather than with respect to the entities themselves). In other words, we shall assume that when people judge two things to be similar those things are (at least temporarily) represented, so that similarity judgments are always made vis-à-vis *representations*. This means that theoretical treatments of representations need to endow them with sufficient richness to allow similarity to perform useful functions. In addition to the perceived similarity that results from attending (only) to highly accessible (typically, so-called perceptual) properties, we need to consider the similarity that results from considering more central (less accessible) conceptual material too, because this deeper aspect of similarity makes an important and sometimes indispensable contribution to cognition. For example, it can account for why people might believe that two things with very different surface properties (e.g., whales and bears) still are instances of the same category and therefore why they might judge them more similar to one another than they would on the basis of surface properties alone.

In this discussion, we consider the implications of the distinction between the more accessible, surface, aspects of representations and the less accessible, deeper, aspects for the nature of similarity and its role in cognition. By surface aspects, we mean the sorts of things people describe when asked to list properties of objects and the sorts of things psychologists have tried to use as the building blocks of concepts. Central to the position that we advocate, which we call *psychological essentialism*, is the idea that these surface features are frequently constrained by, and sometimes generated by, the deeper, more central parts of concepts. Thus there is often a nonarbitrary, constraining relation between deep properties and more superficial ones. We shall argue that, although it can be a powerful heuristic for various cognitive tasks, there are limitations to using similarity with respect only to surface properties and that there are problems with ignoring the relation between surface similarity and deeper properties.

The view we propose is more optimistic about the role of (super-ficial) similarity in cognition than that of Lance Rips but less optimistic than the view proposed by Edward Smith and Daniel Osherson. Rips believes that categorization does not necessarily depend on similarity, although he admits that sometimes it might. He presents arguments and data to support his claim that there are factors that affect judgments of category membership that do not affect judgments of similarity and that there are factors that affect judgments of similarity that do not affect judgments about category membership. If similarity and categorization can vary independently of one another, then neither can determine the other, and, in particular, similarity can be neither necessary nor sufficient for categorization. Smith and Osherson, on the other hand, suggest that similarity has a role not only in categorization but also in decision making. To explain this role they need an approach to similarity that is flexible enough to vary depending on how, whether, and when features are weighted (Tversky, 1977). The other contributors to Part I are more agnostic on the conceptual structure issue as it relates to similarity. Linda Smith argues for a more constrained view of similarity but allows for developmental changes in the aspects of similarity processing that are consciously available. That is, young children may have access only to global, overall perceptual similarity, and may learn only later to identify the components or features that determine it. Ryszard Michalski includes a role for similarity but argues that similarity is constrained by goals (his chapter is covered in the commentaries to Part II). Lawrence Barsalou agrees that similarity is involved in concepts, but a big chunk of the similarity that emerges is apparently context-dependent.

Why are there such divergent views about a matter that one might think should be quite straightforward? As psychologists, we expect a great deal of the construct of similarity. On the one hand, we sometimes treat it as a stable construct. On this view, robins *really are* like sparrows in some absolute observer-independent sense, and it is this objective similarity that underlies our perception of them as similar. In contrast to this strong form of metaphysical realism, at other times psychologists treat similarity as a highly flexible construct grounded not so much in objective reality as in the degree to which shared predicates are judged to be involved. When viewed in this way, similarity becomes more like a dependent variable than an independent variable. If similarity is to be grounded in shared predicates, it is open to the objection that it is not really grounded at all. Indeed, Goodman (1972) and Watanabe (1969) have offered formal proofs of just this point by showing that when similarity is defined in terms of shared predicates all pairs of entities are equally similar. In addition, there is no guarantee that different individuals share the same beliefs about what properties objects have, and contextual factors can have dramatic effects upon the accessibility and salience of different predicates. This need to conceptualize similarity sometimes as fixed and sometimes as flexible poses a dilemma. We require a fixed notion to account for intuitions such as that robins are more like sparrows than they are like sunglasses, whereas we need a flexible notion to account for a whole host of empirical results of the kind presented by Barsalou, for example, and E. Smith and Osherson.

Can this dilemma be resolved? We think that the framework we propose can take us at least part of the way. A first step is to define similarity not in terms of logically possible shared predicates but in the more restricted sense of shared *represented* predicates. For example, both tennis balls and shoes share the predicate *not having ears*, but it is unlikely that this predicate is part of our representation of either tennis balls or shoes. By restricting ourselves to represented predicates we can restrict the predicates that contribute to the determination of similarity. Of course, this leaves unanswered the question of what determines which predicates *are* part of our mental representations. To address this question, we need to take a second step: We suggest that perceptual similarity based on representations of what appear to be more accessible surface properties provides an initial conceptual structure that will be integrated with and differentiated into the deeper conceptual knowledge that is acquired later. Thus properties associated with a concept are linked both within and between levels to produce coherence. The reason that *not having ears* is not a predicate in our mental representation of tennis balls is that it would be an uninformative, isolated fact, unrelated to the rest of our knowledge about tennis balls. Our basic claim is that the link between surface and deep properties serves two functions: It enables surface similarity to serve as a good heuristic for where to look for deeper properties, *and* it functions as a constraint on the predicates that compose our mental representations. Although this constraint need not necessarily be a tight one, it may be enough to allow us to have a notion of similarity that is flexible without being vacuous.

This all suggests that the general way out of the dilemma is to acknowledge, as has been acknowledged in other areas of psychology, that logical and psychological accounts of certain phenomena need not necessarily be compatible. It is now generally accepted that psychologically plausible accounts of certain phenomena are at odds with purely logical analyses. People are not wetware instantiations of formal systems, be they logical or statistical, as a wealth of research on judgment under uncertainty has shown (e.g., Kahneman, Slovic, & Tversky, 1982; Nisbett & Ross, 1980). In the case of similarity, what is needed is a richer account that does more than simply view similarity in terms of lists of matching properties or shared predicates. With this general solution in mind, we shall try to sketch a psychologically plausible view of conceptual structure and then relate it to the chapters that are the subject of our commentary.

What is psychological essentialism?

We consider psychological essentialism to be a psychologically plausible analog of the logically implausible doctrine of metaphysical essentialism. The philosophical problem about essences is this: If one wants to argue that an object has an essence by virtue of which it is that object and not some other object, one has to face the problem, clearly recognized by Aristotle, that what that thing is is not independent of how it is described. The same object might be correctly described as, for example, a piece of rock, a paperweight, or an ashtray. But this means that the same piece of rock under these three different descriptions must have three different essences. In general, the problem is that an object appears to need as many essences as there are possible true descriptions of it.[1] But such a proliferation of essences undermines the very notion of an essence as some unique hidden property of an object by virtue of which it is the object that it is.

Because of observations such as these, the idea that objects might have some (possibly unknown) internal essence that makes them the objects they are is a philosophical orphan, banished to the netherworld of Platonic forms. Justifiable as this exile may be from a philosophical point of view, it is possible, and we think useful, to postulate something that might be called *psychological essentialism*. This would be not the view that *things* have essences, but rather the view that people's *representations* of things might reflect such a belief (erroneous as it may be). Since a major task for cognitive psychology is to characterize knowledge representations, psychological theories about them have to be descriptions of psychological reality, not of metaphysical reality. Thus, if people believe that things have essences, we had better not ignore this fact in our theories of knowledge representation.

We think there is evidence that ordinarily people *do* believe that things have essences. Many people behave as though they believed it, presumably because the assumptions that things have essences is an effective way of viewing the world and making predictions about it. One reason for supposing that people's concepts often embody an implicit belief that things have essences is provided by the third and fourth experiments described by Rips, in which subjects were unwilling to change the way in which they classified objects even though transformations of certain superficial properties of those objects rendered them more similar to exemplars of some other category. In these experiments subjects were behaving as though they believed that category membership depended upon the possession of some "hidden" (Rips calls them "extrinsic") properties of which observable properties are but typical signs. There is another reason that leads us to believe that people typically endorse, at least implicitly, some sort of essentialism. The nature of a great deal of scientific inquiry appears to be focused on trying to get at the "underlying reality" of phenomena rather than merely describing their observable properties. For example, the idea that things have essences was a guiding principle in the development of modern taxonomy by Linnaeus.

We should emphasize again that we are not claiming that objects have essences or that people necessarily believe that they know what these essences are. The point about psychological essentialism is not that it postulates metaphysical essentialism but rather that it postulates that human cognition may be affected by the fact that people believe in it. In other words, we are claiming only that people find it natural to assume, or act as though, concepts have essences.

Psychological essentialism should not be equated with the classical view that concepts are representations of classes of objects that have singly necessary and jointly sufficient conditions for membership. First of all, on our account people may sometimes believe that necessary and sufficient conditions are a *consequence* of the essential nature of the thing in question, rather than that essential nature itself. Furthermore, the essential nature may not generate necessary and sufficient properties at all. For example, it may be part of the represented essence of *bird* that birds fly, even if it happens that not all birds do fly and that people know this. More generally, we propose that the knowledge representations people have for concepts may contain what might be called an *essence placeholder*. There are several possibilities for what is in such a placeholder. In some cases, but by no means in all, it might be filled with beliefs about what properties are necessary and sufficient for the thing to be what it is. In other cases it might be filled with a more complex, and possibly more inchoate, "theory" of what makes the thing the thing that it is (see Murphy & Medin, 1985). It might, additionally, contain the belief (or a representation of the belief) that there are people, experts, who really know what makes the thing the thing that it is, or scholars who are trying to figure out exactly what it is. Just as with theories, what the place-holder contains may change, but the placeholder remains.

Another reason for not equating psychological essentialism with the classical view is based on one particular reading of, or defense of, the classical view. This reading turns on the classical view's distinction between the *core* of a concept, which brings out its relationship to other concepts, and an associated *identification procedure* for identifying instances of the concept (see Smith & Medin, 1981). For example, the core of a concept like *boy* might contain properties such as *male, young*, and *human* that could be used to understand its relation to other concepts like *girl, colt*, and *man*. The identification procedure might consist of processes employing available information about currently accessible properties like hair length, height, characteristic gait, and so on, that can be used to help determine that some person is likely to be a boy rather than a girl or a man. One defense of the classical view is that the typicality effects used to attack it are based on prop-erties involved in the identification procedure rather than on core properties. Insofar as this defense of the classical view can be upheld, however, one might object that it presupposes too great a dissociation between the core properties and the others. Our view is that the more central properties are best thought of as constraining or even gen-erating the properties that might turn out to be useful in identification (see Smith, Medin, & Rips, 1984, for related arguments). Further-more, rather than seeing a sharp dichotomy between core properties and properties that constitute the basis for an identification proce-dure, we conceive of properties as lying on a continuum of centrality ranging from relatively inaccessible, deep properties to more acces-sible, surface ones.

The notion of a continuum of centrality linking deeper and more superficial properties may provide the basis for some structuring of, or coherence in, family resemblance categories. For example, asso-ciated with a person's representation of *male* may be the idea that being male is partly a matter of hormones, which directly influences features such as height and facial hair. In the absence of deeper principles to link more superficial properties, categories constructed only in terms of characteristic properties or family resemblances may not be psychologically coherent. In some recent experiments using artificially constructed category materials, we have clear evidence that providing deeper linkages is sufficient to enable people to find family resemblance categories to be natural or coherent, and suggestive evidence that these linkages may be *necessary* for coherence (Medin, Wattenmaker, & Hampson, 1987). One way to summarize our argument is to say that twins are not twins *because* they are similar; they *are* similar because they are twins. So the second key element in our psychological essentialism is that our mental representations reflect the notion that properties differ in their depth and that deep properties are often intimately linked to the more superficial properties that so often drive our perceptions of and intuitions about similarity. The linkages between surface and deep properties are a function of the theories we have about the deep ones.

So far we have made two main points. First, people act as if their concepts contain essence placeholders that are filled with "theories" about what the corresponding entities are. Second, these theories often provide or embody causal linkages to more superficial properties. Our third tenet is that organisms have evolved in such a way that their perceptual (and conceptual) systems are sensitive to just those kinds of similarity that lead them toward the deeper and more central properties. Thus whales, as mammals that look more like fish than like other mammals, are the exception that proves the rule: Appearances are usually not deceiving. This means that it is quite adaptive for an organism to be tuned to readily accessible, surface properties. Such an organism will not be led far astray because many of these surface properties are constrained by deeper properties. If this view is correct, then the types of category constructions based on global similarities described by Linda Smith will tend to be just those partitionings that will be useful later on as the child acquires more knowledge and begins to develop deeper conceptual representations. In other words, psychological similarity is tuned to those superficial properties that are likely to be causally linked to a deeper level. This is particularly likely to be true with respect to natural kinds.

The question we now want to address is whether or not this way of augmenting the structure of concepts can provide a framework within which to understand the chapters in Part I. We shall suggest that what Rips is actually describing are the kinds of factors that go into *identification* of concepts – his challenge to similarity we take as supporting the general view that similarity of a putative category member to representations of exemplars and prototypes is a fallible heuristic for deciding category membership. We interpret his chapter as showing that the limitations to this heuristic are determined by the degree to which the surface features on the basis of which such judgments are made are constrained by less accessible, deeper features, or psychological essence. Linda Smith's paper provides a developmental perspective according to which infants and young children may have little else to go on than surface features. In the context of the present discussion, this is a profoundly important observation. The very fact that young children seem to classify only in terms of global similarity, rather than by isolating distinct dimensions, may provide them just the stability needed to make it likely that they will construct appropriate and useful categories. This suggests to us that attention to surface features early in development may be an asset rather than a limitation. Edward Smith and Daniel Osherson also present an account of the role of similarity, this time not in judgments of category membership but in decision making and choice. Rather than questioning the theoretical utility of similarity, Smith and Osherson suggest that it may be able to explain more than was previously thought. We suspect, however, that they will ultimately need to supplement their treatment of similarity in terms of representations involving lists of independent features with a view that includes the notion that the predicates in representations are interrelated and may differ in their centrality. On our account of conceptual structure, linkages between deeper features and more superficial features greatly constrain the contexts in which the assumption of independent features will work.

Whereas the Rips chapter and the Smith and Osherson chapter, intentionally or otherwise, are both concerned with the role that similarity plays in some fairly important *processes*, Lawrence Barsalou focuses more on what similarity might tell us about the underlying conceptual representations in terms of which such judgments are presumably made (what we referred to at the beginning of this chapter as the "stuff to which judgments of similarity are applied"). Whether or not you like Barsalou's message about the instability of concepts depends on who you are. We like it because it is consistent with our view that the more central aspects of our concepts are often quite inchoate and not readily accessible. Ryszard Michalski's two-tiered theory of concept representation is somewhat similar both to Barsalou's distinction between context-dependent and context-independent properties and to the general framework we have been developing. Michalski places greater emphasis on cognitive economy (efficient representation) than we do, and he focused on goal-driven rather than theory-driven representation. We think a continuous gradation of depth is more natural than a dichotomy, but we agree with Michalski that categorization may be more like an inference than a similarity computation.

Commentary

Rips's main point seems to be that in many cases properties that we would consider closely linked to the psychological essence (Rips calls them "extrinsic" features) constitute the criteria for category membership, not superficial features. If, as he suggests, the resemblance approach to categorization is limited to the use of superficial properties, then Rips's observations are quite damaging. In principle, however, we see no reason why the resemblance approach should be constrained in this way. It would seem that category members could be judged to be similar *with respect to deeper features*. In Rips's experiments subjects were encouraged to focus on surface or perceptual features for similarity judgments and on other properties for typicality or class membership judgments. For example, the first experiment was set up in such a way as to lead subjects to consider only a single physical dimension (e.g., diameter) of an unknown object relative to that dimension of two potential categories (e.g., quarters and pizzas). This does not rule out the possibility that category membership judgments were also based on similarity, but with more than a single dimension involved (and not necessarily all readily accessible ones at that). Consider the following variant on Experiment 1: Subjects are told that they should bring to mind some object, x, which is 3 inches in diameter, and they are asked, "Is it more likely to be a quarter or a pizza?" They then respond, just as Rips had them respond, presumably by saying that it is more likely to be a pizza. They are then instructed to keep in mind what they imagined x to be, and now they are asked whether that *same* object is more similar to a quarter or a pizza. Our point is that it is necessary to know that subjects made their categorization judgments and their similarity judgments using the same instantiation of the unknown object x. Once we know what x is, the situation with respect to similarity may be radically different. Of course, one would need to be able to explain why people's images are more pizza like than quarter like, so this argument cuts both ways. We agree with Rips that, unless one can specify how similarity is determined, the resemblance approach to similarity is vacuous.

On the other hand, we disagree with Rips's assertion that some of us are committed to the view that (*a*) similarity *determines* the probability that a person will assign some instance to a category and (*b*) that similarity is *responsible* for prototypicality judgments; it is not clear that they are. The assertion that "The probability of classifying exemplar i into category j is an increasing function of the similarity of exemplar i to stored category j exemplars and a decreasing function of the similarity of exemplar *i* to stored exemplars associated with alternative categories" (Medin & Schaffer, 1978) claims no more than the empirical fact that there is indeed a positive correlation, namely, that the more similar *i* seems to stored category *j* exemplars, the more *likely* is *i* to be categorized as a *j*. It doesn't guarantee it; it just makes it more likely. In other words, to say that similarity can play a role in *identification* is not the same as saying that categories (or their corresponding concepts) are *constituted* on the basis of similarity among exemplars. It may be that one heuristic people use for deciding that an *i* is a *j* is similarity to exemplars. Heuristics are not causes, and the fact that a heuristic often works tells us something about the interface between our (selective) perceptual systems and the world. Similarly, Murphy and Medin (1985) suggest that perhaps concepts are like theories in the sense that, if one has a "theory" of what it takes for an *i* to be a *j*, then a decision about a particular case will be based on how well that case seems to "fit" *j*, which is the criterion associated with the theory of *j*-ness. The process of deciding how well it fits may or may not implicate similarity, but it does not *necessarily* do so.

Nevertheless, when all is said and done, we see an important moral in Rips's chapter, although we would give it much more emphasis than he does. We view his arguments and data as supporting the following claim: The criteria for category membership (whatever they are) are not necessarily always apparent on the surface as physical properties of instances of the category. On this reading of Rips, the criteria involve deeper properties that, to varying degrees, may impose constraints on more accessible properties. Sometimes these constraints are strong, although, of course, the issue does not really have to do with categories themselves but has to do with people's representations of them: concepts. So most lay people do not know what the real criteria are for something to be an airplane (although they presumably *do* believe that aeronautical engineers do!). However, even in the absence of such knowledge they assume that these underlying criteria impose strict constraints on some of the accessible features, such as the possession and size of wings, flaps, fins, and other aviation paraphernalia. In cases where the psychological essence imposes strong constraints, similarity to exemplars is likely to be a good heuristic for deciding category membership. Sometimes the constraints are relatively weak, as with many goal-derived categories. Where the constraints are less strong, similarity is likely to be less successful, although in many cases physical properties may be accidentally or indirectly constrained. So, for example, the physical shape of eggs may be indirectly constrained by whatever it is that makes eggs eggs, because the shape is so well suited to protecting the embryo before, during, and after its passage into the outside world. People presumably believe that eggs are oval because the nature of eggs imposes certain constraints on their physical properties rather than because that is the best shape for fitting them into egg cups!

Our first reaction to the Smith and Osherson paper is that the idea of applying notions of similarity to decision-making and judgment tasks is a good one, and although Kahneman and Tversky did not exactly ignore similarity, they did not undertake the systematic analysis that Smith and Osherson attempt. We think that their simplifying assumption that the values of different features are independent, although a convenient starting point, might pose something of a problem for the general case. Their approach seems to treat features as not being linked in any particular way. We think that it is rare for the value of a feature on one dimension not to affect the likely values on other dimensions. For example, finding out that Linda is a feminist bank teller might not simply change the diagnosticity and votes on the property *politics*, it might also change one's ideas about the style of clothing that Linda might wear, her preferences for different forms of recreation, or even the kinds of food she might enjoy. To be fair to Smith and Osherson, the notion of independent dimensions, as we have said, is a simplifying assumption. Our somewhat pessimistic attitude is driven by the exception that, in practice, this assumption just may not hold often enough for it to constitute an adequate basis upon which to build a general analysis. We know that correlated features violate the independence assumption. For example, people rate small spoons as more typical spoons than large spoons, but they rate small *wooden* spoons as *less* typical than large wooden spoons. If correlated features tend to be the rule rather than the exception (as our view implies), then, in general, it seems unlikely that the effects of a property having a particular value can be confined to a single dimension (Rumelhart & Ortony, 1977), and if they cannot, then the independent-dimensions approach is not going to suffice.

The observations on the cab problem and people's failure to use base rate information are interesting and clever. On the other hand, whether this approach will work in general is not clear. It seems to imply that judgments will be based on similarity computations even when the form of similarity is clearly irrelevant. To give an extreme example, suppose the witness testified with 99 percent reliability that the cab had four wheels. Number of wheels has some diagnosticity for differentiating cabs from trucks and motorcycles, and so we wonder what would prevent the similarity computation from running off and leading to a continued failure to use base rate information? (The data seem to go the other way.) Similarity may not always be used in a simple, straightforward way because how one interprets similarity data may depend on one's theory of how that similarity was generated. To use an example based on Einhorn and Hogarth (1985), imagine a set of five eyewitnesses testifying as to the apparent speed of the taxicab. Although credibility might generally be expected to increase with interwitness agreement, suppose in some particular case each of five witnesses testifies that the cab was traveling at exactly 58.2 miles per hour. Does this remarkable similarity increase credibility? It seems to undermine it.

Overall, this incursion of similarity into judgment and decision making is intriguing. Our only reservation is that we think Smith and Osherson are going to need a richer form of knowledge representation and a correspondingly more powerful theory of similarity in order to get it to do what they want it to do.

Linda Smith's analysis reveals that there are nuances associated with modes of similarity processing that undermine the very oversimplified account of development in which young children categorize in terms of superficial similarity whereas older children's categorizations are constrained by deeper aspects of similarity. That is, there appear to be major shifts in how surface similarity is processed at different stages of development. Smith's work appears to conflict with research that shows that young children develop theories that constrain their conceptual behavior (e.g., Carey, 1982; Keil, 1981). Smith's work, however, is with children younger than those used by Carey and by Keil, so that it is not easy to determine the extent of the conflict. There may prove to be a natural integration involving a transition from similarity-based to theory-based categories. Alternatively, it may be that theories are constraining the concepts of even the youngest children and that the similarity-based account of conceptual development is incomplete for all ages.

We agree with Barsalou that there is a great deal of concept instability. However, we think care has to be taken not to equate instability in outputs or behaviors with underlying or internal instability. Might it be that our underlying concepts are in fact stable (whatever that might mean) and that the apparent instability is an artifact of the processes that operate on these stable representations? Given our framework, we would argue that the deeper one goes the more stability one ought to find. So, if we were to ask 200 people on 10 different occasions in 10 different contexts whether dogs are more likely to give birth to puppies than to kittens, we would find remarkable stability. (Of course, Barsalou does not dispute this.) Michalski would probably argue that we should expect stability only for properties that are part of what he refers to as the base concept representation. One might claim that Barsalou is exploring only the fringes of conceptual use while ignoring the huge quantities of knowledge that are so stable we are scarcely aware of them. We have in mind knowledge of the kind that dogs, but not rocks, can take predicates like *sleep* or *eat* (see Keil, 1981). Still, Barsalou convinces us that there *is some* instability, and we think a view of the kind we have proposed is also committed to this conclusion. Clearly, intraperson instability can arise as a result of context-based priming effects. For instance, in making some judgment about some concept, the context in which the judgment is elicited might prime some of the concept's surface features so that the judgment would be more likely to reflect the causal linkages between the psychological essence and such primed features than between the essence and other surface features.

Barsalou's assault on concept stability leads one to ask *where* stability is and what it means to try to measure it. People do not ordinarily walk around making judgments of typicality or providing dictionary definitions, so it is at least relevant to ask how people normally learn about, update, and use concepts, and what stability or instability is associated with *these* functions. We think that Barsalou is correct in his important observation that concept representations often are constructed on the fly. Only in this way can knowledge be tuned to particular contexts. From the traditional contextless view of concepts, the results on context dependence are depressing for what they tell us about concept stability. However, if one thinks of concept representations as frequently being computed, then contexts serve to fix meaning and provide stability *in that context*. So, if one is talking about a "bird on a Thanksgiving platter" the referent is heavily constrained (Roth & Shoben, 1983). Indeed, much of the stability that one might hope for may depend very much on particular contexts. Consider a concept such as *redneck*.[2] If one is asked to list attributes of this concept the potential list is long, and there might well be considerable instability in just what is listed. As more context is added, the situation becomes more like supplying background information needed to generate specific predictions from a theory. Therefore, if people are asked to judge how likely a redneck is to encourage his 17-year-old daughter to date a 39-year-old man of a different race, one can anticipate considerable agreement both across judges and for the same judge at different times. So the notion of deeper properties is perfectly consistent with a considerable amount of instability and a considerable amount of context dependence. In the case of the *redneck* example, the key to successful communication lies not so much in the ability to supply the same definition as it is does in the ability to generate the same predictions in specified contexts. Finally, another aspect of context dependence is that different concepts may interact so as to change the importance of some of their constituent properties (e.g., Barsalou, 1982; Ortony, Vondruska, Foss, & Jones, 1985). This all means that Barsalou's results on concept instability can be taken as evidence for flexibility that paradoxically allows for both *accuracy* and (a fair amount of) stability in particular contexts.

Conclusion

We have proposed that there is often a nonarbitrary relationship between the represented deep properties and the represented surface properties of concepts. This relationship can vary from a strong causal one to a weaker constraining one, but in either case the use of similarity with respect only to relatively accessible surface properties, because they *are* constrained, can serve as a powerful, although fallible, heuristic for various cognitive tasks. It is in this sense that we think Rips perhaps attributes too little power to surface similarity. Knowledge representations have to be construed as having sufficient richness to allow similarity to perform useful functions. Our reservations about the Smith and Osherson chapter hinge on just this point. The model they propose seems to work quite well if one accepts their simplifying assumptions that schemata are unstructured property lists. But if, as they must be, schemata are complex, multivariate representations involving many represented or inferable interdependencies, it is not at all clear that their relatively straightforward analysis can survive.

We started this chapter by suggesting that Wittgenstein's admonition to look rather than to think may have led psychologists to focus too much on superficial similarity with respect to concept representations incorporating only superficial, accessible properties. There are really two issues, the second of which presupposes the first. The first is that the question is a question about *representations*, not about the things that are represented. As such, the issue is not whether birds possess some feature or features by virtue of which they are birds but whether people's *representations* of birds include some such component, explicit or otherwise. Once this point is established, the second point is that we have to examine how the linkages between superficial and deeper properties serve to provide structure to concept representations. We have suggested that if one does this one may discover that there is a meaningful and useful role that can be played by psychological essentialism.

NOTES

Douglas Medin was supported in part by grants from the National Science Foundation, NSF84–19756, and the National Library of Medicine, LM04375. We wish to thank Robert McCauley, Brian Ross, and Ed Shoben for their helpful comments.

1 Locke argued that a distinction between real and nominal essence is needed. The nominal essence for Locke was the abstract idea that constitutes the basis of classification. The real essence he explained as that which some suppose is "the real internal, but generally (in substances) unknown constitution of things, whereon their discoverable qualities depend." Thus both Aristotle and Locke, while accepting some form of essentialism, were forced to deny that the essence of a thing lay in that thing independently of the way it is classified. For Aristotle, the essence of something was bound to the way it was described or conceptualized, and for Locke it had to be bound to a corresponding abstract idea, at least in part because he believed that concepts corresponding to nonexistent entities like unicorns and mermaids had perfectly good essences.
2 We use the term *redneck* to make a purely scientific observation and share Barsalou's opinion regarding the inaccuracy and the prejudice fostered by the use of stereotypes.

REFERENCES

Barsalou, L. W. (1982). Context-independent and context-dependent information in concepts. *Memory & Cognition, 10,* 82–93.
✓ Carey, S. (1982). Semantic development: The state of the art. In E. Wanner and L. Gleitman (Eds.), *Language acquisition: The state of the art* (pp. 347–389). Cambridge: Cambridge University Press.
Einhorn, H. J., & Hogarth, R. M. (1985). Ambiguity and uncertainty in probabilistic inference. *Psychological Review, 92,* 433–461.
Goodman, N. (1972). Seven strictures on similarity. In N. Goodman (Ed.), *Problems and projects.* New York: Bobbs-Merrill.
✓ Kahneman, D., Slovic, P., & Tversky, A. (1982). *Judgment under uncertainty: Heuristics and biases.* Cambridge: Cambridge University Press.
Keil, F. C. (1981). Constraints on knowledge and cognitive development. *Psychological Review, 88,* 197–227.
Medin, D. L., & Schaffer, M. M. (1978). Context theory of classification learning. *Psychological Review, 85,* 207–238.
Medin, D. L., Wattenmaker, W. D., & Hampson, S. (1987). Family resemblance, concept cohesiveness, and category construction. *Cognitive Psychology, 19,* 242–279.

Murphy, G. L., & Medin, D. L. (1985). The role of theories in conceptual coherence. *Psychological Review, 92,* 289–316.

Nisbett, R. E., & Ross, L. (1980). *Human inference: Strategies and shortcomings of social judgment.* Englewood Cliff, NJ: Prentice-Hall.

Ortony, A., Vondruska, R. J., Foss, M. A., & Jones, L. E. (1985). Salience, similes, and the asymmetry of similarity. *Journal of Memory and Language, 24,* 569–594.

Rosch, E. (1973). On the internal structure of perceptual and semantic categories. In T. M. Moore (Ed.), *Cognitive development and the acquisition of language.* New York: Academic Press.

Roth, E. M., & Shoben, E. J. (1983). The effect of context on the structure of categories. *Cognitive Psychology, 15,* 346–378.

Rumelhart, D. E., & Ortony, A. (1977). The representation of knowledge in memory. In R. C. Anderson, R. J. Spiro, & W. E. Montague (Eds.), *Schooling and the acquisition of knowledge* (pp. 99–135). Hillsdale, NJ: Erlbaum.

Smith, E. E., & Medin, D. L. (1981). *Categories and concepts.* Cambridge, MA: Harvard University Press.

Smith, E. E., Medin, D. L, & Rips, L. J. (1984). A psychological approach to concepts: Comments on Rey's "Concepts and stereotypes." *Cognition, 17,* 265–274.

Tversky, A. (1977). Features of similarity. *Psychological Review, 84,* 327–352.

Watanabe, S. (1969). *Knowing and guessing: A formal and quantitative study.* New York: Wiley.

Analogical reasoning

The contributions included in Part II focus on the psychological processes involved in analogical reasoning and discuss how and whether these processes can be captured in computer models. In her chapter, Dedre Gentner outlines a structure-mapping theory of analogy and discusses how this theory can be extended to model other subprocesses in analogical reasoning. John Anderson and Ross Thompson describe a mechanism for doing analogy in problem solving within a production system architecture, and Keith Holyoak and Paul Thagard describe a model of analogical problem solving embedded within a larger computational program of problem solving called PI (for "processes of induction"). In his contribution, David Rumelhart discusses how analogical reasoning might be handled within a parallel distributed processing system. Finally, Philip Johnson-Laird argues that current psychological theories of analogy have underestimated the complexity of analogical phenomena and raises the possibility that profoundly original analogies may depend on classes of algorithms that are not computationally tractable.

There are two discussions of the contributions in Part II. Stephen Palmer offers a critique of the papers by Gentner, Holyoak and Thagard, and Rumelhart, in the context of the Palmer and Kimchi metatheoretical framework for levels of description within information-processing psychology. Gerald DeJong's commentary takes an artificial intelligence perspective, and therefore also includes some reactions to the chapter by Ryszard Michalski in Part I.

7
The mechanisms of analogical learning

DEDRE GENTNER

It is widely accepted that similarity is a key determinant of transfer. In this chapter I suggest that both of these venerable terms – *similarity* and *transfer* – refer to complex notions that require further differentiation. I approach the problem by a double decomposition: decomposing similarity into finer subclasses and decomposing learning by similarity and analogy into a set of component subprocesses.

One thing reminds us of another. Mental experience is full of moments in which a current situation reminds us of some prior experience stored in memory. Sometimes such remindings lead to a change in the way we think about one or both of the situations. Here is an example reported by Dan Slobin (personal communication, April 1986). His daughter, Heida, had traveled quite a bit by the age of 3. One day in Turkey she heard a dog barking and remarked, "Dogs in Turkey make the same sound as dogs in America. . . . Maybe all dogs do. Do dogs in India sound the same?" Where did this question come from? According to Slobin's notebook, "She apparently noticed that while the people sounded different from country to country, the dogs did not." The fact that only humans speak different languages may seem obvious to an adult, but for Heida to arrive at it by observation must have required a series of insights. She had to compare people from different countries and note that they typically sound different. She also had to compare dogs from different countries and note that they sound the same. Finally, in order to attach significance to her observation about dogs, she must have drawn a parallel – perhaps implicitly – between dogs making sounds and humans making sounds so that she could contrast: "As you go from country to country, people sound different, but dogs sound the same." Thus her own experiential comparisons led her to the beginnings of a major insight about the difference between human language and animal sounds.

This example illustrates some of the power of spontaneous remindings. Spontaneous remindings can lead us to make new infer-

199

ences, to discover a common abstraction, or, as here, to notice an important difference between two partly similar situations (e.g., Ross, 1984, this volume). The ultimate aim of this chapter is to trace learning by analogy and similarity from the initial reminding to the final storage of some new information. Spontaneous analogical learning[1] can be decomposed into subprocesses of (a) accessing the base* system; (b) performing the mapping between base and target; (c) evaluating the match; (d) storing inferences in the target; and sometimes, (e) extracting the commonalities (Clement, 1981, 1983; Gentner, 1987; Gentner & Landers, 1985; Hall, in press; Kedar-Cabelli, 1988).

This breakdown suggests that we examine the subprocesses independently. Once this is done, it will become clear that different subprocesses involved in analogical learning are affected by very different psychological factors. Although the chronological first step in an experiential learning sequence is *accessing the potential analog*, I shall postpone the discussion of access until later in this chapter. Instead, I begin with steps 2 and 3: *analogical mapping* and *judging analogical soundness*. This is the logical place to start, because it is these processes that uniquely define analogy and allow us to see distinctions among different kinds of similarity. It turns out that the theoretical distinctions necessary for talking about analogical mapping are also useful for talking about other analogical subprocesses.

The plan of the chapter is, first, to describe the core structure-mapping theory of analogical mapping, using a computer simulation to make the points clear; second, to offer psychological evidence for the core theory of analogical mapping; and, finally, to discuss research that extends the framework to the larger situation of analogical learning.

Analogical mapping

The theoretical framework for this chapter is the structure-mapping theory of analogy (Gentner, 1980, 1982, 1983, 1987; Gentner & Gentner, 1983).[2] As Stephen Palmer (this volume) states, structure-mapping is concerned, first, with what Marr (1982) called the "computational level" and what Palmer and Kimchi (1985) call the "informational constraints" that define analogy. That is, structure-mapping aims to capture the essential elements that constitute analogy and the operations that are computationally necessary in processing

---

* *Editors' note*: The terms "base" and "source" are used interchangeably both in the field in general and in this volume in particular.

analogy. The question of how analogies are processed in real time –
that is, the question of which algorithms are used, in Marr's terminology, or which behavioral constraints apply, in Palmer and Kimchi's
terminology – will be deferred until later in the chapter.

The central idea in structure-mapping is that an analogy is a mapping of knowledge from one domain (the base) into another (the
target), which conveys that a system of relations that holds among the
base objects also holds among the target objects. Thus an analogy is
a way of focusing on relational commonalties independently of the
objects in which those relations are embedded. In interpreting an
analogy, people seek to put the objects of the base in one-to-one
correspondence with the objects in the target so as to obtain the maximum structural match. Objects are placed in correspondence by virtue of their like roles in the common relational structure; there does
not need to be any resemblance between the target objects and their
corresponding base objects. Central to the mapping process is the
principle of systematicity: People prefer to map connected *systems of
relations* governed by higher-order relations with inferential import,
rather than isolated predicates.

Analogical mapping is in general a combination of matching existing predicate structures and importing new predicates (carry-over).
To see this, first consider the two extremes. In *pure matching*, the
learner already knows something about both domains. The analogy
conveys that a relational system in the target domain matches one in
the base domain. In this case the analogy serves to focus attention on
the matching system rather than to convey new knowledge. In *pure
carry-over*, the learner initially knows something about the base domain
but little or nothing about the target domain. The analogy specifies
the object correspondences, and the learner simply carries across a
known system of predicates from the base to the target. This is the
case of maximal new knowledge. Whether a given analogy is chiefly
matching or mapping depends, of course, on the state of knowledge
in the learner. For example, consider this analogy by Oliver Wendell
Holmes, Jr.: "Many ideas grow better when transplanted into another
mind than in the one where they sprang up." For some readers, this
might be an instance of pure mapping: By importing the knowledge
structure from the domain of plant growing to the domain of idea
development they receive a completely new thought about the latter
domain. But for readers who have entertained similar thoughts the
process is more one of matching. The effect of the analogy is then
not so much to import new knowledge as to focus attention on certain
portions of the existing knowledge. Most explanatory analogies are a

combination of matching and carry-over. Typically, there is a partial match between base and target systems, which then sanctions the importing of further predicates from the base to the target.

A clarification may be useful here. A possible misreading is that the systematicity principle implies that the same set of predicates should always be mapped from a given base domain, regardless of the target (Holyoak, 1985). But, by this construal, the interpretation of an analogy would depend only on the base domain, which is patently false, except in the case when nothing is known about the target (the pure carry-over case). In the normal case, when there is information about both base and target, a given base–target pair produces a set of matching predicates. Changing either member of the pair produces a different set of matching predicates. Thus, systematicity operates as a selection constraint: Among the many possible predicate matches between a given base and target, it favors those that form coherent systems of mutually interconnecting relations (see Clement & Gentner, 1988; Gentner & Clement, in press).

To illustrate the structure-mapping rules, we turn to a specific example: the analogy between heat flow and water flow. (See Gentner & Jeziorski, in press, for a discussion of Carnot's use of this analogy in the history of heat and temperature.) Figure 7.1 shows a water-flow situation and an analogous heat-flow situation.

I will go through this analogy twice. The first time I give the analogy as it might occur in an educational setting in which the learner knows a fair amount about water and almost nothing about heat flow. Here the learner is given the object correspondences between water and heat and simply imports predicates from the water domain to the heat domain. This is a case of pure carry-over. The second time, to illustrate the computer simulation, I give the analogy as it might occur with the learner having a good representation of the water domain and a partial representation of the heat domain. Here the analogy process is a combination of matching existing structures and importing new predicates (carry-over).

The heat/water analogy, Pass 1: pure carry-over. Figure 7.2 shows the representation a learner might have of the water situation. We assume that the learner has a very weak initial representation of the heat situation and perhaps even lacks a firm understanding of the difference between heat and temperature. This network represents a portion of what a person might know about the water situation illustrated in Figure 7.1.[3]

The learner is told that heat flow can be understood just like water

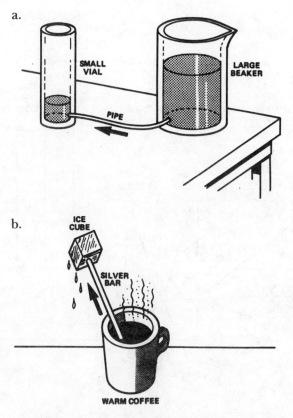

Figure 7.1. Examples of physical situations involving (*a*) water flow and (*b*) heat flow (adapted from Buckley, 1979, pp. 15–25).

flow, with temperature in the heat situation playing the role of pressure in the water situation. The learner is also given the object correspondences

> water → heat; pipe → metal bar;
> beaker → coffee; vial → ice

as well as the function correspondence

> PRESSURE → TEMPERATURE

Now the learner is in a position to interpret the analogy. Even with the correspondences given, there is still some active processing required. In order to comprehend the analogy, the learner must

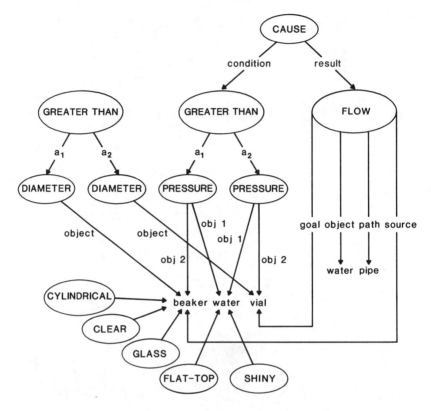

Figure 7.2. A representation of the water situation. Predicates are written in upper case and circled; objects are written in lower case and uncircled.

- ignore object attributes; e.g., CYLINDRICAL (beaker) or LIQUID (coffee)
- find a set of systematic base relations that can apply in the target, using the correspondences given. Here, the pressure-difference structure in the water domain

  CAUSE {GREATER [PRESSURE (beaker), PRESSURE (vial)], [FLOW (water, pipe, beaker, vial)]}

  is mapped into the temperature-difference structure in the heat domain

  CAUSE {GREATER [TEMP (coffee), TEMP (ice)], [FLOW (heat, bar, coffee, ice)]}

- and discard isolated relations, such as

  GREATER [DIAM (beaker), DIAM (vial)]

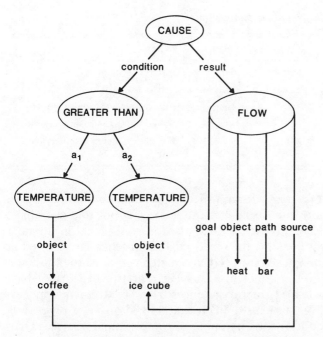

Figure 7.3. A representation of the heat situation that results from the heat/ water analogy.

Figure 7.3 shows the resulting causal representation of heat flow induced by the analogical mapping.

There are several points to note in this example. First, the object correspondences – heat/water, beaker/coffee, vial/ice, and pipe/bar – and the function correspondence PRESSURE/TEMPERATURE[4] are determined not by any intrinsic similarity between the objects but by their role in the systematic relational structure. Systematicity also determines which relations get carried across. The reason that

GREATER [PRESSURE (beaker), PRESSURE (vial)]

is preserved is that it is part of a mappable system of higher-order constraining relations: in this case, the subsystem governed by the higher-order relation CAUSE. In contrast, the relation

GREATER [DIAM (beaker), DIAM (vial)]

does not belong to any such mappable system and so is less favored in the match.

Second, the order of processing is probably variable. Even when the learner is given the object correspondences first, there is no ob-

Table 7.1. *Kinds of domain comparisons*

	Attributes	Relations	Example
Literal similarity	Many	Many	Milk is like water
Analogy	Few	Many	Heat is like water
Abstraction	Few	Many	Heat flow is a through-variable
Anomaly	Few	Few	Coffee is like the solar system
Mere appearance	Many	Few	The glass tabletop gleamed like water

vious constraint on the order in which predicates should be mapped. This is even more the case when the learner is not told the object correspondences in advance. In this case, as exemplified in the next pass through this analogy, the object correspondences are arrived at by first determining the best predicate match – that is, the most systematic and consistent match. I suspect that the order in which matches are made and correspondences tried is extremely opportunistic and variable. It seems unlikely that a fixed order of processing stages will be found for the mapping of complex analogies (see Grudin, 1980; Sternberg, 1977).

Third, applying the structural rules is only part of the story. Given a potential interpretation, the candidate inferences must be checked for validity in the target. If the predicates of the base system are not valid in the target, then another system must be selected. In goal-driven contexts, the candidate inferences must also be checked for relevance to the goal.

Kinds of similarity

Distinguishing different kinds of similarity is essential to understanding learning by analogy and similarity. Therefore, before going through the heat/water analogy a second time, I lay out a decomposition of similarity that follows from what has been said. Besides analogy, other kinds of similarity can be characterized by whether the two situations are alike in their relational structure, in their object descriptions, or in both. In *analogy*, only relational predicates are mapped. In *literal similarity*, both relational predicates and object attributes are mapped. In *mere-appearance matches*, it is chiefly object attributes that are mapped. Figure 7.4 shows a similarity space that summarizes these distinctions. Table 7.1 shows examples of these

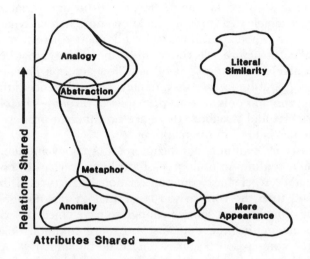

Figure 7.4. Similarity space: classes of similarity based on the kinds of predicates shared.

different kinds of similarity. The central assumption is that it is not merely the relative *numbers* of shared versus nonshared predicates that matter – although that is certainly important, as Tversky (1977) has shown – but also the *kinds* of predicates that match.

Analogy is exemplified by the water/heat example discussed above, which conveys that a common relational system holds for the two domains: Pressure difference causes water flow, and temperature difference causes heat flow. *Literal similarity* is exemplified by the comparison "Milk is like water," which conveys that much of the water description can be applied to milk. In literal similarity, both object attributes, such as FLAT TOP (water) and CYLINDRICAL (beaker), and relational predicates, such as the systematic causal structure discussed above, are mapped over. A *mere-appearance match* is one with overlap in lower-order predicates – chiefly object attributes[5] – but not in higher-order relational structure as in "The glass tabletop gleamed like water." Mere-appearance matches are in a sense the opposite of analogies. Such matches are sharply limited in their utility. Here, for example, little beyond physical appearance is shared between the tabletop and water. These matches, however, cannot be ignored in a theory of learning, because they often occur among novice learners. One further type of match worth discussing is *relational abstraction*.

An example is the abstract statement, "Heat is a through-variable," which might be available to a student who knew some system dynamics. This abstraction, when applied to the heat domain, conveys much the same relational structure as is conveyed by the analogy: that heat (a through-variable) can be thought of as a flow across a potential difference in temperature (an across-variable). The difference is that the base domain contains only abstract principles of through-variables and across-variables and variables; there are no concrete properties of objects to be left behind in the mapping.

These contrasts are continua, not dichotomies. Analogy and literal similarity lie on a continuum of degree-of-attribute-overlap. In both cases, the base and target share common relational structure. If that is *all* they share, then the comparison is an analogy (assuming, of course, that the domains are concrete enough to have object descriptions). To the extent that the domains also share common object descriptions, the comparison becomes one of literal similarity. Another continuum exists between analogies and relational abstractions. In both cases, a relational structure is mapped from base to target. If the base representation includes concrete objects whose individual attributes must be left behind in the mapping, the comparison is an analogy. As the object nodes of the base domain become more abstract and variable-like, the comparison becomes a relational abstraction.

We turn now to the second pass through the analogy. There are two innovations. First, in this pass I describe the way our computer simulation processes the heat/water example. Here we move from informational constraints to behavioral constraints. (See Palmer, this volume.) Second, in this pass I assume that there is some prior knowledge of *both* base and target; thus this pass illustrates a combination of matching and carry-over. Before giving the algorithm, I describe the representational conventions.

Representation conventions. The order of an item in a representation is as follows: Objects and constants are order 0. The order of a predicate is 1 plus the maximum of the order of its arguments. Thus, if x and y are objects, then GREATER THAN (x, y) is first-order. and CAUSE [GREATER THAN (x, y), BREAK(x)] is second-order. Typical higher-order relations include CAUSE and IMPLIES. On this definition, the order of an item indicates the depth of structure below it. Arguments with many layers of justifications will give rise to representation structures of high order.

A typed predicate calculus is used in the representation. There are four representational constructs that must be distinguished: *entities*, which represent individuals and constants, and three types of predicates. Predicates are further subdivided into truth-functional predicates (*relations* and *attributes*) and *functions*. Entities (e.g., *Eddie, side pocket*) are logical individuals: the objects and constants of a domain. Typical entities include pieces of stuff, individual objects or beings, and logical constants. *Attributes* and *relations* are predicates that range over truth values; for example, the relation HIT(cue ball, ball) can be evaluated as true or false. The difference is that attributes take one argument and relations take two or more arguments. Informally, attributes describe properties of entities, such as RED or SQUARE. Relations describe events, comparisons, or states applying to two or more entities or predicates. First-order relations take objects as arguments: for example, HIT(ball, table) and INSIDE (ball, pocket). Higher-order relations such as IMPLIES and CAUSE take other predicates as their arguments: for example, CAUSE [HIT (cue stick, ball), ENTER (ball, pocket)]. *Functions* map one or more entities into another entity or constant. For example, SPEED(ball) does not have a truth value; instead, it maps the physical object *ball* into the quantity that describes its speed. Functions are a useful representational device because they allow either (a) evaluating the function to produce an object descriptor, as in HEIGHT (Sam) = 6 feet, or (b) using the unevaluated function as the argument of other predicates, as in GREATER THAN [HEIGHT(Sam), HEIGHT(George)].

These four constructs are all treated differently in the analogical mapping algorithm. Relations, including higher-order relations, must match identically. Entities and functions are placed in correspondence with other entities and functions on the basis of the surrounding relational structures. Attributes are ignored. Thus there are three levels of preservation: identical matching, placing in correspondence, and ignoring.[6] For example, in the analogy "The wrestler bounced off the ropes like a billiard ball off the wall," the *relations*, such as CAUSE [HIT(wrestler1, wrestler2), COLLIDE(wrestler2, ropes)] must match identically. For *objects* and for *functions*,[7] we attempt to find corresponding objects and functions, which need not be identical: for example, cue ball/wrestler and SPEED(cue ball)/FORCE(wrestler1). Attributes are ignored; we do not seek identical or even corresponding attributes in the billiard ball for each of the wrestler's attributes. To sum up, relations must match, objects and functions must correspond, and attributes are ignored.

It is important to note that these representations, including the distinctions between different kinds of predicates, are intended to reflect the way situations are construed by people. Logically, an *n-*

place relation $R(a,b,c,)$ can always be represented as a one-place predicate $Q(x)$, where $Q(x)$ is true just in case $R(a,b,c,)$ is true. Further, a combination of a function and a constant is logically equivalent to an attribute; for example, applying the function EQUALS [COLOR(ball), red] is logically equivalent to stating the attribute RED(ball). Our aim is to choose the representation that best matches the available evidence as to the person's current psychological representation. As Palmer (this volume) points out, these representational decisions are crucial to the operation of the algorithm. Differences in the way things are construed can cause two situations to fail to match even if they are informationally equivalent. Thus the model would fail to realize that HOTTER THAN(a,b) is equivalent to COLDER THAN(b,a). This assumption may not be as implausible as it initially seems. Empirically, we know that logical equivalence does not guarantee psychological equivalence. Perhaps one reason that people sometimes miss potential analogies (as discussed below) is that their current representations of base and target limit the kinds of analogical matches they can make.

Requiring perfect relational identity in the matching rules allows us to capture the fact that potential analogies are often missed, for the more exactly the representations must match, the less likely analogies are to be seen. More important, the relational identity requirement keeps us from concealing homunculus-like insight in the matcher. As soon as we move away from perfect matching we are faced with a host of difficult decisions: How much insight do we give the matcher? How much ability to consider current contextual factors? How much tolerance for ambiguity? In short, we lose the considerable advantages of having a simple, low-cost matcher. But how can we capture the intuition that people sometimes can use analogy creatively to surmount initially different representations? Burstein (1983) has explored one interesting method: He allows *similar* predicates to match and then generalizes the match. For example, as part of a larger analogy, *inside* in the spatial sense is matched with *inside* in the abstract sense of a variable containing a value. Then a more general notion of containment is abstracted from the match. This is an attractive notion that deserves further study. However, it does run the risk of adding considerable computational ambiguity.

One way to add flexibility without sacrificing the simple matcher is to add some tools for re-representation that are external to the matcher itself. Then, if there were good reason to suspect a possible analogy, a relation currently represented as COLDER THAN(b,a) could be re-represented as HOTTER THAN(a,b). An alternative re-representation would decompose it into GREATER THAN [TEMP(a),TEMP(b)].

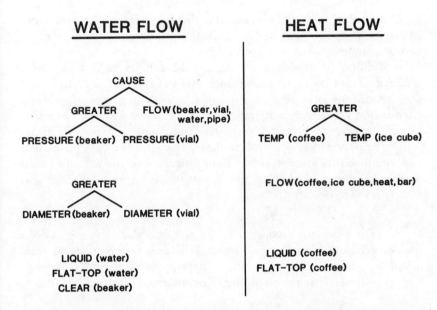

Figure 7.5. Representations of water and heat given to the structure-mapping engine.

In this way a partial analogy could lead to the discovery that two relations hitherto seen as different in fact refer to the same underlying dimension. This would allow us to model the use of analogy in reconstruing one situation in terms of another. An interesting corollary of this approach is that it suggests a way in which analogy could act as a force toward building uniform domain representations, both within and across domains.

The structure-mapping engine. The structure-mapping engine (SME) is a simulation of the structure-mapping process written by Brian Falkenhainer and Ken Forbus (Falkenhainer, Forbus, & Gentner, 1986, in press; Gentner, Falkenhainer, & Skorstad, 1987). Here it is given the representations of the base and target shown in Figure 7.5. As in the previous pass (Figure 7.2), we assume the learner has a fair amount of knowledge about water. In contrast to the previous pass, we now assume some initial knowledge about heat: The learner knows that the coffee is hotter than the ice and that heat will flow from the coffee to the ice. Note, however, that the representations contain many extraneous predicates, such as LIQUID(water) and

LIQUID(coffee). These are included to simulate a learner's uncertainty about what matters and to give SME the opportunity to make erroneous matches, just as a person might.

In addition to modeling analogy, SME can be used with literal similarity rules or mere-appearance rules. Both analogy rules and literal similarity rules seek matches in relational structure; the difference is that literal similarity rules also seek object-attribute matches. Mere-appearance rules seek only object-attribute matches. I will describe the process using literal similarity rules, rather than pure analogy, because this offers a better demonstration of the full operation of the simulation, including the way conflicts between surface and structural matches are treated.

The heat/water analogy, Pass 2: matching plus carry-over. Given the comparison "Heat is like water," SME uses systematicity of relational structure and consistency of hypothesized object correspondences to determine the mapping. The order of events is as follows:

1. Local matches. SME starts by looking for identical relations in base and target and using them to postulate potential matches. For each entity and predicate in the base, it finds the set of entities or predicates in the target that could plausibly match that item. These potential correspondences (*match hypotheses*) are determined by a set of simple rules: for example,

1. If two relations have the same name, create a match hypothesis.
2. For every match hypothesis between relations, check their corresponding arguments; if both are entities, or if both are functions, then create a match hypothesis between them.

For example, in Figure 7.5, Rule 1 creates match hypotheses between the GREATER-THAN relations occurring in base and target. Then Rule 2 creates match hypotheses between their arguments, since both are functions. Note that at this stage the system is entertaining two different, and inconsistent, match hypotheses involving GREATER THAN: one in which PRESSURE is matched with TEMPERATURE and one in which DIAMETER is matched with TEMPERATURE. Thus, at this stage, the program will have a large number of local matches. It gives these local matches *evidence scores*, based on a set of local evidence rules. For example, evidence for a match increases if the base and target predicates have the same name. More interestingly, the evidence rules also invoke systematicity, in that the evidence for a given match increases with the evidence for a match among the parent relations – that is, the immediately governing higher-order relations.

2. Constructing global matches. The next stage is to collect systems of matches that use consistent entity pairings. SME first propagates entity correspondences up each relational chain to create systems of match hypotheses that use the same entity pairings. It then combines these into the largest possible systems of predicates with consistent object mappings. These global matches (called Gmaps) are SME's possible interpretations of the comparison.

An important aspect of SME is that the global matches (Gmaps) sanction *candidate inferences*: predicates from the base that get mapped into the target domain. These are base predicates that were not originally present in the target, but which can be imported into the target by virtue of belonging to a system that is shared by base and target. Thus, associated with each Gmap is a (possibly empty) set of *candidate inferences*. For example, in the "winning" Gmap (as discussed below), the pressure-difference causal chain in water is matched with the temperature-difference chain in heat, and water flow is matched with heat flow. However, you may recall that the initial heat representation lacked any causal link between the temperature difference and the heat flow (see Figure 7.5). In this case, the system brings across the higher-order predicate CAUSE from the water domain to the heat domain. In essence, it postulates that there may be more structure in the target than it initially knew about. Thus the resulting candidate inference in the heat domain is

> CAUSE {GREATER [TEMP(coffee), TEMP(ice)],
> FLOW(heat, bar, coffee, ice)}.

3. Evaluating global matches. The global matches are then given a structural evaluation, which can depend on their local match evidence, the number of candidate inferences they support, and their graph-theoretic structure – for example, the depth of the relational system.[8] In this example, the winning Gmap is the pressure–temperature match discussed above, with its candidate inference of a causal link in the heat domain. Other Gmaps are also derived, including a Gmap that matches diameter with temperature and another particularly simple Gmap that matches LIQUID (water) with LIQUID (coffee). But these are given low evaluations. They contain fewer predicates than the winning Gmap and, at least equally important, they have shallower relational structures.

A few points should be noted about the way the structure-mapping engine works. First, SME's interpretation is based on selecting the deepest – that is, most systematic – consistent mappable structure. Computing a structurally consistent relational match precedes and determines the final selection of object correspondences.

Second, SME's matching process is entirely structural. That is, it attends only to properties such as identity of predicates, structural consistency (including 1–1 object pairings), and systematicity, as opposed to seeking specific kinds of content. Thus, although it operates on semantic representations, it is not restricted to any particular pre-specified content. This allows it to act as a domain-general matcher. By promoting deep relational chains, the systematicity principle operates to promote predicates that participate in any mutually constraining system, whether causal, logical, or mathematical.

Third, as discussed above, different interpretations will be arrived at depending on which predicates match between two domains. For example, suppose that we keep the same base domain – the water system shown in Figure 7.5 – but change the target domain. Instead of two objects differing in *temperature*, let the target be two objects differing in their *specific heats*; say, a metal ball bearing and a marble. Assuming equal mass, they will also have different *heat capacities*. Now, the natural analogy concerns capacity differences in the base, rather than height differences. This is because the deepest relational chain that can be mapped to the target is, roughly, "Just as the container with greater diameter holds more water (levels being greater than or equal), so the object with greater heat capacity holds more heat (temperatures being greater than or equal)."

> IMPLIES {AND (GREATER [DIAM (beaker), DIAM (vial)],
> GREATER [LEVEL (beaker), LEVEL (vial)]),
> GREATER [AMT-WATER (beaker), AMT-WATER (vial)]}

where AMT stands for the amount. This maps into the target as

> IMPLIES {AND (GREATER [H-CAP (marble), H-CAP (ball)],
> GREATER [TEMP (marble), TEMP (ball)]),
> GREATER [AMT-HEAT (marble), AMT-HEAT (ball)]}

where H-CAP stands for heat capacity. This illustrates that the same base domain can yield different analogical mappings, depending on how it best matches the target.

Fourth, SME is designed as a general-purpose tool kit for similarity matching. It can operate with analogy rules, mere-appearance rules, or literal similarity rules, as discussed above.

Fifth, the matching process in SME is independent of the system's problem-solving goals, although the learner's goals can influence the matcher indirectly, by influencing the domain representations present in working memory. Again, this represents a commitment to generality. The view is that analogy in problem solving is a special case of analogy.

An architecture for analogical reasoning

A complete model of analogical problem solving must take account of the context of reasoning, including the current plans and goals of the reasoner (Burstein, 1986; Carbonell, 1983; Holyoak, 1985; Kedar-Cabelli, 1985; Miller, Gallanter, & Pribram, 1960; Schank, 1982; Schank & Abelson, 1977). Indeed, as I discuss in the next section, some researchers have argued that plans and goals are so central in analogical reasoning that the analogy mechanism is built around them. However, analogies can occur outside of a goal-driven context. Further, the very fact that plans and goals influence all kinds of human thought processes, from transitive inference to the use of deductive syllogism, shows that they are not in themselves definitive of analogy. Somehow we need to capture the fact that analogy can be influenced by the goals of the problem solver while at the same time capturing what is specific about analogy.

I propose the architecture shown in Figure 7.6 for analogical reasoning. In this account, plans and goals influence our thinking *before* and *after* the analogy engine but not during its operation. Plans and goals and other aspects of current context influence the analogy process *before* the match by determining the working-memory representation of the current situation. This in turn influences what gets accessed from long-term memory. So, in the heat example, there are many aspects of the heat domain, but only the aspects currently represented in working memory are likely to influence remindings. Once a potential analog is accessed from long-term memory, the analogy processor runs its course. Here too the initial domain representation has strong effects, because it defines one input to the processor; thus it constrains the set of matches that will be found. This leads to "set" effects in problem solving; it is an advantage if we are thinking about the problem correctly and a disadvantage if we are not.

The analogy processor produces an interpretation, including candidate inferences and a structural evaluation. If the evaluation is too low – that is, if the depth and size of the system of matching predicates are too low – then the analogy will be rejected on structural grounds. If the analogy passes the structural criterion, then its candidate in-

216   DEDRE GENTNER

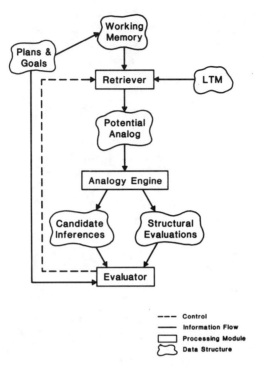

Figure 7.6. An architecture for analogical processing.

ferences must be evaluated to determine whether they are appropriate
with respect to the goals of the reasoner. In terms of the computer
model, this suggests adding a context-sensitive, expectation-driven
module to evaluate the output of SME (Falkenhainer, Forbus, & Gentner, 1986, in press; Falkenhainer, 1987a). This extension is compatible
with the combination models proposed by Burstein (1983) and Kedar-
Cabelli (1985). Thus the key points of this proposed treatment of
plans and goals are that (a) plans and goals constrain the inputs to
the matcher, which is where they have their largest effect; (b) after
the match three separate evaluation criteria must be invoked: structural soundness, relevance, and validity in the target; and (c) the match
itself does not require a prior goal statement.

In the model proposed here, both structural properties and
contextual-pragmatic considerations enter into analogical problem
solving, but they are not equated. The analogy processor is a well-
defined, separate cognitive module[9] whose results interact with other
processes, analogous to the way some natural-language models have

postulated semiautonomous interacting subsystems for syntax, semantics, and pragmatics (e.g., Reddy, Erman, Fennell, & Neely, 1973). This allows us to capture the fact that analogy must satisfy *both* a structural and a pragmatic criterion.

Separating the planning context from the actual analogy processor represents a commitment to identifying processes common to analogy across different pragmatic contexts. It suggests that when comprehending an analogy in isolation, people use many of the same processes as they do to comprehend analogy in a problem-solving context. That is, they use the same structurally guided processor for both situations, simply adding or removing pragmatic context.[10] An advantage of modeling the matching process as structure-driven rather than goal-driven is that it allows for the possibility of finding unexpected matches, even perhaps matches that contradict the learner's initial problem-solving goals. Such unexpected outcomes are important in scientific discovery. For example, the mathematician Poincaré writes about an occasion on which he set out to prove a certain theorem and ended by discovering a class of functions that proved the theorem wrong. If we are ever to model such cases of unexpected creative discovery, the analogy process must be capable of finding matches that do not depend on – and may even contradict – the learner's current goals.

Competing views and criticisms of structure-mapping

Some aspects of structure-mapping have received convergent support in artificial intelligence and psychology. Despite differences in emphasis, there is widespread agreement on the basic elements of one-to-one mapping of objects and carry-over of predicates (Burstein, 1986; Carbonell, 1983; Hofstadter, 1984; Indurkhya, 1986; Kedar-Cabelli, 1985; Miller, 1979; Reed, 1987; Rumelhart & Norman, 1981; Tourangeau & Sternberg, 1981; Van Lehn & Brown, 1980; Verbrugge & McCarrell, 1977; and Winston, 1980, 1982). Further, all these researchers have some kind of selection principle – of which systematicity is one example – to filter which predicates matter in the match. But accounts differ on the nature of the selection principle. Many researchers use specific content knowledge or pragmatic information to guide the analogical selection process, rather than structural principles like systematicity. For example, Winston's (1980, 1982) system favors causal chains in its *importance-guided* matching algorithm. Winston (personal communication, November 1985) has also investigated goal-driven importance algorithms. Hofstadter and his colleagues have developed a connectionist like model of analogical mapping, in which systematicity is one of several parallel influences on the mapping process (Hofstadter, 1984; Hofstadter, Mitchell, & French 1987).

Many accounts emphasize the role of plans and goals as part of the analogical mapping process. For example, some models combine a structure-mapping component with a plans-and-goals component in order to choose the most contextually *relevant* interpretation (e.g., Burstein, 1986; Kedar-Cabelli, 1985). These models use pragmatic context to select and elaborate the relevant predicates and to guide the mapping process. However, although these models have the ability to take contextual relevance into account, they also postulate a set of relatively constant structural processes that characterize analogical mapping. This view contrasts with a very different position, namely, that analogy should be seen as fundamentally embedded in a goal-driven problem-solving system. I now turn to a discussion of this second position.

The pragmatic account: an alternative to structure mapping

Holyoak (1985) proposed an alternative, *pragmatic*, account of analogical processing. Stating that analogy must be modeled as part of a goal-driven processing system, he argued that the structure-mapping approach is "doomed to failure" because it fails to take account of goals. In his proposed account, structural principles played no role; matching was governed entirely by the relevance of the predicates to the current goals of the problem solver. Because of the appeal of such a goal-centered position, I will discuss his arguments in some detail, even though Holyoak and his collaborators are now much less pessimistic concerning the utility of structural principles. I first present Holyoak's pragmatic account of analogy and then consider his critique of structure mapping.[11]

Holyoak states that "Within the pragmatic framework, the structure of analogy is closely tied to the mechanisms by which analogies are actually used by the cognitive system to achieve its goals" (Holyoak, 1985, p. 76). In the pragmatic account, the distinction between structural commonalties and surface commonalties is based solely on relevance. Holyoak's (1985, p. 81) definitions of these terms are as follows:

It is possible, based on the taxonomy of mapping relations discussed earlier, to draw a distinction between *surface* and *structural* similarities and dissimilarities. An identity between two problem situations that plays no causal role in determining the possible solutions to one or the other analog constitutes a surface similarity. Similarly, a structure-preserving difference, as defined earlier constitutes a surface dissimilarity. In contrast, identities that influence goal attainment constitute structural similarities, and structure-violating differences constitute structural dissimilarities. Note that the distinction between surface and structural similarities, as used here, hinges on the relevance of the property in question to attainment of a successful solution. The distinction thus crucially depends on the goal of the problem solver.

Thus a *surface similarity* is defined as "an identity between two problem situations that plays no causal role in determining the possible solutions to one or the other analog," and *structural similarities* are "identities that influence goal attainment." The distinction between surface and structural similarities "hinges on the relevance of the property in question to attainment of a successful solution. The distinction thus crucially depends on the goal of the problem solver."

Holyoak's emphasis on plans and goals has some appealing features. This account promises to replace the abstract formalisms of a structural approach with an ecologically motivated account centered around what matters to the individual. Further, whereas structure-mapping requires both structural factors within the matcher and (in a complete account) pragmatic factors external to the matcher, Holyoak's account requires only pragmatic factors. But there are severe costs to this simplification. First, since structural matches are defined only by their relevance to a set of goals, the pragmatic account requires a context that specifies what is relevant before it can operate. Therefore, it cannot deal with analogy in isolation, or even with an analogy whose point is irrelevant to the current context. By this account, Francis Bacon's analogy "All rising to a great place is by a winding stair," should be uninterpretable in the present context. I leave it to the reader to judge whether this is true.

Holyoak (1985) seems aware of this limitation and states that his pragmatic account is meant to apply only to analogy in problem solving. But this means having to postulate separate analogy processors for analogy in context and analogy in isolation, which seems inconvenient at best. But there are further difficulties with the pragmatic account. Because the interpretation of an analogy is defined in terms of relevance to the initial goals of the problem solver, the pragmatic view does not allow for unexpected outcomes in an analogical match. This means that many creative uses of analogy – such as scientific discovery – are out of bounds. Finally, the pragmatic account lacks any means of capturing the important psychological distinction between an analogy that fails because it is irrelevant and an analogy that fails because it is unsound. In short, a good case can be made for the need to *augment* structural considerations with goal-relevant considerations (though I would argue that this should be done externally to the matcher, as shown in Figure 7.6, for example). However, the attempt to *replace* structural factors like systematicity with pragmatic factors like goal-relevance does not appear tenable.

Holyoak raises three chief criticisms of structure-mapping (Holyoak, 1985, pp. 74, 75). First, as discussed above, Holyoak argues that structural factors are epiphenomenal: What really controls analogical matching is the search for goal-relevant predicates. The higher-order relations that enter into systematic structures "typically are such predicates as 'causes,' 'implies,' and 'depends on,' that is, causal elements that are pragmatically important to goal attainment. Thus, the pragmatic approach readily accounts for the phenomena cited as support for Gentner's theory." There are two problems with this argument. First, as discussed above, people are perfectly capable of processing analogy without any prior goal context, and of interpreting analogies whose point runs contrary to our expectations. Second, it is not correct to state that all higher-order relations are "causal elements pragmatically relevant to goal attainment." For example, *implies* (used in its normal logical sense) is not causal. Mathematical analogies, such as Polya's (1954) analogy between a triangle in a plane and a tetrahedron in space, are clear cases of shared relational structure that is not causal, and that need not be goal-relevant to be appreciated. Hofstadter (1984) provides many examples of analogies based on purely structural commonalities: for example, if $abc \longrightarrow abd$, then $pqr \longrightarrow pqs$.

Holyoak's second point is one of definition. In structure-mapping the distinction between analogy and literal similarity is based on the kinds of predicates shared: Analogy shares relational structure only, whereas literal similarity shares relational structure plus object descriptions. Holyoak proposes a different distinction: that analogy is similarity with reference to a goal. Thus "Even objects that Gentner would term 'literally similar' can be analogically related if a goal is apparent." The problem with this distinction is that although it captures analogy's role as a focusing device, it classifies some things as analogy that intuitively seem to be literal similarity. For example, consider the comparison "This '82 Buick is like this '83 Buick: You can use it to drive across town." By Holyoak's criterion this is an analogy, because a specific goal is under consideration; yet to my ear the two Buicks are literally similar whether or not a goal is involved. But since this is essentially a question of terminology, it may be undecidable.

Holyoak's third set of criticisms is based on the misinterpretation discussed earlier: namely, that in structure-mapping the systematicity of the base domain *by itself* determines the interpretation of an anal-

ogy, so that "the mappable propositions can be determined by a syntactic [structural] analysis of the source analog alone." This is false
except in the rare case where nothing at all is known about the target
(the "pure carry-over" case discussed earlier). This can be seen in the
operation of SME, in which the interpretation arises out of a detailed
match between base and target and not from "a syntactic analysis of
the source analog alone." (See Skorstad, Falkenhainer, & Gentner,
1987, for examples of how SME yields different interpretations when
the same base domain is paired with different targets.) At the risk of
belaboring the point, let us recall that, in structure-mapping, analogy
is seen as a subclass of similarity, and therefore, as with any other
kind of similarity comparison, its interpretation is based on the best
match between base and target. What distinguishes analogy from
other kinds of similarity is that, for analogy, the *best match* is defined
as the maximally systematic and consistent match of relational
structure.

In summary, Holyoak's pragmatic account must be considered a
failure insofar as it seeks to replace structure with relevance. Though
one may sympathize with the desire to take plans and goals into account, discounting structure is the wrong way to go about it. Nonetheless, this work, like that of Burstein (1986), Carbonell (1981, 1983),
and Kedar-Cabelli (1985), has the merit of calling attention to the
important issue of how plans and goals can be integrated into a theory
of analogy.

Separating structural rules from pragmatics has some significant
advantages: It allows us to capture the commonalities among analogy
interpretation across different pragmatic contexts, including analogy
in isolation; it allows for creativity, since the processor does not have
to know in advance which predicates are going to be shared; and it
allows us to capture the difference between relevance and soundness.
However, if the two-factor scheme I propose in Figure 7.6 is correct,
there is still much work to be done in specifying exactly how plans
and goals affect the initial domain representations that are given to
the analogy processor and how they are compared with the output
of this processor in the postprocessing stage.

Psychological evidence for structure-mapping

Ideal mapping rules. Structure-mapping claims to characterize
the implicit competence rules by which the meaning of an analogy is
derived. The first question to ask is how successfully it does so –

whether people do indeed follow the rules of structure-mapping in interpreting analogies. The prediction is that people should include relations and omit object descriptions in their interpretations of analogy. To test this, subjects were asked to write out descriptions of objects and then to interpret analogical comparisons containing these objects. (Gentner, 1980, 1988; Gentner & Clement, in press). They also rated how apt (how interesting, clever, or worth reading) the comparisons were.

The results showed that, whereas object descriptions tended to include both relational and object-attribute information, the interpretations of comparisons tended to include relations and omit object attributes. For example, a subject's description of "cigarette" was as follows:

chopped cured tobacco in a paper roll / with or without a filter at the end / held in the mouth / lit with a match and breathed through to draw smoke into the lungs / found widely among humans / known by some cultures to be damaging to the lungs / once considered beneficial to health.

Note that this description contains both relational and attributional information. Yet, when the same subject is given the metaphor "Cigarettes are like time bombs," his interpretation is purely in terms of common relational information: "They do their damage after some period of time during which no damage may be evident." A second finding was that the comparisons were considered more apt to the degree that subjects could find relational interpretations. There was a strong positive correlation between rated aptness and relationality but no such correlation for attributionality. Adults thus demonstrate a strong relational focus in interpreting metaphor. They emphasize relational commonalties in their interpretations when possible, and they prefer metaphors that allow such interpretations (Gentner & Clement, in press).

Development of mapping rules. The implicit focus on relations in interpreting analogy can seem so natural to us that it seems to go without saying. One way to see the effects of the competence rules is to look at cases in which these rules are not followed. Children do not show the kind of relational focus that adults do in interpreting analogy and metaphor.[12] A 5 year-old, given the figurative comparison "A cloud is like a sponge," produces an attributional interpretation, such as "Both are round and fluffy." A typical adult response is "Both can hold water for some time and then later give it back." Nine-year-olds are intermediate, giving some relational interpretations but also many responses based on common object attributes (Gentner, 1980, 1988; Gentner & Stuart, 1983). The same developmental shift holds for choice tasks and rating tasks (Billow, 1975; Gentner, 1988). Thus there is evidence for a developmental shift from a focus on common object attributes to a focus on common relations in analogical processing.

Performance factors in analogical mapping

As Palmer (this volume) points out, structure-mapping aims first and foremost to capture the essential nature of analogy: what constitutes an analogy and which distinctions are necessary to characterize analogy – what Marr (1982) calls the "computational level" and Palmer and Kimchi (1985) call "informational constraints." Thus structure-mapping is in part a competence theory in that it attempts to capture people's implicit understanding of which commonalities should belong to analogy and which should not. The research described above suggests that under ordinary conditions structure-mapping is also a good approximation to a performance theory, for people's actual interpretations of analogies fit the predictions rather well. But what happens if we make it harder for people to perform according to the rules? Given that the ideal in analogy is to discover the maximal common higher-order relational structure, here we ask how closely people approach the *ideal* under difficult circumstances and what factors affect people's *performance* in carrying out a structure mapping.

Transfer performance. Gentner and Toupin (1986) posed this question developmentally. We asked children of 4–6 and 8–10 years of age to transfer a story plot from one group of characters to another. Two factors were varied: (a) the *systematicity* of the base domain (the original story); and (b) the *transparency* of the mapping (that is, the degree to which the target objects resembled their corresponding base objects). The systematicity of the original story was varied by adding beginning and ending sentences that expressed a causal or moral summary. Otherwise, the stories in the systematic condition were the same as those in the nonsystematic condition. Transparency was manipulated by varying the similarity of corresponding characters. For example, the original story might involve a *chipmunk* helping his friend the *moose* to escape from the villain *frog*.

After acting out the story with the base characters, the child was told to act out the story again, but with new characters. In the high-

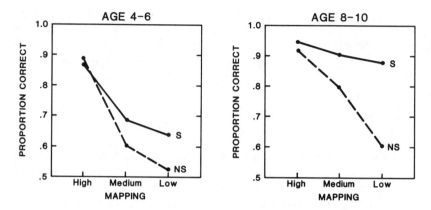

Figure 7.7. Results of the cross-mapping experiment: proportion correct on transfer story given systematic (S) or nonsystematic (NS) original stories, across mappings varying from high transparency to low transparency (Gentner & Toupin, 1986). *High* transparency means similar characters in corresponding roles; *medium*, different characters; and *low*, similar characters in different roles (the cross-mapped condition).

transparency mapping, the new characters would resemble the original characters: for example, a *squirrel*, an *elk*, and a *toad*, respectively. In the medium-transparency condition, three new unrelated animals were used. In the low-transparency (*cross-mapped*) condition, the characters were similar to the original characters but occupied noncorresponding roles: For example, the *chipmunk*, *moose*, and *frog* of the original story would map onto an *elk*, a *toad*, and a *squirrel*, respectively. We expected the cross-mapped condition to be very difficult. More interestingly, we wanted to know how robust the mapping rules are: How firmly can people hold to a systematic mapping when surface similarity pushes them toward a nonsystematic solution?

Both systematicity and transparency turned out to be important in determining transfer accuracy. However the two age groups showed different patterns, Transparency affected both age groups, whereas systematicity affected only the older group. For both ages, transfer accuracy was nearly perfect with highly similar corresponding characters (high transparency), lower when corresponding characters were quite different (medium transparency), and lower still in the cross-mapped condition (low transparency). For the older group, systematicity also had strong effects. As Figure 7.7 shows, 9-year-olds performed virtually perfectly, even in the most difficult mapping conditions, when they had a systematic story structure. This is noteworthy because, as can be seen from their performance in the nonsystematic condition, 9-year-olds found the cross-mapping condition quite difficult. Yet, given a systematic relational structure to hold onto, they could keep their mappings straight. In contrast, the 5-year-olds were affected only by transparency; they showed no significant benefit from systematic relational structure.

How does this happen? Gentner and Toupin (1986) speculated that the benefit comes in part from the way shared systems of relations help guide the mapping of lower-order relations. An error made in mapping a particular relation from base to target is more likely to be detected if there is a higher-order relation that constrains that lower-order relation. Informal observations in our study support this view. The older children, in the systematic condition, would sometimes begin to make an object-similarity-based error and then correct themselves, saying something like "Oh no, it's the *bad* one who got stuck in the hole, because he ate all the food." They were using the systematic causal structure of the story to overcome their local mapping difficulties.

Research with adults suggests that both systematicity and transparency continue to be important variables. Both Ross (1984; this volume) and Reed (1987) have shown that subjects are better at transferring algebraic solutions when corresponding base and target objects are similar. Reed (1987) measured the transparency of the mapping between two analogous algebra problems by asking subjects to identify pairs of corresponding concepts. He found that transparency was a good predictor of their ability to notice and apply solutions from one problem to the other. Ross (1987) has investigated the effects of cross-mappings in remindings during problem solving. He found that, even though adults could often *access* the prior problem, their ability to *transfer* the solution correctly was disrupted when cross-mapped correspondences were used. Robert Schumacher and I found benefits of both systematicity and transparency in transfer of device models, using a design similar to that of Gentner and Toupin (1986), in which subjects transfer an operating procedure from a base device to a target device (Gentner & Schumacher, 1986; Schumacher & Gentner, in press).

The evidence is quite strong, then, that transparency makes mapping easier. Thus literal similarity is the easiest sort of mapping and the one where subjects are least likely to make errors. The evidence also shows that a systematic base model promotes accurate mapping. This means that systematicity is a performance variable as well as a competence variable. Not only do people *believe* in achieving systematic mappings; they *use* systematic structure to help them perform the mapping.

Developmental implications: the relational shift. Like adults, the 9-year-olds in the Gentner and Toupin (1986) study were affected by both systematicity and transparency. But the 5-year-olds showed· no significant effects of systematic base structure. All that mattered to this younger group was the transparency of the object correspondences. These results are consistent with the results reported earlier, and with the general developmental finding that young children rely on object-level similarities in transfer tasks (DeLoache, in press; Holyoak, Junn, & Billman, 1984; Keil & Batterman 1984; Kemler, 1983; Shepp, 1978; L. Smith, this volume; Smith & Kemler, 1977) and in metaphor tasks (Asch & Nerlove, 1960; Billow, 1975; Dent, 1984; Gardner, Kircher, Winner, & Perkins, 1975; Kogan, 1975). These findings suggest a developmental shift from reliance on surface similarity, and particularly on transparency of object correspondences, to use of relational structure in analogical mapping.[13]

Access processes

Now we are ready to tackle the issue of *access* to analogy and similarity. Before doing so, let us recapitulate briefly. I proposed at the start of this chapter a set of subprocesses necessary for spontaneous learning by analogy: (a) accessing the base system; (b) performing the mapping between base and target; (c) evaluating the match; (d) storing inferences in the target; and (e) extracting the common principle. So far we have considered mapping, evaluating, and making inferences. A major differentiating variable in the research so far is *similarity class*: whether the match is one of mere appearance, analogy, or literal similarity. Now we ask how similarity class affects memorial *access* to analogy and similarity.

Accessing analogy and similarity. What governs spontaneous access to similar or analogous situations? Gentner & Landers (1985) investigated this question, using a method designed to resemble natural long-term memory access. (For details of this and related studies, see Gentner & Landers, 1985; Gentner & Rattermann, in preparation; Rattermann & Gentner, 1987.) We first gave subjects a large set of stories to read and remember (18 key stories and 14 fillers). Subjects returned about a week later and performed two tasks: (a) a *reminding* task; and (b) a *soundness-rating* task.

In the reminding task, subjects read a new set of 18 stories, each of which matched one of the 18 original stories, as described below.

Table 7.2. *Sample story set for the access experiment (Gentner & Landers, 1985)*

BASE story
Karla, an old hawk, lived at the top of a tall oak tree. One afternoon, she saw a
  hunter on the ground with a bow and some some crude arrows that had no
  feathers. The hunter took aim and shot at the hawk but missed. Karla knew the
  hunter wanted her feathers so she glided down to the hunter and offered to give
  him a few. The hunter was so grateful that he pledged never to shoot at a hawk
  again. He went off and shot deer instead.

True-analogy TARGET
Once there was a small country called Zerdia that learned to make the world's
  smartest computer. One day Zerdia was attacked by its warlike neighbor,
  Gagrach. But the missiles were badly aimed and the attack failed. The Zerdian
  government realized that Gagrach wanted Zerdian computers so it offered to sell
  some of its computers to the country. The government of Gagrach was very
  pleased. It promised never to attack Zerdia again.

Mere-appearance TARGET
Once there was an eagle named Zerdia who donated a few of her tailfeathers to a
  sportsman so he would promise never to attack eagles. One day Zerdia was
  nesting high on a rocky cliff when she saw the sportsman coming with a crossbow.
  Zerdia flew down to meet the man, but he attacked and felled her with a single
  bolt. As she fluttered to the ground Zerdia realized that the bolt had her own
  tailfeathers on it.

False-analogy TARGET
Once there was a small country called Zerdia that learned to make the world's
  smartest computer. Zerdia sold one of its supercomputers to its neighbor,
  Gagrach, so Gagrach would promise never to attack Zerdia. But one day Zerdia
  was overwhelmed by a surprise attack from Gagrach. As it capitulated the crippled
  government of Zerdia realized that the attacker's missiles had been guided by
  Zerdian supercomputers.

Subjects were told that if any of the new stories reminded them of
any of the original stories, they were to write out the original story
(or stories) as completely as possible. There were three kinds of similarity matches between base and target:

- *mere appearance* (MA): object attributes and first-order relations
  match
- *true analogy* (TA): first-order relations and higher-order relations
  match
- *false analogy* (FA): only the first-order relations match

In all three cases, the base and target shared first-order relations.
Other commonalties were added to create the different similarity

conditions. Table 7.2 shows an example set of four stories: a base story plus one example of each of the three kinds of matches. Each subject received one-third MA, one-third TA, and one-third FA matches, counterbalanced across three groups. After the subjects had completed the reminding task, they performed the soundness-rating task. They were shown their 18 pairs of stories side by side and asked to rate each pair for the soundness or inferential power of the match (with 5 being "sound" and 1 being "spurious").

In the soundness-rating task, subjects showed the predicted preference for true analogies. The mean soundness ratings were 4.4 for true analogy, 2.8 for mere appearance, and 2.0 for false analogy, with the only significant difference being between true analogy and the other two match types. This aspect of the study provides further evidence for the systematicity principle: Common higher-order relational structure is an important determinant of the subjective goodness of an analogy.

The results for access were surprising. Despite subjects' retrospective agreement that only the analogical matches were sound, their natural remindings did not produce analogies. Instead, they were far more likely to retrieve superficial mere-appearance matches. Given mere-appearance matches, subjects were able to access the original story 78% of the time, whereas the true analogies were accessed only 44% of the time, and the false analogies 25% of the time. All three differences were significant, suggesting that (a) surface commonalities have the most important role in access but that (b) higher-order relational commonalties – present in the true analogies but not in the false analogies – also promote access.

We have recently replicated these results, adding a literal similarity condition, and the results show the same pattern (Gentner & Rattermann, in preparation; Rattermann & Gentner, 1987). In access, surface similarity seems to be the dominant factor. Literal similarity and mere-appearance matches are more accessible than true analogies and false analogies. In soundness, systematicity of relational structure is the dominant factor. True analogy and literal similarity are considered sound, and false analogies and mere-appearance matches are not. Interestingly, surface information is superior in access even for subjects who clearly believe that only structural overlap counts toward soundness. It appears that analogical *access* and analogical *soundness* – or at least our subjective estimates of soundness – are influenced in different degrees by different kinds of similarity.

These access results accord with the findings of Gick and Holyoak (1980, 1983) of Reed (1987; Reed, Ernst, & Banerji, 1974), and of

Ross (1984, 1987; Ross & Sofka, 1986). In this research it has reliably been demonstrated that subjects in a problem-solving task often fail to access prior material that is analogous to their current problem. For example, in Gick and Holyoak's (1980, 1983) studies, a substantial number of subjects failed to access a potential analog – and therefore could not solve the problem – yet, when the experimenter suggested that the prior material was relevant, they could readily apply it to solve the problem. This means that (a) they had clearly stored the prior analog; (b) the prior analog contained sufficient information to solve their current problem; but (c) they could not access the prior analog solely on the basis of the current (analogous) problem structure. Thus there is converging evidence for the gloomy finding that relational commonalities often fail to lead to access.

There is also confirmation for the other side of the coin: that surface commonalties do promote access (Holyoak & Thagard, this volume; Novick, 1988; Reed & Ackinclose, 1986; Ross, 1984, 1987, this volume; Ross & Sofka, 1986; Schumacher, 1987). For example, Ross (1984) found clear effects of surface similarity in determining which earlier algebra problems subjects would be reminded of in trying to solve later problems. Reed and Ackinclose (1986) found that perceived similarity, rather than structural isomorphism, was the best predictor of whether subjects solving algebra problems would apply the results of a previous problem to a current problem.[14] Overall similarity, especially surface similarity, appears to be a major factor in accessing material in long-term memory.

Having said all this, we must remember that purely relational reminding does occur. Even young children sometimes experience analogical insights, as attested by Heida's analogy at the beginning of this chapter. As Johnson-Laird (this volume) points out, though remindings between remote domains are relatively rare, their occurrence sometimes sparks important creative advances (Falkenhainer, 1987b; Gentner, 1982; Hesse, 1966; Waldrop, 1987). A correct model of access will have to capture both the fact that relational remindings are comparatively rare and the fact that they occur.

Decomposing similarity

I began this chapter by noting that similarity is widely considered to be an important determinant of transfer (Thorndike, 1903; see Brown, this volume, and Brown & Campione, 1984, for discussions of this issue). The research reviewed here suggests that both *similarity* and *transfer* may be too coarse as variables. A strong theme in this chapter, and indeed a convergent theme across this volume, has been the need to make finer differentiations in the notion of similarity (Collins & Burstein, this volume; Medin & Ortony, this volume; Rips, this volume; Ross, this volume; L. Smith, this volume). The research discussed in this chapter further suggests that *transfer* must be decomposed into different subprocesses that interact differently with different kinds of similarity. Thus the simple statement "Similarity is important in transfer" may conceal an intricate set of interactions between different varieties of similarity and different subprocesses in transfer.

Based on the research presented so far, it appears that different subprocesses are affected by different kinds of similarity. *Access* is strongly influenced by surface similarity and only weakly influenced by structural similarity. *Analogical mapping* is strongly influenced by structural similarity, including shared systematicity; it may also be weakly influenced by surface similarity. *Judging soundness* is chiefly influenced by structural similarity and systematicity. Finally, *extracting and storing the principle* underlying an analogy seems likely to be governed by structural similarity and systematicity. There is thus a relational shift in processing analogy and similarity from surface to structural commonalities.[15]

Similarity-based access may be a rather primitive mechanism, a low-cost low-specificity, high-quantity process, requiring little conscious effort. Analogical mapping and judging soundness are rather more sophisticated. They are often somewhat effortful, they often involve conscious reasoning, and, unlike access, they can be specifically tailored to different kinds of similarity. One can choose whether to carry out a mapping as an analogy or as a mere-appearance match, for example; but one cannot choose in advance whether to *access* an analogy or a mere-appearance match. Access has the feel of a passive process that simply produces some number of potential matches that the reasoner can accept or reject. Finally, one suspects that the processes of mapping and judging soundness are heavily influenced by culturally learned strategies (see Gentner & Jeziorski, in press). In contrast, access processes seem less amenable to cultural influence and training.[16] To the extent that experts differ from novices in their access patterns, I suspect this results chiefly from experts' having different domain representations (e.g., possessing relational abstractions) rather than from their having different access processes.

It is tempting to speculate that similarity-driven access involves something rather like a ballistic process, whereas mapping and judging soundness are more like discretionary processes. In any case, as we move from access to mapping and judging soundness there is a sense of increasing volitional control over the processes. To use an analogy, gaining access to long-term memory is a bit like fishing: The learner can bait the hook – that is, set up the working memory probe – as he or she chooses, but once the line is thrown into the water it is impossible to predict exactly which fish will bite.

The access bias for overall-similarity and surface-similarity matches rather than abstract analogical remindings may seem like a poor design choice from a machine-learning standpoint. But there may be good reasons for a bias toward overall similarity. First, a conservative, overall-similarity bias may be reasonable given the large size of human data bases relative to current artificial intelligence systems. For large data bases, the costs of checking all potential relational matches may well be prohibitive. Second, a conservative matching strategy might be prudent for mobile biological beings, for whom a false positive might be perilous. Third, by beginning with overall similarity the learner allows the relational vocabulary to grow to fit the data. This may be one reason children are better language learners than are adults; paradoxically, their initial conservatism and surface focus may allow the correct relational generalizations slowly to emerge (cf. Newport, 1984; see Forbus & Gentner, 1983; Murphy & Medin, 1985).

These arguments suggest that human access is geared toward literal similarity. But what about the fact that our access mechanisms also retrieve mere-appearance matches? Possibly, this comes about as a by-product of the overall-similarity bias. By this account, it is a design flaw, but perhaps a fairly minor one for concrete physical domains, where appearances tend not to be very deceiving. Very often, things that look alike *are* alike. (See Gentner, 1987; Medin & Ortony, this volume; Wattenmaker, Nakamura, & Medin, 1986.) Where surface matches become least reliable is in abstract domains such as algebra or Newtonian mechanics. The novice who assumes that any new pulley problem should be solved like the last pulley problem will often be wrong (Chi, Feltovich, & Glaser, 1981). Thus our surface-oriented accessor can be an obstacle to learning in abstract domains, where the correlation between surface features and structural features is low.

Implications for learning

Now let's put together these findings and ask how they bear on experiential learning. This discussion is based on that given by Forbus and Gentner (1983). Forbus and Gentner examined the role of similarity comparisons in the progression from early to later representations. A key assumption here is that implicit comparisons among related knowledge structures are important in learning (Brooks, 1978; Jacoby & Brooks, 1984; Medin & Schaffer, 1978; Wattenmaker et al., 1986). We conjecture that much of experiential learning proceeds through spontaneous comparisons – which may be implicit or explicit – between a current situation and prior similar or analogous situations that the learner has stored in memory. We also assume that early representations are characteristically rich and perceptually based. That is, early domain representations differ from more advanced representations of the same domain in containing more perceptual information specific to the initial context of use. What does this predict? First, in terms of *access*, the greater the surface match the greater the likelihood of access. Thus the matches that are likely to occur most readily are literal similarity matches and mere-appearance matches.

Once the base domain has been accessed, the mapping process occurs. To transfer knowledge from one domain to another, a person must not only access the base domain but also set up the correct object correspondences between the base and target and map predicates across. At this level, a mix of deep and surface factors seems to operate. Systematicity and structural similarity become crucial, but so does the transparency of the object correspondences (Gentner & Toupin, 1986; Reed, 1987; Ross, 1987). It appears that, for adults and/or experts, systematicity can to some extent compensate for lack of transparency. The rules of analogy are clear enough and the relational structures robust enough to allow accurate mapping without surface support. But for children and novices surface similarity is a key determinant of success in analogical mapping.

To the extent that children and novices rely on object commonalities in similarity-based mapping, they are limited to literal similarity matches and mere-appearance matches. The disadvantage of mere-appearance matches is obvious: They are likely to lead to wrong inferences about the target. But even literal similarity matches have their limitations. Although adequate for prediction, literal similarity matches are probably less useful than analogies for purposes of explicitly extracting causal principles. In an analogical match, the shared data structure is sparse enough to permit the learner to isolate the key principles. In literal similarity, there are too many common predicates to know which are crucial (Forbus & Gentner, 1983; Ross, this volume; Wattenmaker et al., 1986).

How do learners escape the confines of literal similarity? One way, of course, is through explicit instruction about the relevant abstractions. But there may be ways within experiential learning as well. If we speculate that the results of a similarity comparison become slightly more accessible (Elio & Anderson, 1981, 1984; Gick & Holyoak, 1983; Ortony, 1979; Skorstad, Gentner, & Medin, 1988), then repeated instances of near-literal similarity could gradually increase the salience of the relational commonalities. At some point the relational structures become sufficiently salient to allow analogy to occur. Once this happens, there is some likelihood of noticing the relational commonalities and extracting them for future use. (This conjectural sequence, which is essentially that proposed in Forbus and Gentner, 1983, hinges on the claim that the results of an analogy are sparser and therefore more inspectable than the results of a literal similarity comparison. Hence, the probability of noticing and extracting the common relational structure is greater.) The extracted relational abstractions can then influence encoding. With sufficient domain knowledge, the set of known abstractions – such as *flow rate* or *positive feedback situation* – becomes firm enough to allow relational encoding and retrieval.

The post-access processes can be influenced both by individual training and by local strategies. I suspect that this is the area in which training in thinking skills can be of most benefit. For example, people may learn better skills for checking potential matches and rejecting bad matches, and perhaps also skills for tinkering with potential matches to make them more useful (Clement, 1983, 1986). However, I suspect that some parts of the system will always remain outside direct volitional control. To return to the fishing analogy, we can learn to bait the hook better, and once the fish bites we can learn better skills for landing it, identifying it, and deciding whether to keep it or throw it back. But no matter how accurate the preaccess and post-access processes, there is always uncertainty in the access itself. When we throw the hook into the current we cannot determine exactly which fish will bite. A strategically managed interplay between discretionary and automatic processes may be the most productive technique for analogical reasoning.

Conclusion

In this chapter I have suggested that different kinds of similarity participate differently in transfer. In particular, I have proposed decomposing similarity into subclasses of *analogy, mere-appearance,* and *literal similarity* and transfer into subprocesses of *access, mapping, storing inferences,* and *extracting commonalities.* Although many issues remain to be worked out, it seems clear that this finer-grained set of distinctions will allow a more fruitful discussion of similarity based learning.

NOTES

This research was supported by the Office of Naval Research under Contract N00014–5–K–0559, NR667–551. The developmental studies were supported by the National Institute of Education under Contract 400–80–0031 awarded to the Center for the Study of Reading. I thank Ann Brown, Allan Collins, Judy DeLoache, Ken Forbus, Doug Medin, and Brian Ross for many insightful discussions of these issues, and Cathy Clement, Rogers Hall, Mike Jeziorski, Doug Medin, Andrew Ortony, Mary Jo Rattermann, Bob Schumacher, and Janice Skorstad for their helpful comments on a draft of this paper.

1 For now, I will use the term *analogical learning* to refer to both learning by analogy and learning by literal similarity. Later in the chapter I will distinguish between analogy and similarity.
2 This account has benefited from the comments and suggestions of my colleagues since my first proposal in 1980. Here and there I will indicate some ways in which the theory has changed.
3 The notation in Figure 7.2 is equivalent to a predicate calculus representation; I use it because it emphasizes structural relationships (see Norman & Rumelhart, 1975; Palmer, 1978).
4 In this analogy, the function PRESSURE in the water domain must be mapped onto TEMPERATURE in the heat domain. Like objects, functions on objects in the base can be put in correspondence with different functions in the target in order to permit mapping a larger systematic chain.
5 An ongoing question in our research is whether mere-appearance matches should be viewed as including first-order relations as well as object attributes.
6 The reason that attributes are ignored, rather than being placed in correspondence with other attributes, is to permit analogical matches between rich objects and sparse objects.
7 Adding functions to the representation is a change from my former position, which distinguished only between object attributes (one-place predicates) and relations (two-or-more-place predicates). I thank Ken Forbus, Brian Falkenhainer, and Janice Skorstad for discussions on this issue.
8 Currently, the global evaluation is extremely simple: The match-hypothesis evidence scores are simply summed for each Gmap. Although we have developed more elaborate schemes for computing the goodness of the Gmaps, this simple summation has proved extremely effective. We have tried SME on over 40 analogies, and in every case its highest-ranked Gmap is the one humans prefer.

9 The term *module* here should not be taken in the Fodorian sense. I assume that analogical processing is not innate or hard-wired but, at least in part, learned; nor do I assume that the analogy processor is impenetrable, although its workings may be opaque.

10 As in all top-down expectation situations, comprehension should be easier with a supporting context and harder when context leads to the wrong expectations; but the basic analogy processes do not *require* a context.

11 It should be noted that since this chapter was written Holyoak has revised his position. His recent work incorporates many of the structural constraints discussed here while still postulating a central role for contextual goals (Thagard & Holyoak, 1988).

12 Much of the developmental literature has been couched in terms of *metaphor* rather than *analogy*. Often, the items called *metaphors* are figurative comparisons that adults would treat as analogies.

13 It is not clear whether this shift is due to a developmental change in analytical reasoning skills or simply to an increase in domain knowledge, especially relational knowledge (Brown, this volume; Brown & Campione, 1984; Carey, 1984; Chi, 1978; Crisafi & Brown, 1986; Gentner, 1977a,b, 1988; Larkin, McDermott, Simon, & Simon, 1980, Reynolds & Ortony, 1980; Siegler, 1988; Vosniadou & Ortony, 1986).

14 These results, especially in problem-solving contexts, are problematic for the plan-based indexing view held by many researchers in artificial intelligence. See Gentner (1987) for a discussion.

15 This echoes the relational shift in the development of analogy from an early focus on surface commonalities to the adult focus on relational commonalities. How much we should make anything of this parallel is unclear.

16 We may perhaps learn to guide access by the indirect route of changing the contents of working memory so that a different set of matches arises. However, this is not a very fine-tuned method. I thank Brian Ross for discussions of this issue.

REFERENCES

Asch, S. E., & Nerlove, H. (1960). The development of double function terms in children: An exploratory investigation. In B. Kaplan & S. Wapner (Eds.), *Perspectives in psychological theory*. New York: International Universities Press.

Billow, R. M. (1975). A cognitive development study of metaphor comprehension. *Developmental Psychology, 11*, 415–423.

Brooks, L. (1978). Nonanalytic concept formation and memory for instances. In E. Rosch & B. B. Lloyd (Eds.), *Cognition and categorization* (pp. 169–211). Hillsdale, NJ: Erlbaum.

Brown, A. L., & Campione, J. C. (1984). Three faces of transfer: Implications for early competence, individual differences, and instruction. In M. Lamb, A. Brown, & B. Rogoff (Eds.), *Advances in developmental psychology* (Vol. 3, pp. 143–192). Hillsdale, NJ: Erlbaum.

Buckley, S. (1979). *Sun up to sun down*. New York: McGraw-Hill.

Burstein, M. H. (1986). Concept formation by incremental analogical reasoning and debugging. In R. S. Michalski, J. G. Carbonell, & T. M. Mitchell (Eds.), *Machine learning: An artificial intelligence approach* (Vol. 2, pp. 351–370). Los Altos, CA: Kaufmann.

Carbonell, J. G. (1981, August). Invariance hierarchies in metaphor interpretation. *Proceedings of the Third Annual Conference of the Cognitive Science Society* (pp. 292–295), Berkeley, CA.

Carbonell, J. G. (1983). Learning by analogy: Formulating and generalizing plans from past experience. In R. S. Michalski, J. G. Carbonell, and T. M. Mitchell (Eds.), *Machine learning: An artificial intelligence approach* (Vol. 1, pp. 137–161). Palo Alto, CA: Tioga.

Carey, S. (1984). Are children fundamentally different kinds of thinkers and learners than adults? In S. F. Chipman, J. W. Segal, & R. Glaser (Eds.), *Thinking and learning skills: Current research and open questions* (Vol. 2, pp. 485–517). Hillsdale, NJ: Erlbaum.

Chi, M. T. H. (1978). Knowledge structures and memory development. In R. Siegler (Ed.), *Children's thinking: What develops?* Hillsdale, NJ: Erlbaum.

Chi, M. T. H., Feltovich, P. J., & Glaser, R. (1981). Categorization and representation of physics problems by experts and novices. *Cognitive Science, 5*, 121–152.

Clement, J. (1981). Analogy generation in scientific problem solving. *Proceedings of the Third Annual Conference of the Cognitive Science Society* (pp. 137–140), Berkeley, CA.

Clement, J. (1983, April). *Observed methods for generating analogies in scientific problem solving*. Paper presented at the annual meeting of the American Educational Research Association, Montreal.

Clement, J. (1986, August). Methods for evaluating the validity of hypothesized analogies. *Proceedings of the Eighth Annual Conference of the Cognitive Science Society*, Amherst, MA.

Clement, C. A., & Gentner, D. (1988). Systematicity as a selection constraint in analogical mapping. *Proceedings of the Tenth Annual Conference of the Cognitive Science Society*, Montreal.

Crisafi, M. A., & Brown, A. L. (1986). Analogical transfer in very young children: Combining two separately learned solutions to reach a goal. *Child Development, 57*, 953–968.

DeLoache, J. S. (in press). The development of representation in young children. In H. W. Reese (Ed.), *Advances in child development and behavior* (Vol. 21). New York: Academic Press.

Dent, C. H. (1984). The developmental importance of motion information in perceiving and describing metaphoric similarity. *Child Development, 55*, 1607–1613.

Elio, R., & Anderson, J. R. (1981). The effects of category generalizations and instance similarity on schema abstraction. *Journal of Experimental Psychology: Human Learning and Memory, 7*, 397–417.

Elio, R., & Anderson, J. R. (1984). The effects of information and learning mode on schema abstraction. *Memory & Cognition, 12*, 20–30.

Falkenhainer, B. (1987a). *An examination of the third stage in the analogy process: Verification-based analogical reasoning* (Tech. Rep. UIUCDCS-R86-1302). Urbana-Champaign: University of Illinois, Department of Computer Science.

Falkenhainer, B. (1987b). Scientific theory formation through analogical inference. *Proceedings of the Fourth International Machine Learning Workshop* (pp. 218–229). Los Altos, CA: Kaufmann.

Falkenhainer, B., Forbus, K. D., & Gentner, D. (1986). The structure-mapping engine. *Proceedings of the American Association for Artificial Intelligence* (pp. 272–277), Philadelphia.

Falkenhainer, B., Forbus, K. D., & Gentner, D. (in press). The structure-mapping engine. *Artificial Intelligence*.

Forbus, K. D., & Gentner, D. (1983, June). Learning physical domains: Towards a theoretical framework. *Proceedings of the 1983 International Machine Learning Workshop* (pp. 198–202), Monticello, IL. Also in R. S. Michalski, J. G. Carbonell, & T. M. Mitchell (Eds.), *Machine learning: An artificial intelligence approach* (Vol. 2). Los Altos, CA: Kaufmann, 1986.

Gardner, H., Kircher, M., Winner, E., & Perkins, D. (1975). Children's metaphoric productions and preferences. *Journal of Child Language, 2*, 1–17.

Gentner, D. (1977a). Children's performance on a spatial analogies task. *Child Development, 48*, 1034–1039.

Gentner, D. (1977b). If a tree had a knee, where would it be? Children's performance on simple spatial metaphors. *Papers and Reports on Child Language Development, 13*, 157–164.

Gentner, D. (1980). *The structure of analogical models in science* (BBN Tech. Rep. 4451). Cambridge, MA: Bolt, Beranek & Newman.

Gentner, D. (1982). Are scientific analogies metaphors? In D. Miall (Ed.), *Metaphor: Problems and perspectives*. Brighton: Harvester Press.

Gentner, D. (1983). Structure-mapping: A theoretical framework for analogy. *Cognitive Science, 7*, 155–170.

Gentner, D. (1987). Analogical inference and analogical access. In A. Prieditis (Ed.), *Analogica: Proceedings of the First Workshop in Analogical Reasoning*. London: Pitman.

Gentner, D. (1988). Metaphor as structure-mapping: The relational shift. *Child Development, 59*, 47–59.

Gentner, D., & Clement, C. A. (in press). Evidence for relational selectivity in the interpretation of analogy and metaphor. In G. H. Bower (Ed.), *The psychology of learning and motivation*. New York: Academic Press.

Gentner, D., Falkenhainer, B., & Skorstad, J. (1987, January). Metaphor: The good, the bad, and the ugly. *Proceedings of the Third Conference on Theoretical Issues in Natural Language Processing* (pp. 155–159), Las Cruces, NM.

Gentner, D., & Gentner, D. R. (1983). Flowing waters or teeming crowds: Mental models of electricity. In D. Gentner & A. L. Stevens (Eds.), *Mental models* (pp. 99–129). Hillsdale, NJ: Erlbaum.

Gentner, D., & Jeziorski, M. (in press). Historical shifts in the use of analogy in science. In B. Gholson, W. R. Shadish, & A. Graesser (Eds). *Psychology of Science*. Cambridge: Cambridge University Press.

Gentner, D., & Landers, R. (1985, November). Analogical reminding: A good match is hard to find. *Proceedings of the International Conference on Systems, Man, and Cybernetics*. Tucson, AZ.

Gentner, D., & Rattermann, M. J. (in preparation). Analogical access: A good match is hard to find.

238 DEDRE GENTNER

Gentner, D., & Schumacher, R. M. (1986, October). Use of structure-mapping theory for complex systems. *Proceedings of the IEEE International Conference on Systems, Man, and Cybernetics* (pp. 252–258), Atlanta, GA.

Gentner, D., & Stuart, P. (1983). *Metaphor as structure-mapping: What develops* (Tech. Rep. 5479). Cambridge, MA: Bolt, Beranek & Newman.

Gentner, D., & Toupin, C. (1986). Systematicity and surface similarity in the development of analogy. *Cognitive Science, 10,* 277–300.

Gick, M. L., & Holyoak, K. J. (1980). Analogical problem solving. *Cognitive Psychology, 12,* 306–355.

Gick, M. L., & Holyoak, K. J. (1983). Schema induction and analogical transfer. *Cognitive Psychology, 15,* 1–38.

Grudin, J. (1980). Processes in verbal analogy solution. *Journal of Experimental Psychology: Human Perception and Performance, 6,* 67–74.

Hall, R. (in press). Computational approaches to analogical reasoning: A comparative analysis. *Artificial Intelligence.*

✔ Hesse, M. B. (1966). *Models and analogies in science.* Notre Dame, IN: University of Notre Dame Press.

Hofstadter, D. R. (1984). The Copycat project: An experiment in nondeterministic and creative analogies (Memo 755). Cambridge, MA: MIT, Artificial Intelligence Laboratory.

Hofstadter, D. R., Mitchell, T. M., & French, R. M. (1987). *Fluid concepts and creative analogies: A theory and its computer implementation* (Tech. Rep. 87–1). Ann Arbor: University of Michigan, Fluid Analogies Research Group.

Holyoak, K. J. (1985). The pragmatics of analogical transfer. In G. H. Bower (Ed.), *The psychology of learning and motivation* (Vol. 19, pp. 59–87). New York: Academic Press.

Holyoak, K. J., Junn, E. N., & Billman, D. O. (1984). Development of analogical problem-solving skill. *Child Development, 55,* 2042–2055.

Indurkhya, B. (1986). Constrained semantic transference: A formal theory of metaphors. *Synthese, 68,* 515–551.

Jacoby, L. L., & Brooks, L. R. (1984). Nonanalytic cognition: Memory, perception and concept learning. In G. H. Bower (Ed.), *The psychology of learning and motivation* (Vol. 18, pp. 1–47). New York: Academic Press.

Kedar-Cabelli, S. (1985, August). Purpose-directed analogy. *Proceedings of the Seventh Annual Conference of the Cognitive Science Society* (pp. 150–159), Irvine, CA.

Kedar-Cabelli, S. (1988). Analogy: From a unified perspective. In D. H. Helman (Ed.), *Analogical reasoning: Perspectives of artificial intelligence, cognitive science, and philosophy.* Boston: Reidel.

Keil, F., & Batterman, N. A. (1984). A characteristic-to-defining shift in the development of word meaning. *Journal of Verbal Learning and Verbal Behavior, 23,* 221–236.

Kemler, D. G. (1983). Holistic and analytical modes in perceptual and cognitive development. In T. J. Tighe & B. E. Shepp (Eds.), *Perception, cognition, and development: Interactional analysis* (pp. 77–102). Hillsdale, NJ: Erlbaum.

Kogan, N. (1975, April). *Metaphoric thinking in children: Developmental and individual-difference aspects.* Paper presented at the meeting of the Society for Research in Child Development, Denver, CO.

Larkin, J., McDermott, J., Simon, D. P., & Simon, H. A. (1980). Expert and novice performance in solving physics problems. *Science, 208,* 1335–1342.

Marr, D. (1982). *Vision.* San Francisco: Freeman.

Medin, D. L., & Schaffer, M. M. (1978). Context theory of classification learning. *Psychological Review, 85,* 207–238.

Miller, G. A. (1979). Images and models, similes and metaphors. In A. Ortony (Ed.), *Metaphor and thought* (pp. 202–250). Cambridge: Cambridge University Press.

Miller, G. A., Gallanter, E., & Pribram, K. H. (1960). *Plans and the structure of behavior.* New York: Holt, Rinehart & Winston.

Murphy, G. L., & Medin, D. L. (1985). The role of theories in conceptual coherence. *Psychological Review, 92,* 289–316.

Newport, E. L. (1984). Constraints on learning: Studies in the acquisition of American Sign Language. *Papers and Reports on Child Language Development, 23,* 1–22.

Norman, D. A., Rumelhart, D. E., & LNR Research Group (1975). *Explorations in cognition.* San Francisco: Freeman.

Novick, L. R. (1988). Analogical transfer, problem similarity, and expertise. *Journal of Experimental Psychology: Learning, Memory, and Cognition, 14,* 510–520.

Ortony, A. (1979). Beyond literal similarity. *Psychological Review, 86,* 161–180.

Palmer, S. E. (1978). Fundamental aspects of cognitive representation. In E. Rosch & B. B. Lloyd (Eds.), *Cognition and categorization* (pp. 259–302). Hillsdale, NJ: Erlbaum.

Palmer, S. E., & Kimchi, R. (1985). The information processing approach to cognition. In T. Knapp & L. C. Robertson (Eds.), *Approaches to cognition: Contrasts and controversies* (pp. 37–77). Hillsdale, NJ: Erlbaum.

Polya, G. (1954). *Induction and analogy in mathematics: Vol. 1. Of mathematics and plausible reasoning.* Princeton, NJ: Princeton University Press.

Rattermann, M. J., & Gentner, D. (1987). Analogy and similarity: Determinants of accessibility and inferential soundness. *Proceedings of the Ninth Annual Meeting of the Cognitive Science Society* (pp. 23–34), Seattle.

Reddy, D. R., Erman, L. D., Fennell, R. D., & Neely, R. B. (1973, August). HEARSAY Speech understanding system: An example of the recognition process. *Proceedings of the Third International Joint Conference on Artificial Intelligence* (pp. 185–193), Stanford University.

Reed, S. K. (1987). A structure-mapping model for word problems. *Journal of Experimental Psychology: Learning, Memory, and Cognition, 13,* 124–139.

Reed, S. K., & Ackinclose, C. C. (1986). *Selecting analogous solutions: Similarity vs. inclusiveness.* Unpublished manuscript, Florida Atlantic University, Boca Raton.

Reed, S. K., Ernst, G. W., & Banerji, R. (1974). The role of analogy in transfer between similar problem states. *Cognitive Psychology, 6,* 436–450.

Reynolds, R. E, & Ortony, A. (1980). Some issues in the measurement of children's comprehension of metaphorical language. *Child Development, 51,* 1110–1119.

Ross, B. H. (1984). Remindings and their effects in learning a cognitive skill. *Cognitive Psychology, 16,* 371–416.

Ross, B. H. (1987). This is like that: The use of earlier problems and the separation of similarity effects. *Journal of Experimental Psychology: Learning, Memory, and Cognition, 13,* 629–639.

Ross, B. H., & Sofka, M. D. (1986). *Remindings: Noticing, remembering, and using specific knowledge of earlier problems.* Unpublished manuscript, University of Illinois, Department of Psychology, Urbana-Champain.

Rumelhart, D. E., & Abrahamson, A. A. A. (1973). A model for analogical reasoning. *Cognitive Psychology, 5,* 1–28.

Rumelhart, D. E., & Norman, D. A. (1981). Analogical processes in learning. In J. R. Anderson (Ed.), *Cognitive skills and their acquisition* (pp. 335–339). Hillsdale, NJ: Erlbaum.

✓ Schank, R. C. (1982). *Dynamic memory.* Cambridge: Cambridge University Press.

✓ Schank, R. C., & Abelson, R. P. (1977). *Scripts, plans, goals, and understanding: An inquiry into human knowledge structures.* Hillsdale, NJ: Erlbaum.

Schumacher, R. M. (1987). *Similarity-based reminding: Effects of distance and encoding on retrieval.* Unpublished master's thesis, University of Illinois, Urbana-Champaign.

Schumacher, R., & Gentner, D. (in press). Transfer of training as analogical mapping. *Communications of the IEEE.*

✓ Shepp, B. E. (1978). From perceived similarity to dimensional structure: A new hypothesis about perceptual development. In E. Rosch & B. B. Lloyd (Eds.) *Cognition and categorization* (pp. 135–167). Hillsdale, NJ: Erlbaum.

Seigler, R. S. (1988). Mechanisms of cognitive growth: Variation and selection. In R. J. Sternberg (Ed.), *Mechanisms of cogitive development.* Prospect Heights, IL: Waveland Press.

Skorstad, J., Falkenhainer, B., & Gentner, D. (1987). Analogical processing: A simulation and empirical corroboration. *Proceedings of the American Association for Artificial Intelligence.* Seattle.

Skorstad, J., Gentner, D., & Medin, D. (1988). Abstraction processes during concept learning: A structural view. *Proceedings of the Tenth Annual Conference of the Cognitive Science Society,* Montreal.

Smith, L. B., & Kemler, D. G. (1977). Developmental trends in free classification: Evidence for a new conceptualization of perceptual development. *Journal of Experimental Child Psychology, 24,* 279–298.

Sternberg, R. J. (1977). Component processes in analogical reasoning. *Psychological Review, 84,* 353–378.

Thagard, P., & Holyoak, K. (1988, August). Analogical problem solving: A constraint satisfaction approach. *Proceedings of the Tenth Annual Conference of the Cognitive Science Society,* Montreal.

Thorndike, E. L. (1903). *Educational psychology.* New York: Lemcke & Buechner.

Tourangeau, R., & Sternberg, R. J. (1981). Aptness in metaphor. *Cognitive Psychology, 13,* 27–55.

Tversky, A. (1977). Features of similarity. *Psychological Review, 84,* 327–352.

Van Lehn, K., & Brown, J. S. (1980). Planning nets: A representation for formalizing analogies and semantic models of procedural skills. In R. E. Snow, P. A. Federico, & W. E. Montague (Eds.), *Aptitude, learning, and instruction: Cognitive process analyses* (Vol. 2, pp. 95–137). Hillsdale, NJ: Erlbaum.

Verbrugge, R. R., & McCarrell, N.S. (1977). Metaphoric comprehension: Studies in reminding and resembling. *Cognitive Psychology, 9*, 494–533.

Vosniadou, S. & Ortony, A. (1986). Testing the metaphoric competence of the young child: Paraphrase versus enactment. *Human Development, 29*, 226–230.

Waldrop, M. (1987). Causality, structure, and common sense. *Science, 237*, 1297–1299.

Wattenmaker, W. D., Nakamura, G. V., & Medin, D. L. (1986). *Relationships between similarity-based and explanation-based categorization.* Unpublished manuscript, University of Illinois, Department of Psychology, Urbana-Champaign.

Winston, P. H. (1980). Learning and reasoning by analogy. *Communications of the Association for Computing Machinery, 23*, 689–703.

Winston, P. H. (1982). Learning new principles from precedents and exercises. *Artificial Intelligence, 19*, 321–350.

8

A computational model of analogical problem solving

KEITH J. HOLYOAK and PAUL R. THAGARD

The power of human intelligence depends on the growth of knowledge through experience, coupled with flexibility in accessing and exploiting prior knowledge to deal with novel situations. These global characteristics of intelligence must be reflected in theoretical models of the human cognitive system (Holland, Holyoak, Nisbett, & Thagard, 1986). The core of a cognitive architecture (i.e., a theory of the basic components of human cognition) consists of three subsystems: a problem-solving system, capable of drawing inferences to construct plans for attaining goals; a memory system, which can be searched in an efficient manner to identify information relevant to the current problem; and an inductive system, which generates new knowledge structures to be stored in memory so as to increase the subsequent effectiveness of the problem-solving system.

These three subsystems are, of course, highly interdependent; consequently, the best proving ground for theories of cognition will be the analysis of skills that reflect the interactions among problem solving, memory, and induction. One such skill is analogical problem solving – the use of a solution to a known source problem to develop a solution to a novel target problem. At the most general level, analogical problem solving involves three steps, each of which raises difficult theoretical problems (Holyoak, 1984, 1985). The first step involves accessing a plausibly useful analog in memory. It is particularly difficult to identify candidate analogs when they are concealed in a large memory system, and when the source and target were encountered in different contexts and have many salient dissimilarities. These theoretical issues are closely related to those raised in Schank's (1982) discussion of "reminding." The second step is to adapt the source analog to the requirements of the target problem. Since in realistic analogies the correspondences, or mapping, between the source and target will be imperfect, transfer from the former to the latter must be selective and subject to revision; indeed, the attempted analogy may finally be abandoned as unhelpful. Finally, the third step is to induce new knowledge structures that summarize the useful commonalities between the source and target that have been discovered, a process we will refer to as *schema formation*. The successful use of an analogy provides an opportunity for the induction of general knowledge that will make it easier to solve other similar problems.

In this chapter we will describe a model of analogical problem solving embedded within a cognitive architecture intended to capture some of the flexibility of human intelligence. The analogical problem-solving model is part of a larger effort in which we have been investigating problem solving and learning in the context of a computer program called PI, for *processes of induction* (Holland et al., 1986; Thagard & Holyoak, 1985). The general aim is to integrate a set of learning mechanisms with a set of performance mechanisms for solving problems and generating explanations. This goal is one we share with other investigators, such as Anderson (1983) and Rosenbloom and Newell (1986). As a computational model of analogical problem solving, PI is related to several earlier efforts in artificial intelligence (Burstein, 1986; Carbonell, 1983, 1986; Evans, 1968; Kedar-Cabelli, 1985; Winston, 1980, 1982). We will describe some of the similarities and differences between PI and other models of cognition and analogy as we proceed.

The PI model represents a preliminary attempt to develop a computational account of major aspects of human cognition. We believe that computer simulation will play a crucial role in both the development and the testing of theories that address complex cognitive tasks such as analogical problem solving. Performance of such tasks involves the dynamic interplay of multiple subsystems; the resulting interactions make it extremely difficult to derive the implications of theoretical assumptions by more traditional formal methods. In the case of PI, development of the simulation has been guided by several design principles that we believe characterize the human cognitive system, based on what is known about human problem solving, memory, and induction (Holland et al., 1986). We will first describe these general design principles and then provide an overview of the architecture of PI.

Design principles for a cognitive architecture

Integrated knowledge representations

Analysis of a process as complex as analogical problem solving requires a cognitive architecture with diverse knowledge representations that are nevertheless integrated into a coherent whole. At a minimum, such an architecture needs ways of representing simple factual information corresponding to propositions such as "Lassie is a dog," as well as ways of representing general rulelike information such as "Dogs have fur." In addition, it is necessary to represent general concepts, such as *dog* and *fur* and to provide structures for representing complex problems to be related by analogy.

As we will see in much more detail, PI uses declarative structures called concepts to integrate these kinds of knowledge. For example, both information about what individuals are dogs and rules about the general properties of dogs are stored with the concept *dog*. In addition, problems concerning dogs can be represented by knowledge structures that are associated with the concept *dog*. This form of integrated representation contrasts with both the SOAR system of Rosenbloom and Newell (1986), which represents all long-term knowledge as rules, and the ACT* system of Anderson (1983), which segregates declarative and rule knowledge in separate memory systems. The integrated representations used by PI are intended to allow the operation of specific problem-solving mechanisms, described below, and the generation of new structures by inductive mechanisms.

Bidirectional search

Analyses of problem-solving protocols indicate that people use two basic types of search processes to achieve their goals: forward search from the elements of the problem situation to find possible actions, and backward search from the goal to possible actions and preconditions that could achieve it (Duncker, 1945). The forward-search process corresponds to the question "Given the materials at hand, what could be done with them?" whereas the backward-search process corresponds to the question "Given the current goal, how could it be achieved?" In PI, both forward and backward searches are conducted concurrently using condition–action rules, as will be described below.

Bidirectional search requires some degree of parallelism in the use of knowledge. More generally, in a novel problem situation it is unlikely that any single unit of knowledge will prescribe an optimal solution. Flexible problem solving depends upon the coordination of multiple pieces of knowledge, each of which is to some degree relevant to the current situation. Rule-based systems can allow both complementary and contradictory inferences to emerge in parallel. For example, an instance of the category *dog* might match the rules "If x is a dog, then x is black" and "if x is a dog, then x can bark," which complement each other; in addition, it might also match the rule "If *x* is a dog, then *x* is brown," which contradicts the first inference. When conflicting inferences arise, their resolution can be postponed until the bottleneck in the system, such as competition for control of effectors (i.e., the need to perform some single overt action), forces a decision to be made (Holland, 1986; Rosenbloom & Newell, 1986). PI incorporates simulation of this sort of parallelism in the activity of rules and other knowledge structures, a design feature that is important for flexible retrieval of analogs from memory.

Rule-directed spreading activation

A cognitive architecture must incorporate mechanisms that address two competing requirements: the need for wide-ranging and rapid search of a large body of information in long-term memory, and the need to focus attention primarily on the knowledge most relevant to the current problem. These requirements are particularly evident in the retrieval of candidate analogs. If the initial search is too narrow, useful candidates will be missed; but unless the output of the search is suitably restricted, the system will be swamped with a multitude of potential analogies, virtually all of which would in fact be useless.

PI, like various previous models (Anderson, 1983; Collins & Quillian, 1969), uses a relatively diffuse spreading activation process to retrieve information related to the current situation. However, because of the system's integrated knowledge representations and parallel rule activity, the nature of the postulated activation process differs from most comparable proposals. In systems such as ACT*, activation spreads through a declarative semantic network independently of rule activity. Anderson (1983) argues that this independence is required so that spreading activation does not compete with the use of rules to perform other system functions. Although this argument applies to systems such as ACT* that allow only one rule at a time to fire, it is much less relevant to systems such as PI in which rules can operate in parallel. In PI, activation is passed through the memory system as a side effect of rule activity: When a rule is fired, the concepts mentioned in the rule receive a boost in their activation levels, which is in turn relayed to the rules attached to the newly activated concepts. Since matching is attempted only for activated rules, the activation process sharply reduces the number of rules that must be considered on each cycle as candidates for firing. This feature also contrasts with ACT*, in which matching is performed with all rules in the system on each cycle.

The use of rule-directed activation, similar to the mechanism proposed by Thibadeau, Just, and Carpenter (1982), is intended to increase the expected relevance of activated information to the current problem, since the problem representation will determine the initial rules that are fired and hence the further concepts that are activated. As we shall see, this type of retrieval process allows features of the target problem to serve as retrieval cues for source analogs stored with concepts that can be reached via rules related to the target. An activation criterion is used to "gate" the transmission of activated examples to the mechanism that attempts a mapping with the target. Furthermore, as we shall see, a trace of the activation process is used to initiate mapping, linking the steps of retrieving a source analog and mapping it with the target.

Rule matching augmented with analogical mapping

A design criterion directly related to analogical problem solving within a rule-based system concerns the proper relationship between the use of stored analogical examples to solve problems and the direct use of condition–action rules for this purpose. This issue has generally been evaded in theoretical proposals: Most problem-solving models have given analogy short shrift, which models of analogy have typically returned in kind by dealing with analogy in isolation from other problem-solving mechanisms (exceptions include Carbonell, 1983).

In computational terms, the difference between rule firing and analogy use corresponds to that between matching and mapping. In a rule-based system, a rule is selected for firing when elements in working memory match the elements of the rule's condition (or of its action, in systems such as PI that also use rules for backward search). A match requires either that the elements be identical or that the condition element be a variable of which the working-memory element is an instantiation. In contrast, an analogical mapping requires generation of correspondences between elements that have differences – the elements are neither identical nor in a prespecified instance–variable relation. For example, if a system contains the rule "If x is a cat, then x purrs," and the proposition "Scruffy is a cat" is in working memory, then the rule will be matched and the conclusion "Scruffy purrs" will be inferred. In contrast, suppose the above rule were not available, but a representation of the fact that Fluffy, another cat, is known to purr is stored in memory. In this situation the fact that Scruffy is a cat will not produce a match to a rule about purring; however, the common category may serve as a basis of similarity with

Fluffy (even if Scruffy is black whereas Fluffy is white). If the two instances are perceived as similar, Scruffy could be mapped with Fluffy, and the property *purrs* could be transferred by analogy from the source to the target to yield the same conclusion as above.

Even in such a simple example, it is apparent that analogical mapping is more cognitively demanding than rule matching. The rule made a general claim that cats purr, without referring to any additional properties, such as color. Accordingly, the fact that Scruffy is black was rendered irrelevant to the matching process in advance. In contrast, the mapping between black Scruffy and white Fluffy required that the system first pair the two despite the discrepant property, then tentatively decide (explicitly or implicitly) that color probably does not influence the likelihood that a cat will purr, and finally transfer the property of purring despite the difference between the source and target. The difficulty of the mapping process will be greater when the mapped elements do not belong to salient common categories and only abstract relations are similar, as will be the case for analogies drawn between different domains.

In general, then, we might expect to find that analogical mapping is used as a "backup" mode of problem solving, most likely to be invoked when the problem at hand does not match preexisting generalized rules. We would expect analogy to be used often by the novice in a domain, who may use analogies between highly similar problems in lieu of applicable rules. Analogy is also likely to be used by experts grappling with problems, such as theory development, that go beyond routine problem solving. Because experts will represent their target problems in terms of relatively abstract concepts (Chi, Feltovich, & Glaser, 1981), they may be more likely to activate relatively remote source analogs.

It need not be the case, however, that rule matching will totally override analogical matching when both are possible. If an activated source analog provides a specific and efficient solution procedure, whereas the only matched rules embody a relatively inefficient general solution procedure, use of the analogy may be preferable. It follows that analogical mapping may provide not only a backup mechanism when rule matching fails to find a solution but also a competing mechanism to be continuously exploited. At the same time, the two mechanisms can also complement each other. Often an analogy need not provide a complete solution to the target problem; rather, it is sufficient if some missing component required to achieve a solution can be transferred, allowing the interrupted process of rule firing to restart and possibly succeed. In general, the use of analogy is highly opportunistic, to be invoked when a stored problem becomes highly active as a side effect of the system's attempting to achieve a solution by matching and firing rules. The PI model of analogical problem solving attempts to embody the opportunistic use of analogy within a rule-based system.

Analogy as a trigger for induction

An obvious consequence of the computational advantages of rule matching over analogical mapping is that it is desirable to induce generalized rules that effectively summarize the commonalities between the source and target after an analogy has been used successfully to transfer a problem solution. Winston (1980) introduced the notion that analogy use is an occasion for generalization, and PI maintains this link. In addition to generating new rules by intersecting the categories and properties of mapped elements, PI also forms more general concepts to which the new rules are attached. Representations of specific problem examples, with stored solutions, are used to induce more abstract "problem schemas" along with generalized rules.

The triggering of inductions in the aftermath of analogical problem solving is an instance of a more general design principle: New knowledge structures should be induced in the course of problem solving in response to specific conditions of the system. In order to avoid overloading memory with useless structures it is necessary to constrain induction so that what is induced is likely to contribute to future problem solutions (Holland et al., 1986). If induction is triggered during problem solving, it will be relatively likely that the products of induction are relevant to the system's goals (because certain goals are currently active), and it will be relatively likely that the knowledge on which the induction is based is similarly relevant (because this knowledge has been activated in response to the problem representation).

Problem-solving activity is also a major source of feedback regarding the utility of the knowledge structures currently in the system. PI, like the classifier systems of Holland (1986) and Anderson's (1983) ACT*, represent the utility of rules by a strength parameter that can be revised in accord with feedback. If a rule helps to solve a problem it should be strengthened, so that it is more likely to be used in the future; conversely, a rule that leads to a dead end should be weakened. Given the rule-directed nature of spreading activation, the revision of rule strength will alter the pattern of activation generated during subsequent problem-solving episodes. It follows that feedback regarding the efficacy of rules will serve to "train" the direction of thought indirectly.

The architecture of PI

In this section we will provide a more specific overview of the architecture of the PI system. In PI, various inductive mechanisms are embedded within a problem-solving system. In the course of problem solving, several kinds of inductive inference are performed, including forms of generalization, concept formation, and abduction (inference to explanatory hypotheses). As described above, PI uses an integrated representation scheme, employing both condition–action rules as in such systems as ACT* (Anderson, 1983) and SOAR (Rosenbloom & Newell, 1986), as well as "concepts" similar to Minsky's (1975) frames. The concepts provide a means both of storing simple factual knowledge and of organizing rules together into useful clusters. Thus PI has both declarative and procedural knowledge organized into schemalike units. The propositionlike structures in PI that correspond to the "facts" of ACT* are called "messages" (Holland, 1986) to emphasize that they serve to transmit information within the system. Examples of these structures will follow.

PI simulates parallelism by allowing any number of production rules to fire at once. At any time, however, only a limited number of rules – those attached to active concepts – are active. Activation of concepts spreads in a manner directed by problem solving: Concepts mentioned in actions of fired rules become active, making available rules employing those concepts. The rule-firing process is essentially forward-chaining from starting conditions to goals, but there is also a process of spreading activation of concepts back from the goal via subgoals to the starting conditions, simulating a bidirectional search. Activation spreads through the system by the following cycle:

1. Active concepts make their associated rules and messages available for matching. Initially, the active concepts are those mentioned in the starting conditions and goals of the given problem. For example, if the problem is to get Rover the dog to fetch a newspaper, the concepts of *dog fetch*, and *newspaper* will all be activated, and rules and messages attached to them become available.
2. The conditions of active rules are matched against the active messages, and a preset number are selected for firing. If the number of matched rules exceeds the criterion number, the "best" rules are selected on the basis of three factors: strength, which is a measure of past usefulness; degree of activation, which is a function of the activation of the concepts to which a rule is attached; and direct

relevance to accomplishing a goal, which favors selection of rules with actions that would immediately accomplish a current goal. In addition, effector rules – ones that would lead to some physical action – are checked for conflicts, such as moving to both the right and the left at the same time. In the case of conflicting effector rules, only the one that scores highest on the three factors just mentioned is fired. An effector rule initiates a projection, which indicates that a possible strategy is being explored and that inferences from projected actions are to be made only tentatively.

3. The actions of the selected rules are carried out, creating new messages. For example, if the rule "If x is a dog, then x has a tail" is selected for firing because of its successful match against the message that Rover is a dog, then the message that Rover has a tail will be posted.

4. The new set of messages is checked against the list of goals to be accomplished. If all goals are accomplished, the problem is solved, the rule that started the successful projection is rewarded with an increase in strength. If messages show that a projection has led to violation of one of the goals of the problem, then the projection is stopped and the strength of the rule that initiated it is decreased.

5. The concepts mentioned in the actions of fired rules become active. In the example of Rover, firing the rule that dogs have tails will activate the concept *tail*.

6. Concepts not used on this time step have their degree of activation decremented, and those that drop below a certain threshold become inactive, along with their attached rules.

7. Inductions are triggered, based on the currently active concepts, messages, and rules.

8. Return to 1.

Problem solving in PI involves a continuous process of recategorization, since the activation of new concepts provides new sets of rules that can be applied to the current situation. The set of rules available for firing changes constantly as concepts gain and lose activation. Moreover, the various learning mechanisms can augment the rules and concepts available. By contrast, in ACT* the definition of the search space is constant, since the same set of production rules is always available for firing. SOAR is able to enter multiple problem spaces in the course of a solution attempt, but the problem space for the target problem itself is fixed, except for the possible addition of rules by a mechanism termed *chunking*.

Analogical problem solving in PI

We will now discuss the way in which PI's mechanism of rule-directed spreading activation can be used to model analogical problem solving. The model addresses the three key issues alluded to above: (a) How, in the course of solving a problem, does the system retrieve relevant existing problem solutions? (b) How, once a relevant problem solution is found, does the system exploit the analogy between the source and target? (c) How does the system induce more general knowledge structures from a successful analogical solution?

The radiation problem and convergence analogs

We are currently using PI in an attempt to model a set of experimental results on analogical problem solving obtained by Gick and Holyoak (1980, 1983) using the "radiation problem" first studied by Duncker (1945). The radiation problem consists of figuring out how to use a ray source to destroy a tumor inside a patient, when it is known that radiation at full strength will destroy healthy tissue between the source and the tumor, leading to the death of the patient.

Subjects have great difficulty coming up with a solution to this problem, but their performance is greatly improved when they are first told of an analogous problem. In the "fortress problem" provided in the experimental work of Gick and Holyoak, a general must find a way for his army to capture a fortress when a frontal attack by the whole army is impossible. One solution is to split the army and have it attack the fortress from different sides.

The above solution to the fortress problem suggests an analogous solution for the ray problem, which is to irradiate the tumor with lower-intensity rays from different directions. Gick and Holyoak (1980) demonstrated that variations in an available source analog (a story describing an analogous problem and its solution) can lead subjects to generate qualitatively different solutions to the target. Across many comparable experiments, Gick and Holyoak found that about 75% of college students tested generated the "convergence" solution described above after receiving the corresponding story analog and a hint to apply it. In contrast, only about 10% of students generated this solution in the absence of a source analog, even though most subjects agreed that the solution is an effective one once it was described to them.

Gick and Holyoak also found a striking gap between people's ability to apply the analogy when led to do so by the experimenter and their ability to do so spontaneously. Whereas about 75% of the subjects in a typical experiment are able to generate the convergence solution to the ray problem given a hint to use the prior story, only about 30% generate this solution prior to receiving an explicit hint. The fact that about 10% of subjects produce the convergence solution without any analog indicates that only about 20% of the subjects spontaneously notice and apply the analogy. This finding emphasizes the difficulty of the initial retrieval step for analogies in which there is little surface similarity between the source and target domains.

Solving the radiation problem using PI

We now have running a highly simplified simulation of the solution of the radiation problem using the fortress analogy. The structures used in the simulation include messages, concepts, rules, and problems. For example, the information that an entity called *obj1* is an army is represented by the message:

(army (obj1) true)

Like expressions in predicate calculus, messages can also be used to represent relational facts, such as "obj1 is near obj2." Besides *true*, messages can also include the values *false*, *projected-to-be-true*, and *projected-to-be-false*.

The concept *army* is represented as a set of complex features:

ARMY

data type:	concept
superordinates:	organization
subordinates:	
instances:	(army (obj1) true)
activation:	1
activated by:	
rules:	R1, R2, R3

The superordinate slot indicates that any army is a kind of organization, and the instances slot is used to store the message that obj1 is an army. The rules that are listed in the rules slot includes structures such as the following:

R1

data type:	rule
attached concepts:	army
activation:	1
status:	default
strength:	.8
topic:	movement

conditions:	(army ($x) true)
	(between ($y $x $z) true)
	(road ($y) true)
actions:	· (move-to ($x $z) true effect)

This rule says that, if x is an army and y is a road between x and some z, then x can move to z. As should be apparent, the message (army (obj1) true) can serve to match the condition (army ($x) true). (In simulation with a larger knowledge base, this rule would be replaced by a more general rule about moving groups of people, which would apply following the inference that armies are groups of people.)

CAPTURE FORTRESS

data type:	problem
start:	(army (obj1) true)
	(fortress (obj2) true)
	(road (obj3) true)
	(between (obj3 obj1 obj2) true)
goals:	(capture (obj1 obj2) true)
	(destroyed (obj1) false)
	rules fired in solution
	rules subgoaled in solution
	effectors used in solution
	activation

Given an army, a fortress, and roads between them, the problem is to capture the fortress without destroying the army. In the course of solution attempts, various information is collected concerning what rules and effectors have been used in the solution attempt. Similarly, the problem of destroying a tumor has the following starting conditions and goals:

DESTROY TUMOR

data type:	problem
start:	(radiation (obj4) true)
	(tumor (obj5) true)
	(flesh (obj6) true)
	(patient (obj7) true)
	(alive (obj7) true)
	(between (obj6 obj4 obj5) true)
	(inside (obj5 obj7) true)
goals:	(alive (obj7) true)
	(destroy (obj4 obj5) true)

Our current simulation uses these structures to model analogical problem solving and schema formation in terms of the following seven steps:

1. First, the source problem (here the fortress problem) must be

solved. Initially, the above rule, R1, initiates a projected move of the army directly to the fortress, but an additional rule produces the inference that moving an army to a fortress brings about destruction of the army. So R1 is punished with a decrease in strength, and the projection is stopped. Another rule indicating that armies may be split into divisions that can move separately to a target, is then fired, starting a new projection that leads to solution of the problem. The problem structure CAPTURE FORTRESS is then associated with concepts mentioned in its problem description. In the above example, these include the concepts of *army*, *fortress*, *between*, *road*, and *destroy*. For example, the *army* concept adds the slot: problem solutions: capture fortress. The structure CAPTURE FORTRESS now includes effector actions used to generate the solution; in the case of the fortress problem, these include splitting up the army and moving its divisions separately to the fortress.

2. Second, solution of the target problem (here the radiation problem) is attempted. This initiates rule-directed spreading activation in two directions: forward by rule firing from concepts mentioned in the starting conditions of the target problem, and backward from the concepts mentioned in the goal conditions. If the problem is readily solved by direct use of rules, analogy will not come into play. In our simulation, however, the attempted solution of shooting rays directly at the tumor is found to be unsuccessful, because it results in destruction of intervening flesh and leads to the death of the patient.

3. In the third step of analogical problem solving, the process of rule firing leads to activation of concepts to which the fortress problem has been attached. For example, the concept *between* occurs in the starting conditions of both problems, conferring some activation on the fortress problem that has been stored with it. One association, however, is not sufficient to bring the activation of the fortress problem up to a threshold by invoking analogical mapping. Having such a threshold is essential in order to limit attempts at analogical problem solving to solutions that have a higher degree of potential relevance. PI detects such relevance in the current case because of an association between *destroy* in the tumor problem and *capture* in the fortress problem. This association is found as the result of subgoaling, using rules that produce the following chain of subgoals: Destroying can be brought about by overcoming, which can be brought about by seizing, which can be brought about by capturing. Because the problem CAPTURE FORTRESS is associated with the newly activated concept *capture* as well as the concept *between*, it accumulates sufficient activation to trigger analogical problem solving. (If more than one stored prob-

lem exceeds the activation threshold, the one with highest activation and therefore presumably most relevance is tried first.)

Exploitation of an analogy requires noticing correspondences between the two problems and figuring out how to use key steps in the solution to the source problem to suggest a solution to the target. The fourth and fifth steps involve setting up a mapping between the two problem solutions that highlights the analogous components.

4. PI begins to derive a mapping from the record of spreading activation by determining what concepts were responsible for the activation of any newly activated concept. The mapping between the identical relations in the two problems, *between* and *between,* is immediate; the program also traces back from *capture* to determine that the initial source of activation was *destroy* and therefore postulates that the goal of destroying something in the radiation problem and the goal of capturing something in the fortress problem are analogous elements. The activation path linking *capture* and *destroy* involved intervening concepts, but *destroy* is the only concept that was directly activated as part of the target problem description, and hence it is selected as the element to be mapped with *capture* in the source.

5. In an analogy between problems from disparate domains, it is unlikely that a complete mapping can be recovered by tracing activation records, because only a few similar elements will have contributed to the initial reminding process. In the fifth step, the mapping is extended by using the constraints provided by the initial partial mapping. For example, because the fourth step succeeded in mapping from the concept *capture* to the concept *destroy,* in the fifth step the program maps the corresponding arguments of these relations, for example, the particular army with the particular radiation and the fortress with the tumor.

Here is what PI's output looks like after the above analysis is completed:

> Analogy found between CAPTURE FORTRESS and DESTROY TUMOR
>
> | | |
> |---|---|
> | analogous concepts: | (capture destroy) (between between). |
> | analogous objects: | (obj1 obj4) (obj2 obj5) |
> | source effectors; | (split (obj1) true) |
> | | (move-separately-to (obj1 obj2) true)[1] |
> | new subgoals: | (split (obj4) true) |
> | | (move-separately-to (obj4 obj5) true) |

6. Establishment of the analogous components makes possible the sixth step, performing analogous actions in the target problem. As described above, PI stores with a problem solution a list of effectors

– the actions that were projected to lead to the solution of the problem if they were performed. In the case of the fortress problem, the effectors included the splitting of the army and the separate movements of the resulting groups to the fortress. Using the already established mapping, PI then hypothesizes that a solution to the radiation problem might be found by accomplishing the two subgoals of splitting the focus of the radiation and moving the resulting components separately to the target. At this point, the attempt to solve the radiation problem by the standard processes of rule firing and spreading activation is resumed. The new subgoals now provide a decomposition of the previously ill-structured radiation problem.

Note that the analogy with the fortress problem does not and need not provide a complete solution to the radiation problem. There are important dissimilarities between the two problems: In the fortress problem the constraint is to prevent the army from being destroyed, whereas in the tumor problem the constraint concerns keeping the patient alive. Nonetheless, by triggering generation of new subgoals, the analogy allows the system to recover from an impasse caused by failure to find any possible path toward a solution

PI is currently unable to assess in any detail the degree to which a source analog is contributing to the solution of the target, short of a complete solution being achieved. However, if problem solving is stymied after the analogical transfer, in that no new rules are being fired then the analogy has clearly ceased to be productive. PI then deactivates the source analog and swiches to consideration of the next most active stored problem solution. PI will also switch from one analog to another if spreading activation leads to the second analog becoming more active as the result of additional rule firing and subgoaling. For example, if the attempt to solve the radiation problem eventually led to greater activation of a problem other than the fortress problem, then that new problem would become the focus of analogical problem solving.

7. If an analogy leads to the solution of the new problem, then PI generalizes from the two solutions to form an abstract problem schema. It compares the respective startng points, goals, and effector actions of the two problem solutions in order to see if a more general characterization is possible. The analogical mapping between the radiation problem and the fortress problem suggests a link between (a) using a radiation source to destroy a tumor, and (b) using an army to capture a fortress. PI finds the abstraction: using a force to overcome a target. The abstraction is made by examining analogous concepts and checking to see if they have rules that indicate they have a higher-

order concept in common. For example, the concepts *destroy* and *capture* get generalized to *overcome*, by virtue of rules indicating that both destroying and capturing are kinds of overcoming. Thus PI abstracts from the two problems to produce the following problem schema:

CAPTURE FORTRESS/DESTROY TUMOR

data type:	problem
start:	(between ($y $x $z) true)
goals:	(overcome ($x $z) true)
effectors used	
in solution:	(split ($x) true effect)

In general terms, the above schema states that if you want x to overcome z, and some y is between the two, then you might try splitting x. Once this schema is in place, stored with the concepts *between* and *overcome*, activation of those concepts can lead to future attempts to use the schema analogically. To sum up, Figure 8.1 provides a general schematic view of the process of problem solving in PI.

Limitations of PI

The program PI, which runs in FranzLISP on a Pyramid 90x minicomputer, has proven valuable for developing and testing the basic ideas described above concerning spreading activation, analogy retrieval, and rule formation. But we must stress that the examples on which PI has so far been tested are very small and highly simplified. Our largest simulation of analogical problem solving so far has used only 52 concepts, 53 rules, and 5 problem solutions, capturing only a tiny fraction of the knowledge that people have about armies and tumors. Conspicuously lacking in PI's current knowledge base is an understanding of space and time. For example, PI uses the concept *between*, but its only knowledge of what this means is contained in a rule that says that if x is between y and z, and w is at the same location as x, the w is also between y and z. Other kinds of knowledge, such as that concerning the splitting of armies and of rays, are also highly simplified; such procedures need to be represented in much more detail. Now that the program is running, we plan to construct a much larger and less ad hoc knowledge base that will allow a more thorough test of our model of analogical problem solving.

Comparison with previous models of analogy

We will now compare the PI model of analogical problem solving to some earlier models of analogical reasoning in terms of the three

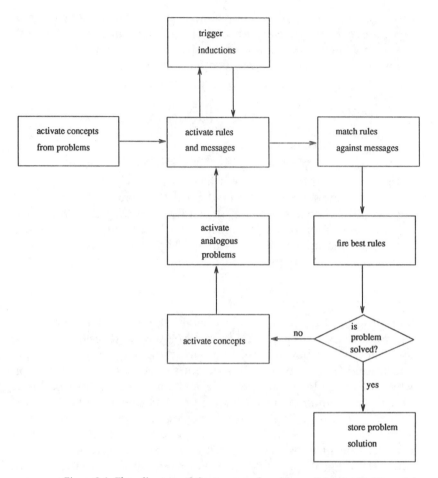

Figure 8.1. Flow diagram of the process of problem solving in the PI model.

broad stages of analogy use: selection of a source analog, adaptation of information provided by the source to the requirements of the target, and subsequent induction of new knowledge structures.

Many models of analogy have evaded serious examination of the initial step, selection of a source analog, by simply assuming that a teacher provides a source analog and indicates its relevance to the target (e.g., Burstein, 1986). Others have, like PI, used the description of the target to guide the search for analogs. Winston (1980), in a discussion of analogies between story scenarios, proposed that source analogs are selected using a similarity metric based on generalizations shared with objects in the target (e.g., if a man appears in the target, then a source that includes a man will be preferred). This scheme appears to lack constraints derived from the goals involved in the target and potential source analogs. Carbonell (1983) suggested that problem analogies are retrieved by an indexing scheme based on initial states, goal states, and solution constraints. PI's retrieval mechanism, which is controlled by activation triggered by concepts used in the representation of the target problem, is akin to Carbonell's proposal. In PI, however, there is no explicit search for source analogs; rather, stored problems related to the current target are activated as a side effect of rule activity directed toward solving the target problem. Because rule activity allows activation to spread forward from individual concepts in the representation of the target, it would appear that PI's activation process is likely to evoke a broader set of associated structures than would a search process based solely on the more constrained indexes suggested by Carbonell (1983).

In the second step in analogy use, adapting the source to the target, most attention has been paid to deciding what information in the source to transfer to the target. In this regard PI's pragmatic approach to analogy use contrasts with the more syntactic approach advocated by Gentner (1983, and this volume). Gentner proposes that the information transferred from a source to a target analog is constrained by a preference ordering based on the syntax of logical form: one-place predicates (i.e., simple features) are not transferred, two-place predicates (relations) tend to be transferred, and higher-order predicates (relations of relations) are most likely to be transferred. Information that participates in a highly interconnected cluster involving higher-order predicates is especially favored for selection (the "systematicity" principle).

In contrast, PI does not base its selection of source elements to be transferred on such syntactic criteria. Rather, the subgoal-transfer mechanism insures that elements of the source problem that proved important in providing a solution are transferred over to the target problem. Especially for interdomain analogies, which do not share surface features, relations will necessarily provide crucial links between the source and target. However, functional relevance to a solution applicable to the source is paramount in selecting information for transfer. Compatible proposals include those of Winston (1980), who emphasized the primacy of causal relations; Carbonell (1983, 1986), who focused on transfer of information derived from solution traces; and Kedar-Cabelli (1985), who suggested that elements of the source linked to its "purpose" provide the basis for transfer. (See Holyoak, 1985, and Johnson-Laird, this volume, for critiques of purely syntactic approaches to analogy.)

PI differs from previous models of analogy in the close connection it postulates between the retrieval of a potential source analog and the initiation of analogical mapping. The activation-tracing mechanism allows the knowledge that led to activation of the source to guide the initial construction of a mapping between its conceptual elements and those of the target. The mapping is developed further by pairing the corresponding arguments in relations that have already been mapped. The mapping can improve as processing continues, because additional activation paths between the source and target may be found through chains of rule firing or subgoaling that take more time to develop than the chains that first established a connection. PI's mapping process uses knowledge-based constraints to eliminate the need for exhaustive tests of possible mappings (Winston, 1980). These constraints are of a more "bottom-up" nature, however, than those postulated in models such as that of Kedar-Cabelli (1985), which use preexisting abstractions in the form of explicit "purposes" to guide the mapping process.

Work on analogical transfer has paid less attention to mechanisms that would allow an imperfect analogy to be adapted to the requirements of the target subsequent to the initial mapping. Burstein (1986) suggested that multiple source analogs may increase a learner's understanding of the target domain, and Carbonell (1983) outlined an array of heuristics for transforming a problem solution generated by analogy. PI's lack of explicit mechanisms for rethinking an analogical mapping and doing explicit causal analysis is undoubtedly a limitation of the current model.

The third and final general step in analogical problem solving is induction of new structures. PI produces problem schemata by abstraction of the mapped concepts in the source and target. Winston (1980) introduced a generalization-by-intersection mechanism of this type to account for learning by analogy. Such generalization from multiple examples contrasts with work in artificial intelligence on generalization from single cases (DeJong, 1982). "Explanation-based" generalization, as the latter type is termed, depends on the exploitation of detailed prior knowledge of the domain. In contrast, PI has so far been used to model the solution of novel types of problems by relatively naive learners who would lack sufficient knowledge to generalize in an optimal fashion from a single case. Empirical studies of college students solving the radiation problem by analogy clearly in-

dicate that multiple examples are very important in producing transfer (Gick & Holyoak, 1983), supporting our focus on generalization
by intersection. However, it seems likely that humans also make use
of more knowledge-dependent constraints on generalization when
such knowledge is in fact available.

A computational framework for empirical findings

We have not yet attempted to simulate the full range of experimental
findings involving the use of analogy to solve the radiation problem.
Nonetheless, it is possible to provide within our computational framework a qualitative account of many findings, including the importance
of hints, the effectiveness of analogical schemata, and the different
processing effects of surface and structural similarities.

The efficacy of hints

As we mentioned earlier, subjects often have much more difficulty in
discovering the relevance of a source analog than in using the analog
once its relevance has been pointed out (Gick & Holyoak, 1980). Why
this is so can easily be explained on the basis of PI's retrieval mechanisms. An explicit hint to use a source analog will eliminate the need
for the diffuse spreading activation process to retrieve the source from
long-term memory; instead, search for a mapping can be initiated
immediately. Without a hint, analogs drawn from different domains
may have few common elements to serve as potential links between
the target and source, so that reminding will often not occur.

Schema formation

Another major class of findings provides evidence that transfer is
facilitated when subjects have the opportunity to form more generalized schematic representations of categories of problems. In particular, analogs drawn from remote domains are more likely to be
noticed spontaneously if multiple source analogs are provided (cf.
Spiro, Feltovich, Coulson, & Anderson, this volume). Gick and Holyoak (1983) had some groups of subjects first read two convergence
stories, whereas other groups read a single convergence story plus a
disanalogous story. All subjects summarized each story and also wrote
descriptions of how the two stories were similar. The latter task was
intended to trigger a mapping between the two stories, which would
have the incidental effect of leading to the induction of an explicit

representation of the shared schematic structure. All subjects then attempted to solve the radiation problem, both before and after a hint to consider the stories. Gick and Holyoak found that subjects in the two-analog groups were significantly more likely to produce the convergence solution, both before and after the hint, than were subjects in the one-analog groups. Gick and Holyoak interpreted these and other more detailed results as indicating that induction of an explicit schema facilitates transfer.

The importance of schemata in mediating transfer across disparate domains can be readily understood in terms of the kind of schema formation performed by PI. A problem schema is a structure of the same sort as the specific problems that give rise to it. It will, however, be more easily retrieved than the specific problems, because of the greater generality of its concepts. The schema formed from the radiation and fortress problems will be activated by new problems that spread activation to the concepts *force*, *target*, and *overcome*, which will be accomplished more easily than spreading activation from a substantially novel problem to more specific concepts such as *army* or *radiation*. Because the schema has eliminated problem-specific details, it will be more similar to individual convergence problems drawn from different domains than such problems will be similar to each other.

Once retrieved, the generalized solution formed in the schema can be applied to suggest a solution to the novel problem. Hence, once a person has induced a schema from initial examples, novel problems that can be categorized as instances of the schema can be solved without directly accessing representations of the initial analogs. Reminding and mapping will both be facilitated by the availability of schemata such as those PI constructs.

Surface and structural similarities

In the absence of a prior schema, relevant source analogs will be difficult to access spontaneously because a remote analog by definition shares few salient surface features of the target. To the extent such features serve as retrieval cues, they will tend to activate competing associations that may block retrieval of more remote analogs. The more the problem solver is able to identify and focus on the aspects of the target problem causally relevant to achieving a solution (Winston, 1980), the greater the probability that a useful but remote analog will be retrieved.

In talking about "surface features" we have implicitly assumed a distinction between surface and structural similarities and dissimilarities (Holyoak, 1985). An identity between two problem situations that play no causal role in determining the possible solutions to one or the other analog constitutes a surface similarity. Similarly, a difference involving a property that plays no causal role in generation of a problem solution constitutes a surface dissimilarity. In contrast, identities that influence goal attainment constitute structural similarities, and differences of this sort constitute structural dissimilarities. In computational terms, structural properties correspond to elements that match rules required to implement a solution (or that block rules that would otherwise have been able to fire and produce a solution).

Ideally, a problem solver would use only the structural properties of the target as retrieval cues, thus avoiding activation of superficially similar but unhelpful situations. In practice, however, the problem solver's ability to distinguish structural from surface properties will be at best imperfect, since full knowledge of which properties of the target are structural depends on knowing the possible solutions – information clearly unavailable at the outset of a solution attempt. Consequently, properties that in fact are functionally irrelevant to a solution to the target problem may affect the solution plan indirectly by influencing the selection of a source analog (Gilovich, 1981).

Once a source analog has been retrieved, surface properties should have less impact on the mapping process than structural ones. Given that multiple constraints determine the appropriate mapping, a single surface difference need not impair subjects' ability to use the analogy. Thus surface properties will tend to have a relatively greater impact on selection of a source analog (since they will influence the reminding process) than on the subsequent mapping process. In contrast, structure-violating differences will diminish not only the probability of selecting the source analog but also the probability of using it successfully once mapping is initiated. In particular, if subgoals are transferred from the source of the target, the source analog will be less useful if it suggests an inappropriate subgoal.

A recent study by Holyoak and Koh (1987) provided evidence in favor of the above analysis of the influence of surface and structural properties on noticing and applying analogies. Their experiments revealed that transfer was significantly impaired if either the surface similarity of the instrument or the structural constraint similarity was reduced. These results indicate that both surface similarities and deeper structural commonalities aid in the retrieval of source analogs. In terms of the PI model, removing either type of shared element will decrease the total activation passed from the target to the source, thus decreasing the probability that activation of the source will exceed the threshold for invoking the mapping procedures. A different transfer pattern, however, was observed once a hint to use the story was provided. Although structural and surface similarity had comparable effects on spontaneous transfer, only the former had a significant impact on total analogical transfer once a hint was provided. These results therefore supported the prediction that surface similarity will have a greater relative impact on retrieval of a source analog than on application of an analog once it is retrieved. (Related findings supporting this conclusion have been reported by Gentner & Landers, 1985.)

From PI's operation, it is clear why structural features will have a greater impact on transfer than surface features. The reason is that the key to transfer, as opposed to retrieval, is using the actions of the source problem to generate useful subgoals for the target problem. Without structural similarities between the source and target, the suggested subgoals will likely be useless for solving the new problem. Structural dissimilarity can thus produce inappropriate subgoal transfer at the mapping stage, even if the elements of the two problems have been successfully mapped. If there are few systematic relations between properties that play a causal role in finding a solution to the source problem and those that are relevant to a solution for the target problem, then the subgoal-construction mechanism that PI employs will send the program off in unproductive directions.

Much work remains to be done to develop the PI program as a detailed model, but we believe it provides a good beginning for an understanding of analogical problem solving.

NOTES

Preparation of this chapter was supported by National Science Foundation Grant BNS–8216068 and Army Research Institute Contract MDA903–86–K–0297. During this period K. Holyoak held a National Institute of Mental Health NIMH Research Scientist Development Award, 1–K02–MH00342–05, and was a Visiting Scholar at the Learning Research and Development Center of the University of Pittsburgh. Phil Johnson-Laird and Andrew Ortony provided valuable comments on earlier versions of this chapter.

1 Here we are simplifying the actual solution trace. After the army has been split, it is not simply the original army (obj1) that moves to the fortress but constituent divisions into which the army has been divided. PI represents these derived entities using existentially quantified variables.

REFERENCES

➤ Anderson, J.R. (1983). *The architecture of cognition.* Cambridge, MA: Harvard University Press.

Burstein, M. H. (1986). Concept formation by incremental analogical reasoning and debugging. In R. S. Michalski, J. G. Carbonell, & T. M. Mitchell (Eds.), *Machine learning: An artificial intelligence approach* (Vol. 2, pp. 351–370). Los Altos, CA: Kaufmann.

Carbonell, J. G. (1983). Learning by analogy: Formulating and generalizing plans from past experience. In R. S. Michalski, J. G. Carbonell, & T. M. Mitchell (Eds.), *Machine learning: An artificial intelligence approach* (Vol. 1, pp. 137–161). Palo Alto, CA: Tioga.

Carbonell, J. G. (1986). Derivational analogy: A theory of reconstructive problem solving and expertise acquisition. In R. S. Michalski, J. G. Carbonell, & T. M. Mitchell (Eds.), *Machine learning: An artificial intelligence approach* (Vol. 2, pp. 371–392). Los Altos, CA: Kaufmann.

Chi, M. T. H., Feltovich, P. J., & Glaser, R. (1981). Categorization and representation of physics problems by experts and novices. *Cognitive Science,* 5, 121–152.

Collins, A. M., & Quillian, M. R. (1969). Retrieval time from semantic memory. *Journal of Verbal Learning and Verbal Behavior,* 8, 240–248.

DeJong, G. (1982). Automatic schema acquisition in a natural language environment. In *Proceedings of the National Conference on Artificial Intelligence* (pp. 410–413). Los Altos, CA: Kaufmann.

Duncker, K. (1945). On problem solving. *Psychological Monographs, 58* (Whole No. 270).

Evans, T. G. (1968). A program for the solution of a class of geometric analogy intelligence questions. In M. Minsky (Ed.), *Semantic information processing* (pp. 271–353). Cambridge, MA: MIT Press.

Gentner, D. (1983). Structure-mapping: A theoretical framework for analogy. *Cognitive Science,* 7, 155–170.

Gentner, D., & Landers, R. (1985). *Analogical access: A good match is hard to find.* Paper presented at the annual meeting of the Psychonomic Society, Boston.

Gick, M. L., & Holyoak, K. J. (1980). Analogical problem solving. *Cognitive Psychology, 12,* 306–355.

Gick, M. L. & Holyoak, K. J. (1983). Schema induction and analogical transfer. *Cognitive Psychology, 15,* 1–38.

Gilovich, T. (1981). Seeing the past in the present: The effect of associations to familiar events on judgments and decisions. *Journal of Personality and Social Psychology, 40,* 797–808.

Holland, J. H. (1986). Escaping brittleness: The possibilities of general purpose machine learning algorithms applied to parallel rule-based systems. In R. S. Michalski, J. G. Carbonell, & T. M. Mitchell (Eds.), *Machine learning: An artificial intelligence approach* (Vol. 2, pp. 593–623). Los Altos, CA: Kaufmann.

Holland, J. H., Holyoak, K. J., Nisbett, R. E., & Thagard, P. R. (1986). *Induction: Processes of inference, learning, and discovery.* Cambridge, MA: MIT Press (Bradford Books).

Holyoak, K. J. (1984). Analogical thinking and human intelligence. In R. J.

Sternberg (Ed.). *Advances in the psychology of human intelligence* (Vol. 2, pp. 199–230). Hillsdale, NJ: Erlbaum.

Holyoak, K. J. (1985). The pragmatics of analogical transfer. In G. H. Bower (Ed.), *The psychology of learning and motivation* (Vol. 19, pp. 59–87). New York: Academic Press.

Holyoak, K. J., & Koh, K. (1987). Surface and structural similarity in analogical transfer. *Memory and Cognition, 15*, 332–340.

Kedar-Cabelli, S. (1985, August). Purpose-directed analogy. *Proceedings of the Seventh Annual Conference of the Cognitive Science Society* (pp. 150–159), Irvine, CA.

Minsky, M. L. (1975). A framework for representing knowledge. In P. H. Winston (Ed.), *The psychology of computer vision* (pp. 211–277). New York: McGraw-Hill.

Rosenbloom, P. S., & Newell, A. (1986). The chunking of goal hierarchies: A generalized model of practice. In R. S. Michalski, J. G. Carbonell, & T. M. Mitchell (Eds.), *Machine learning: An artificial intelligence approach* (Vol. 2, pp. 247–288). Los Altos, CA: Kaufmann.

✓ Schank, R. C. (1982). *Dynamic memory*. Cambridge: Cambridge University Press.

Thagard, P., & Holyoak, K. J. (1985). Discovering the wave theory of sound: Induction in the context of problem solving. *Proceedings of the Ninth International Joint Conference on Artificial Intelligence* (pp. 610–612). Los Altos, CA: Kaufmann.

Thibadeau, R., Just, M. A., & Carpenter, P. A. (1982). A model of the time course and content of reading. *Cognitive Science, 6*, 157–203.

Winston, P. H. (1980). Learning and reasoning by analogy. *Communications of the Association for Computing Machinery, 23*, 689–703.

Winston, P. H. (1982). Learning new principles from precedents and exercises. *Artificial Intelligence, 19*, 321–350.

9

Use of analogy in a production system architecture

JOHN R. ANDERSON and ROSS THOMPSON

Introduction

This is a report on our development of analogy within a production system architecture. A couple of years ago we became persuaded that analogical problem solving was fundamental in the skill acquisition domains we were studying: programming and mathematical problem solving. Students were always resorting to examples from their textbooks or to examples from more familiar domains for solving these problems. We did a number of simulations of this problem solving within the ACT* architecture (Anderson, Farrell, & Sauers, 1984; Anderson, Pirolli, & Farrell, 1988; Pirolli & Anderson, 1985). However, the process of simulating this was awkward within that architecture. It was also ad hoc in the sense that the architecture offered no explanation as to why students were using analogy as their primary problem-solving method. This led us down the path of thinking about how analogy takes place and how it fits into a production system architecture. This is the first report of the new system that we have developed in response to these ruminations.

The term *analogy* is used in multiple senses. We are concerned with how analogy is involved in problem solving and in skill acquisition. That is, how do people call up an analogous experience to help them solve new problems? This experience can come from their own past (when analogy is sometimes called repetition), it might come from looking at the behavior of another (in which case it is sometimes called imitation), or it might come from adapting an example given in a textbook or some other expository medium (in which case it is sometimes called copying). The source for the analogy can be either an explicit experience or a generic or schemalike representation. It also might be from the "same" domain as the problem or from a different domain. It may involve generating a solution to a problem or understanding a solution. This range of phenomena has not always been

267

organized as a single psychological kind. However, they flow from a single mechanism in our theory.

Our mechanism does not address the more literary or mnemonic uses of analogy. For instance, we have nothing to say about the typical use of the solar system to understand the atom. The typical uses of that analogy do not involve any problem solving in our analysis. This is not to say that these are not interesting psychological issues; it is just to define the domain of reference for our chapter.

Our analysis of problem solving sees knowledge organized into *function* and *form*. Generating a solution involves producing a form that will achieve a desired function. Understanding a problem solution involves assigning a function to an observed form. Analogy is a mechanism for achieving the function–form relationships in domains where one has not yet acquired skills for doing so. Skill acquisition involves acquiring productions that circumvent the need to go through the analogy mechanism.

In this chapter we will first describe our knowledge representation, which is factored into a function–form structure. Next we will describe how the analogy process operates on this to fill in missing function and form. Then we will discuss the knowledge compilation process, which operates on the trace of an analogy process to produce new productions (i.e., acquire skill). Finally, we will discuss some issues associated with placing this process into a more general framework of skill acquisition. Before doing any of this, however, we would like to explain a little about the PUPS production system in which the analogy mechanism is implemented.

The PUPS architecture

PUPS (for *PenUltimate Production System*) is intended as an implementation of the theoretical successor to the ACT* theory (Anderson, 1983). This new theory does not yet really exist. We are working on this production system as a means of developing that theory. Therefore, the extent of the difference between the PUPS-based theory and its ACT* predecessor is not clear. Nevertheless, there are a series of problems with the ACT* theory that PUPS intended to remedy.

1. The flow of control in ACT* was implemented by means of a goal stack that yielded top-down, fixed-order traversal of goals. There were two basic problems with this: (a) People can be more flexible in their flow of control. For instance, as Van Lehn (1983) has noted, children doing multicolumn subtraction problems will shift opportunistically among the preferred right-to-left processing of columns,

to a left-to-right processing of columns, to an inside-out processing. Such flexibility is the rule rather than the exception when we watch geometry students develop proofs. (b) The ACT* theory leads to unreasonable expectations about people's ability to remember goals. It also does not predict the fact that people do much better at remembering goals when there is a concrete residue of their problem solving such as marks on a page than when they must solve these problems entirely in their heads. The solution to both of these problems is to abandon the use of goal stacks as separate control structures and let the problem solution itself hold the goals. This ties memory for solution to memory for pending goals as it appears to be. It also makes goals declarative structures and so permits greater flexibility in selection of the goal to follow.

2. In ACT*, generalization and discrimination were automatic processes calculated by the architecture on productions. As a consequence, they were not open to inspection or conscious control. In contrast, it is argued (Anderson, 1986) that people have some access and control over their induction. As we shall see when we discuss analogy and skill acquisition, the new architecture of PUPS enables this less automatic sort of skill induction.

3. Analogy itself was cumbersome to calculate in ACT* because there were not the right representational or processing primitives. In contrast, in every domain of skill acquisition we studied, we found that analogy was the prime mechanism by which students learned to solve new problems. Therefore, it seemed that the architecture had to be reconfigured to permit more natural computation of analogy.

PUPS knowledge representation

Our theory is built around certain assumptions about the organization of knowledge. The basic assumption is that knowledge is represented in schemalike structures. The three obligatory slots for such a structure are a category (isa) slot that specifies the category of which the structure is an instance, a function slot that specifies what function the structure fulfills, and a form slot that specifies the form of the structure. Below is our representation of the LISP function call (+ 2 3):

```
structure1
  isa: function-call
  function: (add 2 3)
  form: (list + 2 3)
  context: LISP
  medium: CRT-screen
  precondition: context: LISP
```

medium: CRT-screen
precondition: context: LISP

This asserts that this is a function call, its function is to add 2 and 3, and its form is literally a list of a +, followed by a 2, followed by a 3. Note there are three optional slots for this structure. The first asserts that this function call is being used in the context of LISP, the second asserts that this is being entered on a CRT screen, and the third asserts that it is critical that the context be LISP for the form to achieve the specified function. Entering this form in other programming languages would not have this effect. On the other hand, the medium is an accidental property of this example and so is not listed as a prerequisite.

The function, form, and prerequisite slots have a certain implicational semantics, which it is useful to set forth at the outset. This implicational semantics is that the form and the prerequisites imply the function.

We can represent this as

(list + 2 3) & context (LISP) → (add 2 3)

As we shall see, analogy creates function and form slots that plausibly create such implications.

There are two complications that greatly enhance the expressive power of our knowledge representation. One is that a structure can serve multiple functions and so have multiple values in its function slot. The second is that one structure can be embedded in another. Consider the following structures that represent the LISP code:

```
(cons (cadr lis) (cons (car lis) (cddr lis)))

structure2
  isa: function-call
  function: (reverse elem1 elem2)
    (insert elem2 lis2)
    (find lis1)
  form: (list cons structure3 structure4)

structure3
  isa: function-call
  function: (extract-second lis)
    (find elem2)
  form: (list cadr lis)

structure4
  isa: function-call
  function: (insert elem1 list3)
  (find lis2)
  form: (list cons structure5 structure6)
```

```
structure5
  isa: function-call
  function: (extract-first lis)
    (find elem1)
  form: (list cadr lis)

structure6
  isa: function-call
  function: (extract-second-tail lis)
    (find lis3)
  form: (list cddr lis)

elem1
  isa: element
  function: (first lis)
    (first lis2)
    (second lis1)
    (value-of structure5)

elem2
  isa: element
  function: (second lis)
    (first lis1)
    (value-of structure3)

lis3
  isa: list
  function: (second-tail lis)
    (second-tail lis1)
    (first-tail lis2)
    (value-of structure6)

lis2
  isa: list
  function: (value-of structure4)
    (first-tail lis1)

lis1
  isa: list
  function: (value-of structure2)
```

This is a fairly elaborate representation of this little piece of LISP code, and we do not mean to imply that all LISP programmers always have as rich a representation. However, we will see that success in problem solving can turn on the richness and correctness of such structure representations.

Analogy

There are number of distinct cases of analogy that need to be considered. The one that is most basic in our work is the filling in of a

missing form slot in a structure that has a filled-in function slot. For
example, consider the structures below:

```
structurex
    isa: function–call
    function: (extract-first (a b c))
    form: ???
```

```
structurey
    isa: function-call
    function: (extract-first (p q r s))
    form (list car '(p q r s))
```

Structurex above has a functional specification that it gets the first
element of the list (*a b c*), but there is no form specification. This is
how we represent a goal in PUPS – a structure with a filled-in function
but missing form. *Structurey* is a structure with a form filled in that
achieves an analogous goal.

The analogy we solve to fill in the form slot is the following:

function(structurey) : form(structurey) :: function(structurex) : ???

or

(extract-first (p q r s)):(list car '(p q r s)) :: (extract-first (a b c)) : ???

The solution of course is to put (*list car '(a b c)*) in the form slot of
structurex. This is produced by creating the following mapping between elements of the form slot of the two structures:

```
list            → list
car             → car
'               → '
(p q r s)       → (a b c)
```

Three of these elements map onto themselves, and the other uses a
correspondence established between the functions of the two structures. The first element in the form slot (*list*, in this case) is always
special and maps onto itself. The symbols *car* and ' are mapped onto
themselves and (*p q r s*) is mapped onto (*a b c*). Momentarily, we will
explain how we decide which symbols can be mapped to themselves
and which must be mapped onto new symbols from the target domain.

The mappings are obtained from the function slots. For an analogy
to be considered successful the first elements in the two function slots
(*extract-first*, in this case) must correspond. The remaining elements
are put into correspondence (just (*p q r s*) and (*a b c*) in this case) and
are available for the mapping in the analogy.

It is worthwhile to identify the inductive inference that is contained in this analogy. Going back to our implicational analysis of the relationship between function and form we can represent the content of structure*y* as:

(list car '(p q r s)) → (extract-first (p q r s))

What we have done in making the analogy is to make the generalization:

(list car '*x*) → (extract-first *x*),

thus, variabilizing the nonterminal (*p q r s*). Given this, we can derive the structure*x* as a special case. This inductive inference step we have called the *no-function-in-content* principle. That is, the actual content identities of nonterminal symbols like (*p q r s*) are not critical to the function achieved by the form in which they appear.

Note that the necessary and sufficient condition for an analogy is that all the terms in the consequent of the above implication be variabilized (except the first special terms). Then, by producing an instantiation of the antecedent we can derive the consequent. Said another way, the necessary and sufficient condition is that mappings be found for all terms in the function slot. It is all right if terms are left unmapped in the form slot as they are in this example (car and '). They are simply mapped onto themselves in the target domain. This determines which constants can be left and which must be mapped in building up a new form.[1]

In the preceding example the mapping for (*p q r s*) could be obtained by simply comparing the function slots of the target and the goal. However, this is not always possible. Consider the following example of how someone encodes a call to the LISP function *quotient* by analogy to the LISP function *difference*:

    Example
      isa: function-call
      function: (perform subtraction 6 2)
      form: (list func1 6 2)

    func1
      isa: LISP-function
      function: (implement subtraction)
      form: (text difference)

    goal
      isa: function-call
      function: (perform division 9 3)
      form: ??

    func2
        isa: LISP·function
        function: (implement division)
        form: (text quotient)

This represents the knowledge state of someone who knows what
both *difference* and *quotient* do but has seen only the syntax for *difference*
and is trying to figure out the syntax for *quotient*. In looking at the
function slot of this example to make the correspondences for the
analogy, we get the following:

        subtraction   → division
        6   → 9
        2   → 3

However, this does not provide a specification about how to map the
term func1 that appears in the form slot of the example. But if PUPS
looks at the function slot of func1, it will find that it implements
subtraction. Knowing that subtraction corresponds to division, it
knows it wants the name of a function that implements division. Because it knows *quotient* is such a function, it writes (LIST quotient 9 3)
into the form slot of *goal*.

If we return to our implicational analysis we can see what assumptions are involved in making this step. The analysis of the example
would be

        (list difference *y z*) → (perform subtraction *y z*)

We have replaced the constants 6 and 2 by *y* and *z* to reflect the no-
function-in-content principle. However, this will not match the function slot of *goal* because of the unmapped element subtraction. However, if we replace difference by its functional specification we get

        (LIST (implement subtraction) 6 2) → (perform subtraction 6 2)

Applying the no-function-in-content principle to this example, we get
the following variabilized expression:

        (list (implement *x*) *y z*) → (perform *x y z*)

This essentially says, if we create a list of the function name that
implements an operation and two arguments, we will apply that operation to the arguments. In replacing difference by its functional
specification we are assuming that the critical thing about *difference*
was its functionality and not its identity. If there is another function
that implements subtraction (as there is), then it would work the same
way. This is another inductive principle, which we have called *sufficiency of functional specification*.

These two inductive principles, *no function in content* and *sufficiency of functional specification* can in combination produce rather elaborate problem solutions by analogy. To take one example, we were able to get the mechanism to code the function *summorial* by (10 iterations of) analogy to the function *factorial*, both of which are given below:

```
(defun factorial (n)
  (cond ((zerop n) 1)
      (t (times n (factorial (sub1 n))))))

(defun summorial (i)
  (cond ((zerop i) 0)
      (t (plus i (summorial (sub1 i))))))
```

Factorial calculates the product of the integers to *n* whereas *summorial* calculates the sum. Both are given recursive definitions.

Although we haven't space to go through this whole analogy process in detail, it is worth going through a few key steps. First, the following gives some of the original encoding of the example and the problem:

```
fact.ex
    isa: LISP.function
    function: (calculate fact.algorithm)
    form: (LIST defun fact.name fact.args fact.body)

fact.algorithm
    isa: algorithm
    function: (algorithm-for fact.ex)
    form: (compute product (range zero fact-arg))

fact.arg
    isa: variable
    function: (parameter-for fact.algorithm)
    form: (text n)

fact.name
    isa: function.name
    function: (name-of fact.algorithm)
    form: (text factorial)

fact.args
    isa: param.list
    function: (enumerate-args fact.ex)
    form: (list fact.arg)

fact.body
    isa: LISP.code
    function: (body-for fact.ex)
    form: (LIST cond case1 case 2)

sum.goal
    isa: LISP.function
```

```
function: (calculate sum.algorithm)
form: ???
```

sum.algorithm
  isa: algorithm
  function: (algorithm-for sum.goal)
  form: (compute sum (range zero sum.arg))

sum.arg
  isa: variable
  function: (parameter-for sum.algorithm)
  form: (text i)

sum.name
  isa: function.name
  function: (name-of sum.algorithm)
  form: (text summorial)

The first task that is solved by analogy is to determine the top level of the *summorial* code. To follow the analogy process, it starts with a representation of the implicational structure of fact.ex:

```
(list defun fact.name fact.args fact.body)
  → (calculate fact.algorithm)
```

In this form it does not allow for any variabilization; however, by replacing terms with their functional specification (applying the sufficiency-of-functional-specification principle) we get:

```
(list defun (name-of fact.algorithm) fact.args fact.body)
  → (calculate fact.algorithm)
```

This expression could be variabilized and mapped to the target. Note *fact.args* and *fact.body* would not be variabilized and would be directly copied to the target structure. This would represent a subject who thought that it was sufficient to change the name of function and it would change its behavior. Clearly, this is not acceptable. Thus, we have a third principle, which we call *maximal functional elaboration*. This principle is that, if there are unvariabilized terms in the form (left-hand side), arguments in the function (right-hand side) of the implication will be embellished with their functions as long as the sufficiency-of-functional-specification principle can apply. In this case, we embellish *fact.algorithm* with its functional specification (*algorithm-for fact.ex*). This creates another element *fact.ex* on the right-hand side, which will invoke elaboration of *fact.args* and *fact.body* and lead to a form that can have greater variabilization:

```
(list defun (name-of fact.algorithm) (enumerate-args fact.ex)
  (body-for fact.ex))
  → (calculate fact.algorithm  =(algorithm-for fact.ex))
```

This can now be variabilized using the no-function-in-content principle to give:

(list defun (name-of *x*) (enumerate-args *y*) (body-for *y*))
→ (calculate *x* = (algorithm-for *y*))

Instantiating this with the *summorial* function we get

(list defun (name-of sum.algorithm) (enumerate-args sum.goal)
 (body-for sum.goal))
→ (calculate sum.algorithm = (algorithm-for sum.goal))

Thus we need to fill in the form slot of the *summorial* function with a list consisting of *defun*, the name of *summorial*, the list of arguments, and the body for the function. There is already a name for the *summorial* function. In cases where a structure serving the function exists, analogy will use the existing structure rather than creating a new one. However, it has to create new PUPS structures, *goal.args* and *goal.body*, to fill the last two slots. So the following structure is inserted into the form slot of *sum.goal*:

(list defun sum.name goal.args goal.body),

and the following two data structures are created to describe *goal.args* and *goal.body*.

goal.args
    isa: param.list
    function: (enumerate-args sum.goal)
    form:???

goal.body
    isa: LISP. code
    function: (body-for sum.goal)
    form: ???

These structures act as goals to invoke further problem solving. Thus we have spawned two subgoals as the by-product of solving this analogy. In our simulation, these goals were themselves solved by analogy. The *goal.body* structure spawned a rich set of goals corresponding to all the levels of the recursive code for summorial.

There are a couple of interesting moments in the subsequent analogy problem solving, one of which occurred when it came time to generate the code that would correspond to the recursive action: (plus *i* (summorial (sub1 *i*))). The example and the *goal* at this point were:

fact.rec.value
    isa: LISP.expression
    function: (recursive-value fact.algorithm)
    form: (list times fact.arg fact.recursive.call)

times
   isa: LISP.primitive
   function: (compute product)
   form: (text times)

fact.recursive.call
   isa: recursive.call
   function: (recurse-on fact.ex)
   form: (list fact.name fact.rec.arg)

sum.rec.value
   isa: LISP.expression
   function: (recursive-value sum.algorithm)
   form: ???

Again, the implicational structure of the example, *fact.rec.value*, is:

(list times fact.arg fact.recursive.call)
   → (recursive-value fact.algorithm)

The terms in this can be rewritten to become:

(list (compute product) (parameter-for fact.algorithm)
(recurse-on fact.ex))
   → (recursive-value fact.algorithm = (algorithm-for fact.ex) &
(compute product (range zero (parameter-for fact.algorithm))))

What is noteworthy about this is that we have rewritten *factorial* by its form slot as well as its function. This gives us the term product that corresponds to *sum* in the specification of *summorial*.

Variabilized, the expression becomes:

(list (compute *x*) (parameter-for *y*) (recurse-on *z*))
   → (recursive-value *y* = (algorithm-for *z*) &
(compute *x* (range zero (parameter-for *y*)))),

which, applied to the *summorial* case, causes us to create the form:

(list plus sum.arg goal.recursive.call)

Plus is recognized as the function that computes *sum*; *sum.arg* is recognized as the argument for summorial; and *goal.recursive.call* is a goal structure created to calculate the form of the recursive call.

Extending the analogy model

Analogical filling of function slots

So far we have discussed how analogy is used to map a form from an example to a target using correspondences set up in mapping the function. However, analogy can also be used to do the reverse; that is, to map a function from an example using correspondences set up in mapping the form. In this we are dealing with a situation where

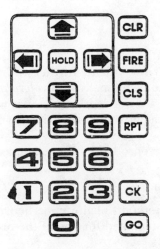

Figure 9.1. Keypad on the toy tank used by Shrager (1985).

the form slot is filled but the function slot is not. In an experiment by Shrager (1985), subjects were presented with a toy tank that had the keypad in Figure 9.1. They determined that the key labeled with the up-arrow moved the tank forward, and they had to figure out what the keys with the down-arrow and left-arrow did. Below we have PUPS structures that purport to represent their states of knowledge.

```
example
   isa: button
   function: (move forward)
   form: (labeled up-arrow)

up-arrow
   isa: symbol
   function: (points forward)
   form: (image thing1)

problem1
   isa: button
   function: ???
   form: (labeled down-arrow)

down-arrow
   isa: symbol
   function: (points backward)
   form: (image thing2)

problem2
   isa: button
   function: ???
   form: (labeled left-arrow)
```

```
left-arrow
  isa: symbol
  function: (points leftward)
  form: (image thing3)
```

The example is encoded as an up-arrow with the further information that an up-arrow is a symbol that conventionally means *forward*. The functions of the other two buttons are not represented, but we have represented the conventional knowledge that down-arrows symbolize *backward* and left-arrows *left*.

We can represent the knowledge encoded by the example by the following variabilized expression:

$$\text{(labeled (points } x)) \rightarrow \text{(move } x)$$

This implication represents the operation of the same heuristics as we saw before. This can now be instantiated for one of the problems as:

$$\text{(labeled (points backward))} \rightarrow \text{(move backward)}$$

Hence, we can infer that the function of the problem1 button is to move backward. Similarly, we can infer that the function of the problem2 button is to move left. As it turned out, only the first inference was correct. The left-arrow button did not actually move the tank in the left direction but only turned it in that direction. This is an example of where the no-function-in-content assumption was violated. Some buttons moved the tank in the specified direction, and some turned. One simply had to learn which did which. The actual identity of the direction determined the function of the button. This just proves that analogy has the danger of any inductive inference. The important observation is that human subjects also made this misanalogy.

Refinement

Though each structure can have one form slot, it can serve multiple functions. This leaves open a third and important kind of analogy: the filling in of a second function by analogy to a first.[2] This kind of analogy is very important in problem solving because the key to finding the form for solving a problem might be to represent correctly the function of a structure. This process of producing a new functional slot (or new views on the structure) is what we call refinement. Its usefulness is illustrated in the following example, which comes quite close to what subjects originally do when they initially reason about how to call LISP functions.

Consider how someone might analogize from an example of *car* to determining the value of (*cdr* '(*x y*)). Suppose, they had an example of (*car* '(*a b c*)) = *a*. They might encode this:

    example
      isa: LISP.call
      function: (show-value exp1 value1)
      form: (string exp1 = value1)

    exp1
      isa: LISP.expression
      function: (calculate first arg1)
      form: (list car ' arg1)

    car
      isa: LISP.function
      function: (calculate first)
      form: (text car)

    value1
      isa: sexpression
      function: (first arg1)
              (value-of exp1)
      form: (text *a*)

    arg1
      isa: list
      function: (hold (a b c))
      form: (list a b c)

The problem would be encoded:

    problem
      isa: LISP.call
      function: (show-value exp2 goal2)
      form: (string exp2 = goal2)

    exp2
      isa: LISP.expression
      function: ???
      form: (list cdr ' arg2)

    cdr
      isa: LISP.function
      function: (calculate rest)
      form: (text cdr)

    goal2
      isa: sexpression
      function: (value-of exp2)
      form: ???

    arg2
      isa: list

```
function:???
form: (list x y)
```

This represents an encoding where the subject has not yet figured out the function of *arg2* or *exp2* from the cdr example, and the goal is to figure out the form of *goal2*, which corresponds to figuring out the value of the *cdr* example. Using form-to-function analogy, the function slot of *arg2* is filled in as (*hold* (*x y*)), and the function slot of *exp2* is filled in (*calculate rest arg2*). However, the important task of filling in the form slot of *goal2* remains unsatisfied. We can form an analogy between the two function slots of *value1* and the one function slot of *goal2* to create a second functional description of *goal2*: (*rest arg2*). This is an example of goal refinement; *goal2* now has the form:

```
goal2
    isa: sexpression
    function: (value-of exp2)
        (rest arg2)
    form: ???
```

This cannot be solved by analogy to the *car* example, because it has no illustration of the *rest* relationship. However, given this refinement the system can look to its other, non-LISP knowledge for an analog. So we might have the following encoding of a state when we were sending out invitations to a list of people to attend a meeting:

```
new3
    isa: list
    function: (rest arg3)
        (hold (Mary Tom))
    form: (list Mary Tom)

arg3
    isa: list
    function: (hold (John Mary Tom))
        (invitees meeting1)
    form: (list John Mary Tom)
```

By analogy to this example, we can fill in the form slot of *goal2* by (*list b c*).

This example illustrates the characteristic scenario of what might be called creative problem solving. We start with a problem that we cannot solve but refine its function so that it has a different description. Now we can call on an extradomain analogy to solve the problem. This is one example of many where multiple models can be combined to solve a problem. The resulting solution is inherently more "novel" than if a single model has been mapped.

Selecting examples for use in analogy: spreading activation

What we have discussed so far is a method by which a person in a novel situation can solve a problem by analogy. There are three major complications to this, which we will discuss in the next three major sections of this chapter. This section will consider how examples are selected for use as models in the analogy, the section "Knowledge Compilation" will consider how knowledge compilation replaces analogy with learned productions, and the section "Discrimination Learning" will consider discrimination of overly general knowledge.

Our idea of how analogs are selected is no different than the proposal put forth in Anderson (1983, chap. 5), that analogs are chosen in the the process of matching productions. Basically, analogy is controlled in the PUPS system by productions of the form:

IF	there is a target structure needing a form serving a specified function
	and there is a model structure containing a form that serves that function
THEN	try to map the model form to the target form

Thus analogy is an action that can be called on the right-hand side of a production. This is a "bare-bones" selection production in that the only criterion for selecting a model is that the model serve the same function. It is possible to have more heuristic versions of this production, which used domain-specific tests to look for likely analogs. However, this complication does not really eliminate the problem of choosing from multiple possible candidates. It means only that in certain cases the set of possible candidates might be reduced.

The critical issue for selecting a model is how the second condition of the above production is matched. The actual PUPS code representing this production is:

```
(p draw-analogy
   =target: isa =object
      function ( =rel)
      form nil
   =model: isa =object
      function ( =rel)
      form (group! <> nil)
   →
analogy! = model = target form)
```

The terms =*model* and =*rel* are variables. This production looks for any structure (which will be bound to =*model*) for which the first term in the function slot is the same as for the target goal (this test is enforced by the appearance of the same variable in the function slots of the goal and the model). Of course, the arguments of the function slot can be different and will be put into correspondence for purpose of analogy. What is important is that the first, predicate, terms are the same, indicating similar function. PUPS will calculate all instantiations of this production and so find all the possible models. The issue is how it selects among these instantiations. This is the issue of conflict resolution.

Our view is that conflict resolution is determined by the same activation-based pattern-matching mechanisms that solved this problem in the ACT* model. Thus, basically, the most active model structure will be the one selected. There are a lot of things that seem right about this suggestion. Activation of a structure basically reflects the strength of that structure and the number of network pathways converging on it from active elements. The first factor, strength, means that the subject is likely to use recent and frequently studied examples. The dominance of recency and frequency in example selection is pretty apparent in our research on analogy in problem-solving domains like LISP and geometry. Research such as Ross's (1984, this volume) points to the importance of feature overlap in analogy selection. He found that the number of features an example shared with the current problem determined the probability of selecting the example, whether the features are relevant to the problem or not. We have argued a similar point (Anderson, 1983) for the domain of geometry but without the benefit of careful data like Ross's. Thus, in contrast to the analogy computation itself, which carefully examines the functionality of the problem features, the criterion for selecting among possible models is quite superficial.

Knowledge compilation

Knowledge compilation is motivated to deal with the computational costs of problem solving by analogy. Analogy is expensive to compute and requires having an example at hand and holding a representation of the example in working memory. Knowledge compilation is the process that inspects the trace of analogy and builds productions that directly produce the effect of analogy without having to make reference to the example. Our view is that this knowledge compilation process occurs simultaneously with the first successful analogy. Subsequent occasions where the knowledge is required show the benefit of the compiled production. This corresponds to the marked improvement in speed and accuracy from first trial to second in a typical problem-solving situation. We typically see more than 50% improvement and a concomitant marked decrease in any verbalization, indicating that the analogy is being computed (Anderson, 1982, 1987b). Thus analogy is something done only the first time the knowledge is needed (see also Holyoak & Thagard, this volume).

We have adapted the knowledge compilation process (Anderson, 1986) to operate in PUPS. It compiles productions from the trace of the analogy process. Thus, after writing the summorial function by analogy to factorial, PUPS compiled a set of productions that represented the transformations being computed by analogy. For instance, it formed the following production:

IF	the goal is to write a LISP function y
	which calculates an algorithm x
THEN	create the form (list defun name args body)
	where name is the name of algorithm x
	and args enumerate the arguments for function y
	and body is the body for function y

This is basically an embodiment of the abstract implicational structure that we extracted in doing the analogy:

(list defun (name-of x) (enumerate-args y) (body-for y))
→ (calculate x = (algorithm-for y))

Thus, knowledge compilation stores away the implication that we had to induce to perform the analogy. The availability of that implication saves us from having to calculate it a second time.

The other thing that knowledge compilation will do is to collapse a number of steps of problem solution into a production that produces the same effect in a single step. To consider an example, suppose we start with the goal to code the second element of a list:

goal
    isa: function-call
    function: (extract-second lis)
    form: ???

Suppose this has its function slot refined by analogy or an existing production to have the additional specification (*extract-first lis1*) where *lis1* is the tail of the list. The structure *lis1* is specified as:

lis1
    isa: list
    function: (extract-tail lis)
    form: ???

The form slots for *goal* and *lis1* can then be solved by analogy or existing productions. The form slot for *goal* becomes (*list car lis1*) and for *lis1* becomes (*list cdr lis*). In all, three steps were involved, refining the function slot of *goal* and filling in the two structure slots:

A production can be composed to summarize this computation:

IF   the goal is to code a function call *x*
         which calculates the second of lis *y*
THEN create a form (list car struct)
         where struct is a function call that calculates the tail of lis *y*
         and has form (list cdr *y*)

This is just the composition of the implication structures of the two PUPS structures *goal* and *lis1*. This is an interesting observation: Compilation of productions can be defined on the PUPS structures involved without actually inspecting the productions that fired. That is, we do not need a procedural trace to define compilation as in the ACT* theory. It can be extracted directly from the PUPS structures. It is more realistic to propose that the learning mechanism simply inspects declarative traces and not procedural traces. Declarative PUPS structures are already there and are by definition inspectable. Procedural traces were an invention in earlier theory just for the purposes of learning.

Another advantage of this is that we do not have to require that the productions to be composed fire contiguously in time or that they be invoked by a single ACT* goal. They only have to produce a contiguous fragment of the problem solution. In this way we have modified composition to deal with the problem of noncontiguous compositions first noted by Lewis (1981).

Discrimination learning

In the terminology of ACT*, analogy is a mechanism for generalization. It is a way of going beyond a particular single experience to rules of broader generality. The production rules produced as compilations of the analogy process are, in fact, basically the generalized rules produced by the older ACT generalization mechanisms. There are some advantages to the current PUPS formulation. The formulation of the mechanism is more uniform. Developed from the semantics of PUPS structures, the mechanism also has a well-worked-out rationalization and is not a purely syntactic process. By changing the PUPS encodings, one can change the direction of generalization, and so we do not have the same inflexible mechanism that existed in

ACT where the same generalization would emerge independent of context. Also, by anchoring analogy in declarative structures, we enable the subject to have conscious access to the basis for these generalizations – again, something subjects seem to have access to.

It was necessary to have a countervailing discrimination process in the ACT* theory. Generalizations can miss critical features about why examples work and so produce overgeneralizations. A process was required to look back and try to discover critical features to restrict a generalized rule that was overapplying.

The same dilemma exists in the PUPS theory although its character is a little different. Overgeneralizations arise because the original examples are not adequately encoded in PUPS. There may be preconditions to the successful operation of a rule that were missed in the encoding. For instance, suppose a subject has the following encoding of the LISP call in FranzLISP (*mapcar 'sub1 lis*), which subtracts 1 from a list of numbers:

> Example:
>   isa: function-call
>   function: (apply neg-op lis)
>   form: (list mapcar ' sub1 lis)
>   context: FranzLISP
>
> sub1
>   isa: LISP.function
>   function: (implement neg-op)
>   form: (text sub1)

Now suppose the person wants to add 1 to each number in a list but is working in INTERLISP. Below is the PUPS encoding of the new goal:

> goal
>   isa: function-call
>   function: (apply pos-op lis2)
>   form: ???
>   context: INTERLISP
>
> add1
>   isa: LISP.function
>   function: (implement pos-op)
>   form: (text add1)

The analogy process would calculate the following implication from the example:

> (list mapcar '(implement x) y) $\rightarrow$ (apply x y),

which leads to the inference that (*mapcar 'add1 lis2*) will do the trick. Unfortunately, the correct argument order is (*mapcar lis2 'add1*) – as we will suppose the student determines by experimenting and testing the opposite order after the first attempt fails. Now we have a circumstance where the student must try to make a discrimination. We assume that the student does this by the same correspondence process that underlies making analogies. The student tries to put the elements in the example and the problem into correspondence, looking for some feature that cannot be mapped. There are features such as that the first example involved *sub1* and the current example involved *add1*, but these are already in the implication that led to the analogy. The most immediate feature that does not map is the context, which is FranzLISP in the former example and INTERLISP in the current example. Therefore, the hypothesis is made that this is the critical feature, and we add as a precondition to example that the context be FranzLISP and to the current goal that the context be INTERLISP. The implication for the example now becomes:

context (FranzLISP) & (list mapcar '(implement x) y) → (apply x y)

Given that INTERLISP cannot be mapped onto FranzLISP, the analogy is now blocked from going through in the future. On the other hand, the INTERLISP example (with (*list mapcar lis2 'add1*) as a form slot) is available for future analogy, and that analogy can be compiled into an INTERLISP-specific rule.

A frequent context for performing discriminations is to add heuristic constraints to overgeneral rules. Consider the example in Figure 9.2 of a geometry problem that a student faced with the geometry tutor. Students when they encounter this problem know only the side-side-side postulate and the side-angle-side postulate. One student, not atypical, was observed to think about using first the side-side-side postulate and then the side-angle-side postulate but not to be able to apply either directly. Then the student tried to apply some of the rules he knew would work. He applied the definition of congruence to infer that the measure of segment $\overline{AD}$ is congruent to the measure of the segment $\overline{CD}$. Then he applied the reflexive rule to infer that $\overline{AD}$ was congruent to itself. These last two gave him legal inferences that led nowhere. His final step in this floundering was to apply the reflexive to infer $\overline{BD}$ was congruent with itself. With this in place the student was finally able to apply the side-side-side rule to infer that the triangles were congruent.

The student had created two examples for himself of the use of the reflexive rule – one involving $\overline{AD}$, which had been unsuccessful,

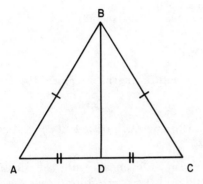

Given: $\overline{AB} \cong \overline{BC}$

$\overline{AD} \cong \overline{DC}$

Prove: $\triangle ABD \cong \triangle CBD$

Figure 9.2. A geometry problem that invokes discrimination of the appropriate situation in which to employ the reflexive rule of congruence.

and one involving $\overline{BD}$, which had been successful. Let us consider how the student represented these two inferences and formed a discrimination between the two of them:

inference1
  isa: geometry-inference
  function: (help-prove goal)
  form: (rule diagram reflexive statement1)

goal
  isa: geometry-statement
  function: (to-be-proven problem1)
  form: (statement triangle*ABD* congruent triangle*CBD*)

statement1
  isa: geometry-statement
  function: (conclusion-of inference1)
  form: (statement segment*AD* congruent segment*AD*)

segment*AD*
  isa: segment
  function: (part-of triangle*ABD*)
  form: (segment *A D*)

inference2
  isa: geometry-inference

    function: (help-prove goal)
    form: (rule diagram reflexive statement2)

statement2
    isa: geometry statement
    function: (conclusion-of inference2)
    form: (statement segment*BD* congruent segment*BD*)

segment*BD*
    isa: segment
    function: (shared-part triangle*ABD* triangle*CBD*)
    form: (segment *B* *D*)

In comparing the successful inference2 with the unsuccessful inference1 the student would add the precondition that segment *BD* is shared by two triangles. This would then lead to a rule that would have the student infer that shared segments of triangles are congruent, and the application of this rule would not depend on the context in which the rule was evoked – side-side-side, side-angle-side, angle-angle-side, hypotenuse-leg, and so forth. This is in fact the behavior we observe of our students; their use of this rule is not restricted to proving triangles congruent by side-side-side as in this example.

The astute reader will note another feature of this rule, which is that it does not require (but should) the shared sides to be parts of to-be-proven congruent triangles. About half of the students we have observed appear to have induced the rule in the above form and will inappropriately apply the reflexive rule in one of the later problems that involved triangles with shared sides where the triangles are not to be proven congruent. From this, subjects learn an additional precondition by the same discrimination mechanism.

The interesting question concerns the other half of the students, who appear to learn this "part of to-be-proven congruent triangles" precondition from the first example, which does not seem to create the opportunity for learning it. That is, the successful and unsuccessful examples are not discriminated by this feature. We can only speculate, but it seems plausible to us that a good student might try to create an example that satisfies the precondition (shared parts of triangles) but does not serve the function (help to prove the problem). Such examples are easy to come by, and these self-generated examples would serve to force the desired discrimination.

It should be noted that even the constraint of shared segments of to-be-proven congruent triangles is not logically sufficient to guarantee that the rule is a necessary part of the proof. However, there are no proof problems that occur in high school geometry texts that create situations that bring this out. So we have not been able to observe what high school students do. However, informally passing such problems among ourselves we have found that we have an irresistible urge at least covertly to make the reflexive inference. This seems to indicate that the acquisition of preconditions is not based on a formal analysis of logical necessity or sufficiency. Rather, as it is implemented in the PUPS system, it is based on empirical comparisons of cases where an example does or does not work.

A major feature of this discrimination mechanism is that the preconditions are stored as declarative embellishments along with the example. This means that a student can in principle examine them for their adequacy and reject or embellish preconditions that are inadequate. This potential for conscious filtering of proposed preconditions makes the PUPS discrimination mechanism much more satisfactory than the ACT discrimination mechanism or other mechanisms, which are automatic comparison procedures whose results cannot be inspected because they immediately become embodied as productions.

Comparison to related work

It may be instructive to look at how our theory compares with other work on analogy and related topics. There are several similar projects.

Mitchell's generalization

Mitchell (Mitchell, Keller, & Kedar-Cabelli, 1986) forms descriptions of a concept based on a single example, and without a problem-solving context. The system is given a high-level description of the target concept (the *goal concept*), a single positive instance of the concept (the *training example*), a description of what an acceptable concept definition would be (the *operationality criterion*), and a list of facts about the domain. Included in these facts are abstract rules of inference about the domain. An EBG (explanation-based generalization) algorithm tries to find a proof that the training example satisfies the goal concept. To do this it simply expands the terms in a high-level description until all the terms in the description meet the operationality criterion. If disjuncts are ever found in a term's expansion, the disjunct corresponding to the training example is used (for example, if *graspable* means either *has-handle* or *small-diameter*, and the training example is *has-handle*, then the expansion of *graspable* will be *has-handle*). After a proof is generated that the training example satisfies the goal concept, the proof is generalized to form a rule that is capable of matching any instance of the goal concept that meets this same low-level description. Note that this generalization is in general more restrictive than the goal concept, reflecting the choices made at any disjuncts encountered during the expansion process. Since the entire tree of expansions is saved during this process, a side effect is that the system can explain why the training example is an instance of the goal concept: It can point to specific features of the example that fulfill the various criteria specified in the high-level concept description (Mitchell et al., 1986).

The expansions done by the EBG method are not unlike the elaborations done by the PUPS system. The essential difference is that, whereas the EBG system blindly expands until it reaches a dead end or the (apparently ad hoc) operationality criterion is met, the PUPS system has an implicit operationality criterion, which is that the expansion is sufficiently elaborate for the no-function-in-content principle to apply. A second difference is that PUPS need not be given abstract rules of inference for the domain. It tries to infer these directly from its encoding of examples. Thus EBG starts out with a strong domain theory and essentially composes new rules; whereas PUPS discovers the rules hidden in its examples. A third difference is that the EBG method simply characterizes the way in which a single object instantiates a concept, whereas PUPS draws analogies in order to further problem-solving efforts.

Kedar-Cabelli's purpose-directed analogy

Kedar-Cabelli (1985) developed an analogy system based on EBG. Her system is typically given an object description and the task of answering a question such as "Does this object serve function x?" In order to answer the question, the system searches its knowledge base for model objects that serve function x and tries to "prove" that the model object serves the function. Then it tries to use this proof to prove that the target object serves the specified function. If the proof is successful, a generalization is formed that could essentially answer this question directly, without the analogy process.

Kedar-Cabelli's system is like ours with the differences already noted with respect to Mitchell's system. It is basically the obvious application of EBG to analogy. The major difference in the way it treats analogy is that whereas she asks questions of the form "Is it true that A serves function x?" we ask questions of the form "What function does A serve?" Another difference is the extent of the elaboration; Kedar-Cabelli elaborates her examples until she cannot elaborate further, whereas PUPS simply elaborates as far as is necessary for the no-function-in-content principle to apply.

Winston's analogy

Winston's ANALOGY system (Winston, Binford, Katz, & Lowry, 1983) is very similar to the work of Mitchell and Kedar-Cabelli. The major difference is that the rules of inference are stored with the examples and not stored separately, and thus the example serves the additional function of providing rules of inference. The system starts off with a description of the target concept and a description of a single positive instance. The system elaborates the description of the example, making inferences about physical properties that are not explicitly represented in the input description of the example. Once the elaboration is complete (i.e., no more elaboration can take place), the system attempts to show that the elaborated description of the example meets the description of the target concept. ANALOGY does this using "precedents" in order to provide functional descriptions of various features of the example. For example, if the target example has a flat bottom and the system knows that bricks are stable because they have flat bottoms, then the system concludes that the example is stable as well and that the purpose of its flat bottom is stability. Assuming that this proof attempt is successful, a generalization, describing the way in which the current example fulfills the description of the concept, is built in the form of a rule that could apply in a situation similar to the current one.

One of the big differences between ANALOGY and PUPS is that ANALOGY seems capable only of filling in *function* slots. That is, ANALOGY would not be able to generate an example that served a specific function. Indeed, this observation could be made of all the research we have looked at, except for Carbonell's work (which is capable only of finding form that fills a particular function and not the reverse). PUPS is the only system we know of that can draw analogies in either direction.

Rumelhart and Norman's analogy

Rumelhart and Norman (1981) discuss a method for drawing analogies that consists of generating a description of the differences between the model and the goal and writing new form that observes those differences. Their algorithm would compare functional descriptions of the model and the goal and notice that the goal is "just like the target, except that you use x for y." Using this information, the algorithm would then copy the structure of the model exactly, except for making the appropriate substitution of y wherever an x appeared in the model.

What is specified in this model is very like our own work, but there are a number of things in PUPS that correspond to nothing in Rumelhart and Norman's model. There is no discussion of the problems of model selection, and they make no mention of any kind of generalization process. They also do not discuss elaboration in detail, so it is difficult to know exactly what the termination condition of the elaboration process is.

Gentner's structure-mapping

Gentner's (1983, this volume) theory distinguishes among various types of features of the model. In particular, there are *attributes*, which are predicates taking one argument, and *relations*, which are predicates of two or more arguments. In an analogy, one is concerned only with mapping relations. From this assumption, she distinguishes in a natural way those features that should map when comparing the solar system to an atom. For instance, the relationship between electrons and the nucleus should be mapped, but the features specific to the sun (e.g., hot, yellow) do not. An analogy that maps a large number of attributes is called a *literal similarity*. An analogy in which the model is an abstract description rather than a physical object is called an *abstraction*. The method for selection of what features will map to the target domain involves a causal analysis of the domains. The *systematicity principle* says that those relations that are central to the functional description of the domain are much more likely to be mapped than those that are not. So, for instance, the fact that the sun is more massive than a planet in some way *causes* the planet to orbit the sun. Thus this relation is more likely to be mapped to the domain of atoms than the assertion that the sun is *hotter* than the planets (which doesn't cause anything). This causal analysis is similar to Winston's (1979) model. The central idea is that, if you cannot show a reason for a relation to be mapped, then you should not map it.

Carbonell's derivational analogy

Carbonell's (1985) work is different in kind than the systems so far discussed. His basic strategy is to take a worked-out solution for a problem and convert it to the current task. The problem solution may be represented at any level of abstraction (corresponding to various points along the problem-solving continuum) as a list of operators along with an elaborate description of the dependencies among the operators and the parts of the problem domain. These dependencies are then evaluated with respect to the current problem, and various editing operations are performed to convert the solution to one appropriate for the current problem. The editing operations include changing the order of the operators, inserting new operators, or deleting old ones. When enough related instances of a problem solution exist at one level, they are combined by a learning/generalization process into a more general solution.

A major difference between Carbonell's work and our own is that he represents problem solutions as a whole and requires that the entire solution be transported (modulo certain possible transformations) into a solution to the current problem. In our work, each operator application is done by a separate step (which may be either a learned rule or an analogy), and our solutions may therefore potentially borrow from many different examples. Also, since the generalizations we learn describe an individual step in a problem solution rather than the entire solution, these generalizations are more widely applicable (our theory predicts more transfer to novel problems). We think this more piecemeal approach is closer to the human use of analogy.

Conclusion

A general framework for analogy might have the following steps of processing:

1. Obtain a goal problem.
2. Find an example similar to the problem.
3. Elaborate the goal.
4. Generate a mapping between the goal and the example.
5. Use the mapping to fill in the goal pattern.
6. Check the validity of the solution.
7. Generalize and form a summarization rule.

It is apparent that the systems we have discussed by and large fit with this framework. The differences between the systems lie in how they accomplish the steps and in the order in which the steps are done. For instance, in PUPS the elaboration of the goal is done in parallel with an elaboration of the example. The consequence of this is that the mapping is a by-product of the elaboration and thus trivial to find. By contrast, Winston's (Winston et. al., 1983) system does the elaboration before it searches for the example and must generate the mapping explicitly.

Another way in which we can contrast the systems is by looking at the kind of questions the systems attempt to answer. There are systems (such as Winston's and Mitchell's) in which the object is to take an example form and determine whether or not it serves a particular function. Carbonell's system is given a functional description (in terms of a goal that needs to be accomplished) and provides a structure that serves that function (in terms of a problem solution). PUPS, by contrast, can do both of these tasks.

NOTES

This research is supported by Contract MDA903–85–K–0343 from the Army Research Institute and the Air Force Human Resources Laboratory. We would like to thank Kazuhisa Niki for his comments on various drafts of the manuscript.

1 This discussion differs slightly from the implementation.
2 The logical justification for this derives from the fact that the relationship among multiple functions is assumed to be biconditional – if one function is satisfied, then all are.

REFERENCES

Anderson, J. R. (1982). Acquisition of cognitive skill. *Psychological Review, 89*, 369–406.
✓ Anderson, J. R.. (1983). *The architecture of cognition*. Cambridge, MA: Harvard University Press.
Anderson, J. R. (1986). Knowledge compilation: The general learning mechanism. In R. S. Michalski, J. G. Carbonell, & T. M. Mitchell (Eds.), *Machine Learning: An artificial intelligence approach* (Vol. 2, pp. 289–310). Los Altos, CA: Kaufmann.
Anderson, J. R. (1987a). Methodologies for studying human knowledge. *Behavioral and Brain Sciences, 10*, 467–505.
Anderson, J. R. (1987b). Production systems, learning, and tutoring. In D. Klahr, P. Langley, & R. Neches (Eds.), *Self-modifying production systems: Models of learning and development*. Cambridge, MA: MIT Press (Bradford Books).
Anderson, J. R., Farrell, R., & Sauers, R. (1984). Learning to program in LISP. *Cognitive Science, 8*, 87–129.
Anderson, J. R., Pirolli, P., & Farrell, R. (1988) Learning recursive programming. In M. Chi, M. Farr, & R. Glaser (Eds.), *The nature of expertise* (pp. 153–183). Hillsdale, NJ: Erlbaum.
Carbonell, J. G. (1985, March). *Derivational analogy: A theory of reconstructive*

problem solving and expertise acquisition (Tech. Rep. CMU-CS-85-115). Pittsburgh: Carnegie-Mellon University, Computer Science Department.

Gentner, D. (1983). Structure-mapping: A theoretical framework for analogy. *Cognitive Science, 7,* 155–170.

Kedar-Cabelli, S. (1985, August). Purpose-directed analogy. *Proceedings of the Seventh Annual Conference of the Cognitive Science Society* (pp. 150–159), Irvine, CA.

Lewis, C. (1981). Skill in algebra. In J. R. Anderson (Ed.), *Cognitive skills and their acquisition* (pp. 85–110). Hillsdale, NJ: Erlbaum.

Mitchell, T. M., Keller, R. M., & Kedar-Cabelli, S. T. (1986). Explanation-based generalization: A unifying view. *Machine Learning, 1,* 47–80.

Pirolli, P. L., & Anderson, J. R. (1985). The role of learning from examples in the acquisition of recursive programming skill. *Canadian Journal of Psychology, 39,* 240–272.

Ross, B. H. (1984). Remindings and their effects in learning a cognitive skill. *Cognitive Psychology, 16,* 371–416.

Rumelhart, D. E., & Norman, D. A. (1981). Analogical processes in learning. In J. R. Anderson (Ed.), *Cognitive skills and their acquisition* (pp. 335–339). Hillsdale, NJ: Erlbaum.

Shrager, J. C. (1985). *Instructionless learning: Discovery of the mental device of a complex model.* Unpublished doctoral dissertation, Department of Psychology, Carnegie-Mellon University, Pittsburgh.

Van Lehn, K. (1983). *Felicity conditions for human skill acquisition: Validating an AI-based theory* (Tech. Rep. CIS-21). Palo Alto, CA: Xerox Parc.

Winston, P. H. (1979, April). *Learning by understanding analogies* (Tech. Rep. AIM 520). Cambridge, MA: MIT Artificial Intelligence Laboratory.

Winston, P. H., Binford, T. O., Katz, B., & Lowry, M. (1983, August). Learning physical descriptions from functional definitions, examples, and precedents. *Proceedings of the American Association of Artificial Intelligence,* Washington, DC.

10

Toward a microstructural account of human reasoning

DAVID E. RUMELHART

For the past several years my colleagues and I have been analyzing what we call parallel distributed processing (PDP) systems and looking at what we call the microstructure of cognition (cf. McClelland, Rumelhart, & the PDP Research Group, 1986; Rumelhart, McClelland, & the PDP Research Group, 1986). In this work we developed computational models of cognitive processes based on principles of "brain-style" processing. The major focus of this work has been in perception, memory retrieval, and learning. The question remains as to how this work extends to the domains of "higher mental processes." We have made one attempt to show how our PDP models can be used to account for schemalike effects (Rumelhart, Smolensky, McClelland, & Hinton, 1986). This chapter is designed to push those ideas further and to sketch an account of reasoning from a PDP perspective. I will proceed by first describing the basic theoretical structure of the PDP approach. I will then give a brief account of the reasoning process and finally show how it can be seen as resulting from a parallel distributed processing system.

Parallel distributed processing

Cognitive psychology/information processing has become the dominant approach to the understanding of higher mental processes over the past 25 years or so. The computer has provided, among other things, the primary conceptual tools that have allowed cognitive psychology to succeed. These tools have been powerful and have offered a conceptualization of mind that has proven both more rigorous and more powerful than any that have preceded it. There have, however, been some drawbacks. Because we have, by and large, worked with serial, digital, stored-program, symbol-processing Von Neumann-type computers, we have (perhaps inadvertently) carried much of the baggage of the Von Neumann computer into the "computer meta-

298

phor" and thence into our formal theories and into our intuitions. The argument is not that we should abandon the computational approach to the study of cognitive processes. Viewing the human cognitive system as a computational system is surely valuable, but, I believe, we have been drawing our insights from the wrong kind of computer. It is clear that brains are very different kinds of computers from the Von Neumann systems with which we have gained so much experience. The PDP approach suggests that we should ask the question directly about what kind of computer the brain might be, experiment with "brainlike" computers, and then draw our inspiration from these computational systems. In short, we want to replace the computer metaphor with the brain metaphor for cognitive systems.

Our work builds on the classical work on neural networks (cf. Grossberg, 1976), associative memories (cf. Anderson, 1977; Kohonen, 1977, 1984), and the work on Perceptrons and other self-organizing machines from the artificial intelligence literature from the late 1950s and early 1960s (cf. Minsky & Papert, 1969; Rosenblatt, 1962). We have tried to take these developments, understand their import for the nature of mental processing, develop our own variations on these ideas, evaluate the formal characteristics of such systems, build concrete models of specific psychological processes, and develop new kinds of networks for application to the particular problems that have seemed most important.

PDP models, like brains, consist of very large networks of very simple processing units, which communicate through the passing of excitatory and inhibitory messages to one another. All units work in parallel without a specific executive. The results emerge from a relaxationlike interaction among the relatively homogeneous processing units. Knowledge resides only in the connections, and all learning involves a modification of the connections.

Thinking and reasoning

One of the areas that has been least touched by our work on PDP models is that of reasoning and problem solving. Some believe that the existence of inferences implies a kind of logical system similar to that employed in conventional symbol-processing models. I have become increasingly convinced that much of what we call reasoning can better be accounted for by processes such as pattern matching and generalization, which are well carried out by PDP models.

If the human information-processing system carries out its computations by "settling" into solutions as the PDP perspective suggests rather than applying logical, symbolic operations as we might have thought, why are humans so intelligent? How *do* we make inferences? How do we know how to respond to new situations? How can we do science, mathematics, logic, and so on? In short, how can we do logic if our basic operations are not logical at all? We can begin to see an answer to these questions, I believe, with a careful look at reasoning tasks and the cognitive processes involved in them.

There are, it seems to me, three common processes for reasoning about novel situations.

- *Reasoning by similarity*, in which a problem is solved by seeing the current situation as similar to a previous one in which the solution is known (generalization and analogical reasoning fall in this category).
- *Reasoning by mental simulation*, in which a problem is solved by imagining the consequence of an action and making the knowledge that is implicit in our ability to imagine an event explicit.
- *Formal reasoning*, in which a formal symbolic system, such as mathematics, is employed in the solution of a problem.

The major point of this chapter will be to make these types of processes explicit and to show how PDP systems can naturally account for these three types of behavior.

The basic idea is that we succeed in thinking and logical problem solving by making the problems we wish to solve conform to problems we are good at solving. People seem to have three essential abilities which together allow them to come to logical conclusions without being logical. It is these three abilities that underlie the three reasoning strategies mentioned above. These abilities are:

- *Pattern matching*: We seem to be able to "settle" quickly on an interpretation of an input pattern. This is an ability that is central to perceiving, remembering, comprehending, and reasoning by similarity. Our ability to pattern-match is probably not something that sets humans apart from other animals but is probably *the* essential component to most cognitive behavior.
- We are good at modeling our world. That is, we are good at anticipating the new state of affairs resulting from our actions or from an event we might observe. This ability to build up expectations by "internalizing" our experiences is probably crucial to the survival of all organisms in which learning plays a key role. This is the fundamental ability that underlies our ability to imagine and to perform mental simulations.
- We are good at manipulating our environment. This is another version of man-the-tool-user, and I believe that this is perhaps the crucial skill that allows us to think logically, do mathematics and science, and in general build a culture. Especially important here is our ability to manipulate the environment so that it comes to represent some-

thing. This is what sets humans and their intellectual accomplishments apart from other animals.

In the following sections I will outline the PDP mechanisms that allow for these abilities and show how they may result in the reasoning categories postulated above.

Reasoning by similarity

Most everyday reasoning probably does not involve much in the way of manipulating mental models. It probably involves even less in the way of formal reasoning. Rather, it probably involves assimilating the novel situation to other situations that are in some way similar – that is, reasoning by similarity. Now, it is possible to see a continuum of possible situations for reasoning by similarity involving at one pole what might be called *remembering* and at the other what might be called *analogical reasoning*. In between, we have such processes as *generalizing*, *being reminded*, and *reasoning by example*.

There are, within the framework of PDP models, ideal mechanisms for accounting for a large portion of these phenomena. To see this, it is useful to conceptualize a PDP system as a content-addressable memory system (cf. McClelland & Rumelhart, 1985). The simplest way to do this is to imagine a memory system consisting of a very large number of processing units. These units are rather densely interconnected, and for simplicity we imagine that each unit has a potential connection to each other unit in the memory. Each unit receives input from outside the memory system (either from the external world or from other modules in the information-processing system itself). The memory system in turn sends outputs to other modules. The units themselves can be seen as microfeatures. A particular situation is represented by turning on those microfeatures that constitute a description of the represented situation. Certain collections of microfeatures might represent the physical characteristics of the situation, such as the color or size of an object being viewed, whether some particular object is present, and so on. Other microfeatures represent more abstract relational aspects of a situation, such as whether or not two objects are the same shape. An experience is assumed to result in a particular pattern of activation impinging on the memory units. Retrieval is assumed to occur when this previously active pattern is reinstated over the set of memory units. Information is stored in the memory by strengthening the connections among those units that co-occur and weakening the connections between pairs of units in which one is on and the other is off.[1] Although the exact values of the weights connecting any two units in the memory system will differ depending on exactly the rule employed for changing the weights, to a first-order of approximation, the connection strengths will be a function of the correlation between the two units. If they are positively correlated, their connection strengths will be positive. If they are negatively correlated, the connection strengths will be negative. If they are uncorrelated, the connection strengths will be near zero. Retrieval involves pattern completion. The memory is given a probe in which the activation of a subset of the units of the memory system is set and the system is allowed to settle into a stable state of activation. Such a memory system can be shown to have the following characteristics:

- When a previously stored (i.e., familiar) pattern enters the memory system, it is amplified and the system responds with a stronger version of the input pattern. This is a kind of recognition response.
- When an unfamiliar pattern enters the memory system, it is dampened and the activity of the memory system is shut down. This is a kind of unfamiliarity response.
- When part of a familiar pattern is presented, the system responds by "filling in" the missing parts. This is a kind of recall paradigm in which the part constitutes the retrieval cue and the filling in is a kind of memory reconstruction process. This is a content-addressable memory system.
- When a pattern similar to a stored pattern is presented, the system responds by distorting the input toward the stored pattern. This is a kind of assimilation response in which similar inputs are assimilated to similar stored events.
- Finally, if a number of similar patterns have been stored, the system will respond strongly to the central tendency of the stored patterns – even though the central tendency itself was never stored. Thus this sort of memory system automatically responds to prototypes even when no prototype has been seen.

McClelland and I have studied this sort of memory system in some detail (McClelland & Rumelhart, 1985) and have shown how this model can be applied to a range of memory phenomena. It should be noted that this is a substantially different view of memory than that suggested by the traditional *place* metaphor for memory. In this model an experience corresponds to a pattern of activation over the memory units. A memory trace corresponds to the specific set of weight changes that occur in response to a particular experience. A distributed model of this sort leads naturally to the suggestion that semantic memory may be just the residue of the superposition of episodic traces. Consider, for example, the representation of a pattern encountered in several different contexts, and assume for the moment that the context and content are represented by different units. Over repeated experience with the same pattern in different contexts, the pattern will remain in the interconnections of the units relevant to the content subpattern, but the particular associations to particular contexts will wash out. However, material that is encountered only in one particular context will tend to be somewhat contextually bound. So we may not be able to retrieve what we learn in one context when we need it in other situations.

The heart of this proposal, which makes it so useful for our present purposes, is that the memory access is determined by the similarity between the input patterns and the stored patterns. At the same time that it is considered a content-addressable store, the memory can be seen as a device for making generalizations to novel situations. Note that what is really being stored is the degree to which one microfeature predicts another. Thus, if there are regularities in the stored patterns such that whenever a certain configuration of microfeatures is present a certain other set of microfeatures is present, these regularities are as much stored as the particular instance. In this way, the system can respond correctly in the face of novel situations. Consider, for example, a memory system in which we store patterns one part of which represents the pronunciation of the root form of a verb and another part of which represents the past-tense form of the verb. Since there are regularities between the present-tense and past-tense forms of the verb, these regularities are stored. Subsequently, when a probe is given consisting of a representation of a completely novel root form of a verb, the system will construct the correct form of the past tense (cf. Rumelhart, McClelland, & the PDP Research Group, 1986). This generalization is stored just as much as the patterns that were actually observed (unless, of course, the novel verb is irregular – in which case the memory will "over-regularize").

Similarly, reminding "falls out" of the structure of this system. If the current situation is similar to a previously encountered situation, it is then possible that the previous situation will be evoked in the face of the current situation. It should be noted that the dimension of similarity on which the match occurs may be of any sort. It may be primarily on the basis of object similarity, in which case the situation of which you are reminded would bear a good deal of surface similarity to the current situation, or it could depend primarily on more abstract relational microfeatures. In this case, the system could well settle into a state that constituted a memory for a situation that was quite different on the surface but that had a similar abstract structure. Generally, of course, reminding would depend on a mix of relational and more concrete microfeatures.

Analogical reasoning is a small step from being reminded of a situation on the basis primarily of relational microfeatures. Essentially, I imagine the following situation. The microfeatures are ordered somehow in terms of abstractness from most concrete to most abstract and relational. I imagine that upon encountering a novel situation certain aspects of the situation come to attention and serve as the "retrieval cue" for the system. There are now a number of possible situations. It might happen that we had encountered a very similar situation in the past. In this case, the system would settle on an "interpretation" of the present situation that would amount to remembering a similar situation and filling in the missing microfeatures based on this situation. It might also happen that there is no close match wholly consistent with the input features. In this case, I imagine that the input "constraints" would gradually be weakened. Normally, in these systems we "clamp" the inputs, requiring that the final state of the system be consistent with the retrieval cue. Now consider a case in which the retrieval cue itself is gradually weakened. Suppose that, first, the most concrete inputs are released. Progressively more abstract microfeatures are released until an acceptable match is reached on the subspace containing as many as possible of the more relational features. The system could then generalize based on this subspace and, in that way, come to conclusions about the present situation based on another set of stored patterns that have the same basic relational structure as the current situation. In short, the system would do analogical reasoning.

Figure 10.1 gives a more concrete illustration of the process. We assume that we have a set of microfeatures ordered, in some way, according to their "abstractness." The most concrete features are indicated on the left and the more abstract on the right. A reasoning situation begins with the observation of some set of features. These features are "clamped." Some of the clamped features are concrete surface features, and others are more abstract relational aspects of the novel situation. Once these features are clamped, the system begins the process of filling in the missing features. The filling in is done in such a way as to maximize a "goodness" function (see Rumelhart, Smolensky, McClelland, & Hinton, 1986). The system will always find a maximum of this goodness-of-fit function (that is, a function that measures the degree to which the reconstructed information is consistent with the stored information). Normally, when retrieval occurs,

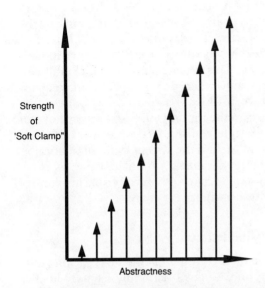

Figure 10.1. Memory features organized from most concrete to most abstract from left to right. The inputs may either clamp certain features on or simply provide a constant input to certain of the units.

the overall fit will be good. The system will be able to find a minimum that corresponds to some stored experiences, and the result will be retrieval. Other times, however, the overall goodness will be not as great but still adequate. This case may correspond to a case of generalization or, perhaps, the memory of an unusual situation. Finally, it can sometimes happen that the resulting goodness measure is very low indeed. This corresponds to a situation in which the memory contains no close matches to the probe situation. In this case, we can "release" the clamp on the leftmost microfeature and see if a good fit will occur after ignoring this input feature. If not, the next feature can be released, and so on. This process can continue until a satisfactory fit is discovered. When such a fit is discovered, it will constitute the discovery of a situation that shares the same abstract structural features as the current situation – namely, an analogous situation.

Ideally, one would like to find a state that matched as many of the input features as possible, giving greater weight to the relational features but generally preferring more matches to fewer. Moreover, it would be nice if we did not need an explicit mechanism for monitoring the level of the goodness function and deciding that it was time to release a feature. Fortunately, it is possible to solve both problems simultaneously by introducing the idea of a "soft clamp." Rather than clamp inputs on, we can simply have an input line deliver a constant amount of activation to an input unit. The lower that constant, the more easily the system can override the input constraint. The size of the smallest input determines the goodness threshold before it overrides *any* of the input features. This system can find the overall best fit, overriding input features only when doing so will lead to a sufficiently good fit to make it worthwhile to give up the goodness contribution given by conforming to the input. Under this scheme of soft clamps, we would make the weight of the concrete features the least and the abstract features the most, and the system will "automatically" go from merely retrieving to generalizing, to analogizing, as is required by the problem. This will occur without any specific control process determining which to do when.

Mental models and mental simulation

Reasoning by similarity is the most common method of reaching conclusions, but it is not the only one. Much of reasoning seems to involve imagination. It seems that to some degree we can solve problems by imagining situations and "seeing" what would happen. Broadly, I take it that the term *mental model* refers to our knowledge of some domain that allows us to reason about it by stepping through a sequence of operations and imagining what would happen. Thus, for example, when we answer the question of how many windows our home has by imagining ourselves walking through it and counting the windows, I take this to be the application of a mental model of our home. Similarly, when we imagine what would happen as a result of some action, say, throwing a cup of water on a desk or sitting on a salt shaker, we are employing mental models to reason about the consequences of our actions. How can we account for such phenomena in the context of PDP models? When discussing the normal PDP interpretation system above, I suggested that the system simply received a set of inputs and then settled to a state that amounted to the best account of the input, a standard "comprehension" assumption. When we reason through the application of mental models, however, we carry out a sequence of mental activities – not a single settling. How can that sequence be represented and controlled in a PDP model?

Suppose, for argument's sake, that the system is broken into two pieces, two sets of units. One piece is the one that we have been discussing – it receives inputs and relaxes to an appropriate state that includes a specification of an appropriate action, which will, in turn, change the inputs to the system. The other piece of the system is similar in nature, except it is a "model" of the world on which we are acting. This consists of a relaxation network that takes as input some specification of the actions we intend to carry out and produces an interpretation of "what would happen if we did that." Part of this specification would be expected to be a specification of what the new stimulus conditions would be like. Thus one network takes inputs from the world and produces actions; the other takes actions and predicts how the input would change in response. This second piece of the system could be considered a mental model of the world events. This second portion, the mental model of the world, would be expected to be operating in any case, inasmuch as it is generating expectations about the state of the world and thereby "predicting" the outcomes of actions.

Now, suppose that the world events did not happen. It would be possible to take the output of the mental model and replace the stimulus inputs from the world with inputs from our model of the world. In this case, we would expect that we could "run a mental simulation" and imagine the events that would take place in the world when we performed a particular action. This mental model would allow us to perform actions entirely internally and to judge the consequences of our actions, interpret them, and draw conclusions based on them. In other words, we can, it would seem, build an internal control system based on the interaction between these two modules of the system. Indeed, we have built a simple two-module model of tic-tac-toe that carries out exactly this process and can thereby "imagine" playing tic-tac-toe (cf. Rumelhart et al., 1986). Figure 10.2 shows the relationships among the interpretation networks, the inputs, the outputs, and the network representing a model of the world and the process of mental simulations. There are a variety of applications of mental simulation in PDP models. For example, it should be possible to have the system carry out "mental rotations" by applying a rotation model to some perceptual inputs. It also should be possible to build a system capable of doing mental arithmetic by imagining doing arithmetic with pencil and paper (see discussion of formal reasoning in the next section).

Formal reasoning

Roughly speaking, the view is this: We are good at "perceiving" answers to problems. Unfortunately, this is not a universal mechanism for solving problems and thinking, but as we become more expert we become better at reducing problem domains to pattern-matching tasks

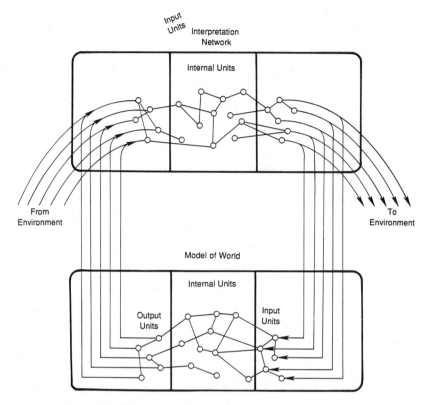

Figure 10.2. The relationships among the model of the world, the interpretation network, the inputs, and the outputs for the purpose of mental simulations.

(of the kind best accomplished by PDP models). Thus chess experts can look at a chess board and "see" the correct move. This, I assume, is a problem strictly analogous to the problem of perceiving anything. It is not an easy problem, but it is one that humans are especially good at. It has proven to be extraordinarily difficult to duplicate this ability with a conventional symbol-processing machine. However, not all problems can be solved by immediately "seeing" the answer. Thus, few (if any) of us can look at a three-digit multiplication problem (such as 343 times 822) and see the answer. Solving such problems cannot be done by our pattern-matching apparatus; parallel processing alone will not do the trick; we need a kind of serial processing mechanism to solve such a problem. Here is where our ability to manipulate our environment becomes critical. We can, quite readily, learn to write down the two numbers in a certain format when given such a problem.:

343
<u>822</u>

Moreover, we can learn to see the first step of such a multiplication problem (viz., that we should enter a 6 below the 3 and 2):

343
<u>822</u>
6

We can then use our ability to pattern-match again to see what to do next. Each cycle of this operation involves first creating a representation through manipulation of the environment, then processing this (physical) representation by means of our well-tuned perceptual apparatus, which leads to a further modification of this representation. By doing this we reduce an abstract conceptual problem to a series of concrete operations at which we can become very good. Now, not only does this apply to solving multiplication problems, it applies as well to solving problems in logic (e.g., syllogisms), in science, in engineering, and so on. These dual skills of manipulating the environment and processing the environment that we have created allow us to reduce very complex problems to a series of very simple ones. This ability allows us to deal with problems that are otherwise impossible. This is *real* symbol processing and, I am beginning to think, the primary symbol processing that we are able to do. Indeed, on this view, the external environment becomes a key extension to our minds.

There is one more piece to the story. This is the tricky part and, I think, the part that fools us. Not only can we manipulate the physical environment and then process it, we can also learn to internalize the representations we create, "imagine" them, and then process these imagined representations – just as if they were external. As I said before, I believe that we are good at building models of our environment so that we can anticipate what the world would be like after some action or event takes place. As we gain experience with the world created by our (and others') actions, we develop internal models of these external representations. We can thus imagine writing down a multiplication problem and imagine multiplying the numbers together. If the problem is simple enough, we can actually solve the problem in our imagination; similarly for syllogisms. Consider, for example, a simple syllogism: All *A* are *B* and no *C* are *B*. We could solve this by drawing a circle for *A*, a larger circle including all of the *A*'s around the first circle to represent the *B*'s, and a third disjoint

310 DAVID E. RUMELHART

circle standing for the C's. We could then "see" that no A's are C. Alternatively, we need not actually draw the circles; we can merely imagine them. I believe that this ability to do the problem in our imagination is derived from our ability to do it physically, just as our ability to do mental multiplication is derived from our ability to do multiplication with pencil and paper. The argument that external representations play a crucial role in thought (or, say, in solving syllogisms) is sometimes challenged on the grounds that we do not really *have* to draw Venn diagrams (or whatever) to solve them since we *can* solve them in our head. I suspect that the major way we can do that is to imagine doing it externally. Since this imagination is dependent on our experience with such representations externally, the argument that we *can* solve them mentally loses its force against the view that external symbols are important for thought processes.

It is interesting that it is apparently difficult to invent new external representations for problems we might wish to solve. The invention of a new representation would seem to involve some basic insight into the nature of the problem to be solved. It may be that the process of inventing such representations is the highest human intellectual ability. Perhaps simply creating an external representation sufficient to support problem solving of a particular kind is evidence of a kind of abstract thinking outside of the simpleminded view sketched here. That may be, but it seems that such representational systems are not very easy to develop. Usually they are provided by our culture. Usually they have evolved out of other, simpler such systems and over long periods of time. Newer ones, when they are developed, usually involve taking an older system and modifying it to suit new needs. One of the critical aspects of our school system would seem to be teaching such representational schemes. The insights into the nature of the problem become embedded in the representations we learn to use to solve the problems.

Language plays an especially interesting role in all of this. Perhaps the internal/external issue is not too important with language. The notion here is one of "self-instruction." This follows Vygotsky's (1934/ 1962) view, I believe. We can be instructed to behave in a particular way. Responding to instructions in this way can be viewed simply as responding to some environmental event. We can also remember such an instruction and "tell ourselves" what to do. We have, in this way, internalized the instruction. I believe that the process of following instructions is essentially the same whether we have told ourselves or have been told what to do. Thus, even here, we have a kind of internalization of an external stimulus (i.e., language). I do not want to make too much of this point because I recognize that the distinction between external and internal when we ourselves produce the external representation is subtle at best, but I do not really think it differs too much from the case in which we write something down and therefore create a real, physical viewable representation. Saying something aloud creates a hearable representation. Imagining saying something aloud creates a representation that can be processed just as if someone else had said it.

Before leaving this topic, we should note one more important aspect of external representations (as opposed to internal representations). External representations allow us to employ our considerable perceptual/motor abilities in solving abstract problems. This allows us to break problems into a sequence of relatively simple problems. Importantly, once an external representation is created, it can be reinterpreted without regard to its initial interpretation. This freedom allows us to discover solutions to problems without "seeing" our way to the end. We can inspect intermediate steps and find alternative solutions that might be better in some ways. In this way, we can discover new features of our representations and slowly extend them and make them more powerful.

Conclusion

I have tried to show that three of the most common aspects of reasoning can be naturally and simply produced by distributed memory systems. I have argued that the memory system naturally supports reasoning by similarity. I have argued that such a memory system coupled with a prediction system offers an account of reasoning by mental simulation. Finally, I have argued that formal reasoning is essentially the product of carrying out a sequence of perceptual/motor operations on external representations. I have suggested that these external representations may only be imagined on any particular occasion. It should be noted that these are all methods of coming to valid conclusions without the need of an internal logic – natural or otherwise.

NOTE

1 There are actually a number of important details to the memory storage procedures that determine the detailed behavior of such systems. The rule described in the text is a variant of the so-called Hebbian learning rule. Although this rule is simple, it is not adequate in many cases. A more

complex version of the rule for learning, which I call the generalized delta rule or sometimes the back-propagation rule, would be required in a realistic situation. For present purposes it is sufficient to think of the Hebbian learning rule.

REFERENCES

Anderson, J. A. (1977). Neural models with cognitive implications. In D. LaBerge & S. J. Samuels (Eds.), *Basic processes in reading: Perception and comprehension* (pp. 27–90). Hillsdale, NJ: Erlbaum.

Grossberg, S. (1976). Adaptive pattern classification and universal recoding: 1. Parallel development and coding of neural feature detectors. *Biological Cybernetics, 23*, 121–134.

Kohonen, T. (1977). *Associative memory: A system theoretical approach*. New York: Springer.

Kohonen, T. (1984). *Self-organization and associative memory*. Berlin: Springer-Verlag.

McClelland, J. L., & Rumelhart, D. E. (1985). Distributed memory and the representation of general and specific information. *Journal of Experimental Psychology: General, 114*, 159–188.

McClelland, J. L., Rumelhart, D. E., & the PDP Research Group. (1986). *Parallel distributed processing: Explorations in the microstructure of cognition: Vol. 2. Psychological and biological models*. Cambridge, MA: MIT Press (Bradford Books).

Minsky, M. L., & Papert, S. (1969). *Perceptrons*. Cambridge, MA: MIT Press.

Rosenblatt, F. (1962). *Principles of neurodynamics*. New York: Spartan.

Rumelhart, D. E., & McClelland, J. L. (1986). On learning the past tenses of English verbs. In J. L. McClelland, D. E. Rumelhart, & the PDP Research Group, *Parallel distributed processing: Explorations in the microstructure of cognition: Vol. 2. Psychological and biological models* (pp. 216–271). Cambridge, MA: MIT Press (Bradford Books).

Rumelhart, D. E., McClelland, J. L., & the PDP Research Group. (1986). *Parallel distributed processing: Explorations in the microstructure of cognition: Vol. 1. Foundations*. Cambridge, MA: MIT Press (Bradford Books).

Rumelhart, D. E., Smolensky, P., McClelland, J. L., & Hinton, G. E. (1986). Schemata and sequential thought processes in PDP models. In J. L. McClelland, D. E. Rumelhart, & the PDP Research Group, *Parallel distributed processing: Explorations in the microstructure of cognition: Vol. 2. Psychological and biological models* (pp. 7–57). Cambridge, MA: MIT Press (Bradford Books).

Vygotsky, L. S. (1962). *Thought and language* (E. Hanfmann & G. Vakar, Eds. and Trans.). Cambridge, MA: MIT Press. (Original work published 1934.)

11

Analogy and the exercise of creativity

PHILIP N. JOHNSON-LAIRD

Introduction

Analogies are tools for thought and explanation. The realization that a problematical domain (the target) is analogous to another more familiar domain (the source) can enable a thinker to reach a better understanding of the target domain by transporting knowledge from the source domain. A scientific problem can be illuminated by the discovery of a profound analogy. A mundane problem can similarly be solved by the retrieval of the solution to an analogous problem. An analogy can also serve a helpful role in exposition: A speaker attempting to explain a difficult notion can appeal to the listener's existing knowledge by the use of an analogy. A psychological theory of analogies must accordingly account for three principal phenomena: (a) the discovery or retrieval of analogies of various sorts from the profound to the superficial, (b) the success or failure of analogies in the processes of thinking and learning, and (c) the interpretation of analogies that are used in explanations.

My main purpose in this chapter is to establish that psychological theories of analogy have so far failed to take the measure of the problem. The processes underlying the discovery of profound analogies are much harder to elucidate than is generally realized. Indeed, I shall argue that they cannot be guaranteed by any computationally tractable algorithm. But my goals are not entirely negative; I want to try to establish a taxonomy of analogies and to show that there are some forms of analogy that can be retrieved by tractable procedures. I shall begin with an area that has undergone considerable psychological investigation: the role of analogies in problem solving.

Transfer: an analogy that worked and an analogy that failed

There are many cases in which an analogy can help people to solve a difficult problem. In a series of studies, Gick and Holyoak (1980,

313

1983) have demonstrated the phenomenon using as a target Duncker's celebrated X-ray puzzle. The problem is to think of a way in which to use X-rays to destroy an internal tumor without at the same time damaging the healthy surrounding tissue. The solution is to use many sources of weak X-rays harmless to normal tissue but to direct their beams so that they converge on the tumor. Few people discover the solution spontaneously in the context of a laboratory experiment. What Gick and Holyoak have established is that many more subjects produce the solution if they have already encountered an analogous problem, and its solution, in a story. The story recounts that it is impossible for an army to capture a fortress in a single frontal attack, but the army can succeed if it is divided into separate bands that attack the fortress from all sides. Merely hearing the story before encountering the X-ray problem leads subjects to a modest improvement in performance; a major improvement occurs if the subjects are given an explicit hint to make use of the story. The analogy works when subjects' attention is drawn to it.

A striking failure of an analogy occurred in an experiment on reasoning that my colleagues and I carried out many years ago (see Johnson-Laird, Legrenzi, & Legrenzi, 1972). Our starting point was the well-known difficulty of Peter Wason's "selection" task (see, e.g., Wason & Johnson-Laird, 1972). In the original version of this task, the subjects are presented with four cards lying on a table, which bear, respectively, the letter A, the letter B, the number 2, and the number 3. The subjects know that each card has a number on one side and a letter on the other side. The experimenter gives them a general rule, "If a card has an A on one side, then it has a 2 on the other side," and asks them to select just those cards that they need to turn over in order to find out whether the rule is true or false. The task seems trivial, but it is deceptive. The majority of subjects select either the cards bearing the A and the 2 or else just the card bearing the A. They say they have chosen the A card because if it has a 2 on the other side the rule is true, and that they have chosen the 2 card for the converse reason. Strictly speaking, the selection of the 2 card is unnecessary because even if it did not have an A on its other side it would not falsify the rule. The surprising and more serious error is one of omission: an almost universal failure to select the 3 card. If it has an A on its other side, then there is a decisive falsification, since the combination of A and 3 is plainly incompatible with the rule.

Although there is still no definitive explanation for the subjects' oversight, it soon became apparent that its immediate cause was the reluctance or inability of the subjects to search for falsifying evidence

– contrary to a central claim made by Piaget and his colleagues about adult logical competence. Paolo and Maria Legrenzi and I therefore carried out an experiment in which we used an analog of the selection task designed to overcome this problem. We made two small but significant changes in the task. The first change was in the materials. Instead of using an arbitrary rule about letters and numbers, we introduced a realistic rule, which was a variation on a then current and familiar postal regulation. Our rule was:

If a letter is sealed, then it has a 50-lire stamp.

The subjects were British, and in Britain at that time a sealed letter cost more to mail than an unsealed one. The array from which the subjects made their selections consisted of actual envelopes: Two were facedown, one sealed and the other unsealed, and two were faceup, one bearing a 50-lire stamp and the other bearing a 40-lire stamp. (There was a fifth envelope I shall ignore here.) The second change in the experiment concerned the subjects' task. Instead of asking them to select those items they needed to turn over to find out whether the rule was true or false, we asked them to imagine they were sorting letters to determine whether or not they violated the postal rule.

Each subject had two trials with the postal rule and two trials with the original arbitrary rule (and envelopes bearing letters and numbers): If a letter has an *A* on one side, then it has a 2 on the other side. As we had predicted, the new version of the task led to a large improvement in performance: 22 out of the 24 subjects made at least one correct selection with the realistic materials. However, although the subjects carried out one sort of trial directly after the other, and there was every opportunity for transfer from the realistic to the abstract materials, none occurred significantly. Only 7 out of the 24 subjects made at least one correct selection with the original abstract materials.

The two tasks have an almost identical structure, yet the subjects persisted in the standard failure to select the potentially falsifying instance. The analogy had failed. The question I am going to address is what this failure can tell us about the nature of analogy, but first I shall consider some theories of the psychology of analogies.

A formal theory of analogy

Could there be a purely formal theory of analogy? One might suppose that an analogy must be able to convey new information and that if theorists try to specify semantic or conceptual criteria for an analogy, such as Dedre Gentner's (1983) demand that there should be a match of high-level semantics, they will rob analogies of this power. This argument, however, is nonsequitur. Consider a parallel case. Many inferences are a source of new information. Suppose, for example, that I tell you: "The victim was stabbed to death in a cinema during the afternoon showing of *Bambi*. The suspect was on an express train to Edinburgh when the murder occurred." Your immediate conclusion is likely to be "The suspect is innocent." But, if I ask you whether you are certain, you are likely to raise such questions as:

> Are there cinemas on express trains to Edinburgh?
> Did the suspect have an accomplice?
> Could there have been a knife hidden in the seat of the cinema?

These are just the sorts of scenarios that subjects invented in some unpublished experiments that Tony Anderson and I have carried out. What they show, of course, is first, that commonsense inferences lead to informative conclusions (e.g., the suspect is innocent) and, second, that such inferences are based on semantic and factual considerations (e.g., a person is a physical object; a physical object cannot be in two places at the same time; there are no cinemas on express trains to Edinburgh). Hence, a procedure that leads to new information need not be based on formal principles alone. This possibility of a purely formal theory of induction was likewise refuted by Goodman (1955).

There are other, more direct, difficulties for a formal theory of analogy. It cannot explain the failure of the realistic postal regulation to act as a helpful analog and to enable subjects to make a correct selection with the arbitrary rule. The two tasks have exactly the same formal structure of objects and relations, the trials occurred alternately, and the subjects certainly appreciated that they were similar – some even thought that they had made the same selections in both. Yet the analogy failed. Where the tasks differ, however, is in their meaning, and one is bound to conclude that this difference inhibited the setting up of the appropriate mappings and the transfer of relevant knowledge.

Another difficulty for a formal theory will arise from its ontology, if it needs to distinguish objects, properties, and relations. This ontology is not directly reflected in natural language. As has long been observed, nouns can refer to objects, properties, or relations, and adjectives and verbs can refer to properties or relations. Hence, before any purely formal principles can be used, it is crucial that the representations of the domains properly reflect the intended ontology.

In order to decide that a noun used in the description of the source domain refers, say, to an object, it is necessary to carry out some essential semantic work. Formal principles can be properly applied only after this semantic process.

Yet another difficulty is to insure that the same domain can be used as an analogy for different target domains, particularly where the same sets of objects are mapped from source to target in both cases. For example, if you ask people in what way a clock is analogous to the solar system, then, from my anecdotal observations, they are likely to respond: "Both involve a revolution: The hands of the clock go around just as the planets go around the sun." Or, more profoundly: "The hands of the clock rotate just as the earth rotates with respect to the sun: A clock tells you, in effect, your current position in relation to the sun." The danger is that a purely formal and deterministic account of analogy will be unable to yield different analogies if the object mappings are the same.[1] Thus, given the respective object mappings from the source to two target domains,

Atom target	Source	Clock target
nucleus ⟵——— sun	———⟶	center
electrons ⟵——— planets	———⟶	hands

the theory must avoid transferring the same structural relations in both cases. Unlike the case of the atom, the higher-order relation; "The sun's attraction of the planets causes them to revolve around it," must not be carried over in an inference about clocks: "The center's attraction of the hands causes them to revolve around it."

This conclusion is obviously false, but matters of fact are precisely what formal theories must *not* rely on.

The "structure-mapping" theory of analogy

The dictionary tells us that an analogy is "A relation of likeness *between* two things ... consisting in the resemblance not of the things themselves but of two or more attributes, circumstances, or effects ... its specific meaning is a similarity of *relations*." This idea has been elevated by Gentner (1983, and in this volume, where she presents a slightly revised theory) into a provocative theoretical framework for thinking about analogy. She argues that the mere similarity of features shared by the source and target domains cannot possibly account for an analogy. What matters is that a *relational structure* can be carried over from source to target. To clarify this idea, we need to consider the "ontology" of everyday life. Ordinarily, people think of the world as containing objects, their properties, and relations among them. There are also recursive constructions that make it possible to think (and to talk) about higher-order types, such as relations between relations, for example, causation.

Granted that the source of the analogy and the target domain can both be represented by semantic networks (but cf. Johnson-Laird, Herrmann, & Chaffin, 1984), Gentner argues that an analogy maps the nodes representing objects in the source domain onto the nodes representing objects in the target domain. Three rules apply to create the analogy:

1. The properties of the objects in the source are ignored, since they do not have to match. In the latest version of the theory, these properties include functions that take an object as argument, for example, the temperature of a liquid.
2. The semantic relations among the objects in the source are, if possible, preserved.
3. Higher-order semantic relations (between relations) are preserved at the expense of lower-order relations.

Gentner calls the last rule the principle of "systematicity." Because higher-order relations enforce connections between lower-order relations, the principle enables a whole structure to be carried over from the source to the target domain. A cardinal point of the theory is that the mapping process is not guided by any specific semantic agenda, such as always looking for the same causal relation to carry over from one domain to the other. It merely looks for the highest order of semantic relations that are the same in both domains.[2]

Gentner (1983) illustrated her theory by considering the analogy between the solar system and Rutherford's model of the atom. The sun maps onto the nucleus, and the planets map onto the electrons. The properties of the sun, such as its yellowness, are dropped, but the higher-order relations are carried over. For example, "The sun's attraction of the planets causes them to revolve around it" yields the inference, "The nucleus's attraction of the electrons causes them to revolve around it." The reader should note that the recent computer model (Falkenhainer, Forbus, & Gentner, 1986) works the other way around. The best global mapping of systematic structure is established and is then used to set up the corresponding object matches.

What is particularly appealing about Gentner's framework is that it accommodates other types of comparison between domains: A statement of *similarity* involves mapping all sorts of predicates including properties; an *abstraction* depends on a source that is itself an abstract relational structure containing nodes denoting superordinate and abstract entities; a *simile* such as "The sunflower is like the sun" calls for mapping of properties rather than relations.

There is an important insight lying behind Gentner's principle of systematicity: Analogies really do appear to rest on high-level relations. Moreover, as we have seen, there are no grounds for supposing that they cannot be established on the basis of knowledge and meaning. There is, however, an alternative theory that assumes that matters of *fact* play an essential role in the establishment and interpretation of analogies, and I want now to consider this theory.

A factual theory of analogy

Keith Holyoak and Paul Thagard (this volume) have proposed a theory of analogy that takes into account matters of fact and meaning (see also Thagard and Holyoak, 1985). The theory has been modeled as part of a more general computer program for problem solving and induction, which is called PI (for "processes of induction"). It will be easier to delineate the underlying theory if I first outline the way the program works. I shall simplify certain of its features, including the syntactic format of expressions.

PI employs three main sorts of data structure in its representation of problem domains: (*a*) concepts, such as *army, capture, move*, which roughly correspond to predicates in the first-order predicate calculus; that is, they can be properties, relations, or functions; (*b*) propositions about specific individuals, such as "Object 122 is an army," which roughly correspond to assertions about entities denoted by constants in the predicate calculus; and (*c*) content-specific rules of inference, such as "for any x, if x is an army, then x fights," which roughly correspond to universally quantified assertions, or meaning postulates, in the predicate calculus. Concepts are represented in the program by names (LISP atoms) and among the list of property values attached to them are the names of relevant rules of inference. Thus one of the rules attached to the concept of *army* will indeed be the rule above that captures the fact that armies fight. Such rules are represented as condition–action pairs in the familiar format of production systems (see, e.g., Newell & Simon, 1972). The program is controlled by levels of activation that are attached to concepts, and hence both rules of inference and propositions about specific individuals (which are called "messages") are always attached to concepts. The attachment is by way of names that function as "pointers" from the concept to the rule or proposition.

The human user of the program feeds in an initial set of definitions of the various concepts and rules of a particular domain (such as the fortress problem described earlier) together with a statement of one or more specific problems. The solution of these problems is a goal for the program to achieve. The initial concepts are all "active," and thus the rules associated with them are also active. When the program is running, it stimulates three main parallel processes:

1. Inferences. These are made by matching a proposition about a specific individual (which is active because it is attached to an active concept) to the condition of a rule (which is active because it is attached to an active concept). For example, if the proposition, "Object 122 is an army," is matched to the rule, "For any x, if x is an army, then x fights," then the rule yields a new specific fact: "Object 122 fights." This proposition is added (via a pointer) to the concept *fights*. Only a preset number of such inferences can be made in each cycle of the program, and the ones that are selected are those with rules that are highly active and that have been frequently used with success in the past. One sort of inference yields new facts as I have illustrated; another sort yields hypothetical actions, for example, "Object 122 moves to the fortress." Such an action is again associated with the relevant concept by way of a name that acts as a pointer. Some actions may turn out to be mistaken and thus they will have to be undone: The program explores blind alleys. Ultimately, however, the solution to a problem depends on the generation of an appropriate sequence of actions.

2. Inductive learning. Various processes of inductive learning occur. They include the production of new rules of inference by generalizing from a small number of specific instances or by forming a more general category that allows two rules to be collapsed into one. There are also processes that generate explanations and combine concepts. I shall say no more about these matters because they are discussed by Holyoak and Thagard (this volume) and, in any case, do not play an essential role in the theory of analogy.

3. The creation of subgoals. On each cycle, the program checks whether it has achieved its current goals, that is, solved the problems that it has been set, by testing whether they correspond to currently active specific propositions that have been inferred. Once PI has discovered a solution, it attaches a statement of it to each of the concepts that occur in the formulation of the problem (by the use of a name that acts as a pointer). If a solution has not been obtained, the program uses its rules of inference to create subgoals. For example, given the goal of establishing "Object 104 fights," then the rule of inference, "For any x, if x is an army, then x fights," can be used to argue backward from the action part of the rule to the condition so as to establish the subgoal: "Object 104 is an army." The main purpose of creating such subgoals, however, is not to generate the solution to the problem by working backward from the goal (cf. the backward-chaining of such rules used in PLANNER and its many descendants; see, e.g., Winograd, 1972) but rather to activate those concepts that occur in subgoals.

After each cycle of inference, learning, and subgoal creation, the levels of activation of the concepts are revised: Those that occur in the actions of rules that have been executed are activated, and those that have played no part in the cycle have their level of activation reduced – they may drop below threshold and become totally inactive.

How does PI deal with analogies? Once again, the central mechanism depends on the activation of concepts. Given that the program has solved the source problem (e.g., the fortress problem), the solution will be attached to each concept in the formulation of the problem. The program then attempts to solve the target problem (e.g., the X-ray problem). If it fails, then the analogical mechanism comes to life. In the current implementation, the mechanism depends on the user defining rules that relate the concepts in the target problem to those of the source problem, for example, rules that relate *rays* to *force* to *weapon* to *army*. The idea is that such rules could, in principle, be acquired by the program as a result of learning. When at least two concepts of the source problem are activated in this way, it itself becomes activated; that is, the name of the problem is active. By determining what led to this activation the program is able to establish a mapping from one domain to the other; for example:

Target domain		Source domain
ray	⟵⟶	army
tumor	⟵⟶	fortress
destroy	⟵⟶	capture

This mapping, in effect, sets up the conditions for the exploitation of the solution of the source problem in an attempt to solve the target problem: The analogy mechanism transfers the actions from the solution to the source problem to the target problem. Thus, since the fortress problem was solved by actions that split up the army and moved the separate units to the fortress, the program carries out the hypothetical actions of splitting up the ray and moving its components separately to the tumor. Once the corresponding concepts of *splitting* and *moving* have been activated, the normal sequence of problem-solving steps can be resumed.

If you stand back from the details of its implementation, the PI theory makes three major claims about successful analogical transfer. First, the theory has an ontology corresponding to the predicate calculus. There are specific individuals picked out by constants, and there are variables that range over the individuals in the domain of discourse. There is no significant difference in the theory between properties (monadic predicates) and relations (predicates with more than one argument). Hence, the initial step in discovering an analog depends on mapping any sort of predicate from one domain to another. Mappings between specific entities do not occur directly. Second, the discovery of the mappings depends on content-specific rules of inference, that is, on a knowledge of facts and meanings. These rules are triggered by concepts in the target problem when the problem-solving system has been unable to solve it. The theory makes the pragmatic claim that the goals of the target problem control the mapping process: Different goals lead to different mappings from the same source domain. At present, the program needs to be provided with these rules, because it cannot construct them for itself. Third, what is transferred in the successful exploitation of an analogy is a sequence of actions that was originally generated by the rules of inference triggered during the solution of the source problem.

This theory can explain the failure of the solution to the postal problem to transfer to the arbitrary selection task. The concepts that appear to be critical in the postal problem do not have any corresponding concepts likely to activate them in the arbitrary problem. Thus, although there is the following theoretical mapping,

Arbitrary problem	Postal problem
envelope $\longleftrightarrow$	envelope
has an A $\longleftrightarrow$	is sealed
has a 2 $\longleftrightarrow$	has sufficient postage (50-lire stamp)

there is nothing about the concepts of *sealing* or *sufficient postage* that is likely to lead to such a mapping. Moreover, because the arbitrary problem does not appear to be difficult, the subjects readily advance what they take to be its solution. Hence, the theory offers a twofold explanation of the failure of the analogy: No search for a detailed analog is made because the problem appears to be solved, and there are no obvious and precise factual mappings between the two domains.

Does the PI theory of analogy resolve all the theoretical puzzles? Hardly surprisingly, there remain a number of troubling issues, some of which can be characterized at the level of *what* is computed and others of which concern *how* the program computes them. At the computational level, PI offers an account of how certain analogies might be discovered and then exploited in the process of trying to solve a problem. The theory is not intended to account for the use of analogies in exposition or, perhaps, for the discovery of profound analogies or the creation of scientific theories or works of art. In the final sections of this chapter, I shall consider these aspects of analogy in order to motivate some further suggestions about the psychology of analogy.

The interpretation of expository analogies

Here is a typical example of an expository analogy: "The Westland helicopters affair has transformed Mrs. Thatcher into the Richard Nixon of British politics." The core of the analogy is simple, provided one knows about Westland and Watergate: Mrs. Thatcher (allegedly) called for the leaking of a government document, and she subsequently attempted to cover up this misdemeanor. When the analogy was made, its point was that the Westland affair might do to Thatcher what Watergate did to Nixon. The likely sequence of processes leading to this inference is as follows: First, the assertion itself calls for a mapping between Thatcher and Nixon and asserts that the analogy between the two has been brought about by the Westland affair. Second, the reader must retrieve the essential facts of the Westland affair or of Nixon's career (or both). A reader who is unfamiliar with either set of facts will be unable to understand the analogy. Third, the information that is retrieved must then be given a superordinate characterization. The Westland affair can thus be characterized: "A politician commits a misdemeanor and then attempts to cover it up." A salient feature of Nixon's career can be given the same superordinate characterization, to which can be added the fact that his political career was finished when the events came to light. Fourth, this additional information must be transferred to Mrs. Thatcher as a possible outcome. Someone who knows about Watergate but not about

Westland may still be able to transfer the superordinate information and to infer that the Westland affair involves some sort of cover-up that may jeopardize Thatcher's position. Someone (per impossibile!) who knows about Westland but not about Watergate may be able to transfer its superordinate characterization to Nixon and thus will infer that he was involved in some failed attempt to cover up a misdemeanor.

This example highlights two aspects of expository analogies (both of which create problems for the current version of PI). First, an important role can be played by mappings between specific individuals and entities. A restriction to mappings between predicates is particularly implausible in the case of expository analogies, which often assert a direct link between individuals, for example, "Stravinsky is the Picasso of music." By individuals here, I mean those entities denoted by individual constants in the first-order predicate calculus. Of course, one could define an individual as a set of all sets of which the individual is a member, but that would call for a theory outside the current version of PI. Second, the PI theory is correct to emphasize the pragmatic role of failure in a target problem – it is that failure which triggers the analogical mechanism, but expository analogies can work in either direction. The norm may be for the source to be mapped onto the target and then for information from the source to be transferred to the target. In practice, however, a quite different sequence is possible. Even people who are familiar with all the facts relevant to an expository analogy may interpret it in a variety of different sequences. One person may work from source to target, another from target to source, and yet another in alternate directions, in order to establish the initial mappings.

The discovery of profound analogies

Innovations in science and art often arise as a result of analogical thinking (see Hesse, 1966). Such analogies, however, call for genuinely creative thought. An act of creation, I assume, yields a product that is novel for the individual who produced it (though not necessarily for society as a whole), that is not constructed by rote or by some other deterministic process, and that satisfies some existing criteria or constraints. One creates pictures, poems, stories, sonatas, theorems, theories, principles, procedures, inventions, games, jokes, problems, puzzles, and so on and on. There are criteria about what counts as members of these categories, and even the creation of a new genre must meet certain criteria. Anything that lies outside all constraints is likely to be deemed uncategorizable and not the product of a creative process.

The only problematical condition in this working definition of creativity is the notion that it is nondeterministic. In the theory of computation, a nondeterministic device is one that can yield different outcomes from the same state. Real computers can simulate nondeterminism by borrowing a technique from the casino in Monte Carlo; they make a random choice. The claim that human creativity is nondeterministic is open to several interpretations. It could be taken to mean no more than that we are ignorant of the true causes of a particular choice. The reason that a scientist happens to think of *this* idea rather than *that* may depend on some minuscule aspect of the environment, the state of his or her digestive system, or some otherwise quite unrelated event. On this interpretation, creativity is deterministic, but ignorance forces us to treat it as nondeterministic. Another interpretation is that the mind is able to make arbitrary decisions. It may not be good at making truly random choices, but nevertheless it can choose between alternatives by the mental equivalent of spinning a biased coin, in which the trials are not independent. Yet another possible interpretation is that the brain is intrinsically nondeterministic, much as events in the quantum domain are nondeterministic.

There is a basis for choosing among these alternatives (see Johnson-Laird, 1988), but for present purposes we can be agnostic about them. The crucial point is that the relevant facts about a domain place constraints on what can be thought about that domain, but they still allow an indefinite number of possible thoughts, just as, for example, the rules of a language place constraints on what counts as an expression in the language but still allow an indefinite number of different sentences. If the constraints on thinking about a domain allowed only one possible continuation at each step in grappling with a problem, then the process of discovering a solution would be either trivial or impossible. There would be no choice about what to do next. Hence, a theory of creativity is forced to introduce an element of nondeterminism.

Given that creativity calls for something that is novel for the individual, that is not merely a result of deterministic or calculative procedure, and that meets certain constraints, then, as I have argued elsewhere (see Johnson-Laird, 1988), there are three main classes of algorithms that can yield a creative product. First, there are "neo-Darwinian" algorithms. They make some random, or quasi-random, constructions out of existing elements so as to generate a vast number of putative products; and then they use a set of constraints to filter out those products that are not viable. Some theorists have argued that such algorithms are the only mechanism for creativity (see, e.g., Skinner, 1953). Second, there are "neo-Lamarckian" algorithms. They form initial constructions under the guidance of all the constraints in the domain, where these constraints may suffice to guarantee viability; and then they select at random from the set of viable alternatives generated in this way. The final selection has to be at random because by definition all the constraints have been taken into account in the first stage. Third, there are "multistage" algorithms. They make use of some constraints in the initial generative process; and then they use other constraints to act as filters. Since the complete set of constraints does not pinpoint a unique product, the final stage calls for a random selection from among the set of viable alternatives.

Undoubtedly, the most efficient algorithms are those constructed on a neo-Lamarckian design, and it can be shown that a particular task that calls for creativity in real time – musical improvisation – can be modeled in computer programs that realize such an algorithm (see Johnson-Laird, 1988). The requirements for a neo-Lamarckian algorithm are that there is a set of constraints that define only viable products and that this set is represented in the mind. Musicians improvising in a particular genre have a tacit grasp of the principles defining the genre, and they can use them to generate music that lies within the genre. If they have an inadequate grasp of these principles, they will produce unacceptable music and fail to find gainful employment – at least as improvisers. In the case of a major innovation in science or art, however, there are grounds for doubting whether there even exist principles that define only viable products. On the one hand, there are too few instances of a major revolution within a particular domain. On the other hand, it is hard to see what the instances might have in common that could be captured by principles that would generate nothing but successful innovations. What substantive constraints, for example, are common to both the transition to Newtonian mechanics and the transition to the special theory of relativity? Indeed, it hardly needs to be said that even the best of scientists may try out many bad ideas before discovering a good one.

If there are no constraints that underlie all and only the successful innovations in a domain, there can be no neo-Lamarckian algorithm for the discovery of new ideas or new analogies. It follows that, at best, scientists must use a multistage algorithm, which employs some constraints on the initial generation of ideas. But these constraints are not sufficient to guarantee the viability of the product, and thus the initial generation of ideas is likely to be highly wasteful. A scientist searching for an explanation of some perplexing phenomenon may try out many putative analogs and many novel combinations of ideas.

The creation of a profound analogy is unlikely to depend on preexisting rules that establish mappings between the source and target domains. The innovation indeed depends on the invention of such rules. (It is the provision of these rules and only a limited number of potential source domains that enables PI to work efficiently.) Once one has found the appropriate analog, there are presumably fewer degrees of freedom about what information should be transferred from it to the target problem. To establish a mapping is accordingly a process that resembles the construction of a complex proposition that links an element in one domain with an element in another domain. If we think of all domains of knowledge – knowledge of the solar system, of atoms, of waves, of clocks, and so on – as constituting a vast epistemic "space," then the task of creating a profound analogy consists initially in establishing a mapping from one domain to another. The more remote the two domains are from one another (prior to the construction of the analogy), the larger the number of potential source domains and the longer the chain of links that will have to be established from the right source to the target domain. Granted that at each point in the construction of the chain there are a number of different possible continuations, then the mapping is like the construction of a novel sentence – a sentence that captures the content of the mapping. Plainly, the number of possible sentences increases exponentially with the length of the sentence, and likewise the number of possible mappings increases exponentially with the number of links. The problem is a member of the class of NP problems; that is, it could be solved by a nondeterministic automaton in a time proportional to some polynomial of the number of links in the chain. If there were some efficient way of simulating nondeterminism, then the problem would be tractable. Failing that, however, it is intractable: No algorithm for searching for the correct mapping can run in a realistic time beyond a certain number of links. The more constraints that can be brought to bear on the search process, the larger the number of links that can be tractably handled. However, sooner or later the number of links will call for an impossibly long search time.

Certain algorithms, such as simulated annealing (see Kirkpatrick, Gelatt, & Vecchi, 1983), are helpful with NP problems, such as the classic "traveling salesman" problem (to find the shortest route by which to travel to a number of towns once only and to return to base).

Such algorithms work by a process of gradual stochastic optimization through a succession of many minute changes in a vast number of variables. The procedure is useful if the goal is to deliver not the best solution but one that is reasonably optimal. Unfortunately, such algorithms and their variants in "connectionist" schemes (see, e.g., Rumelhart, this volume) are unlikely to discover profound scientific analogies as a matter of course. One cannot find the right analog by way of a large number of successive approximations to the correct mapping. There are many variables, but a small change in just one of them may make all the difference in establishing the correct mapping.

Of course, there are computer programs that have produced novel proofs of theorems, interesting mathematical conjectures, and original works of art and music. Their success depends on operating in highly constrained domains, using a neo-Lamarckian procedure or assistance from the user. Even trial and error will work if you are prepared to carry out billions of experiments over millions of years and to countenance a high proportion of failures. The point of my argument is that there can be no tractable algorithm that is guaranteed to make profound analogies as a matter of course.

Finally, I should note that the PI program is not intended to cope with the problems of the exponential increase in the size of the search space. The number of possible mappings that it could construct is kept under control by the user insuring that the number of different domains and the number of mapping rules are kept to a tractable size. In reality, of course, a tractable domain will exclude the possibility of discovering a really deep analog. However, there is no reason to suppose that the mental algorithm that human beings use for solving problems is in general tractable. The task of discovering a profound analogy defeats all but a handful of individuals: The number of concepts that might be relevant is too large for us to be able to consider all their implications. The exceptional thinker has mastered more constraints – to be used generatively as opposed to merely critically – and thus has a greater chance of making the required mapping.

Conclusion

Analogies are tools for thought and explanation, but they do not form a unitary class. Expository analogies and those that are exploited in mental tests can be grasped by tractable algorithms. A test item such as

sluice is to *water* as which of the following pairs:
gate : pasture
jet : gas
dam : channel
bulwark : fortress
turbulence : air

can be solved by an appropriate variation on the procedure that I described for expository analogies, provided, of course, that the requisite knowledge is available. Thus the first step is to recover from memory a semantic relation between the initial terms; for example, a sluice controls the flow of water. The next step is to examine each of the potential answers to determine whether there is a unique pair of items that has the same semantic relation: x controls the flow of y. In this instance, there is such a pair (jet : gas). Since there are always alternative relations, such as superordinate ones, that hold between pairs, the initially selected relation may be satisfied by more than one potential answer. If so, it is necessary to find an alternative relation, for example, by examining the difference between the possible answers. The essential point, however, is that when the source and target are known, as in an expository analogy, or when there are only a small number of potential analogs as in an analogy test, then, given access to the relevant knowledge, the analogy can be grasped using a neo-Lamarckian algorithm that is tractable.

At the heart of the algorithm is a process that recovers a semantic relation between the objects or predicates of a domain, and this relation may call for the construction of a superordinate or subordinate of the relation initially recovered. The semantic relation is then transferred from the source to the target, or, in certain cases, the relation may be recovered from the target and transferred to the source.

The use of analogies to solve problems relies on a similar transfer of semantic relations – schematic models that capture the structure of the domain (cf. Johnson-Laird, 1983) – but there are additional and more critical steps. First, the target problem must fail to yield to conventional inferential approaches. If it seems to have been solved, then people are unlikely to look for an analog, as was the case with the arbitrary rule in the selection task. Second, the relevant source domain has to be found. This step, as I have implied, lies at the heart of all profound analogies. But, like many search problems, it turns out that there is no tractable algorithm that is guaranteed to succeed. The more constraints that individuals can bring to the task – the more they know about potentially relevant domains – the more likely they are to find the illuminating source. With an increase in the number of potential sources, however, any search algorithm runs into intractable difficulties.

As previous theorists have emphasized, the search for an analogy is engendered by pragmatic reasons; it is established on the basis of fact and meaning; and, if possible, it exploits large-scale systematic structures. What, perhaps, has not been noted before are the computational consequences of the exercise of creativity in the discovery of original analogies.

NOTES

I am grateful to Paul Thagard for some very helpful conversations on PI and analogy and for his criticisms of an earlier draft of this chapter. My thanks also for their help and support to Joel Cooper, Sam Glucksberg, Steve Hanson, George Miller, Charlie Rosenberg, Sue Sugarman, and other members of the Department of Psychology, Princeton University, where this was written. I am also indebted to Dedre Gentner for pointing out my misinterpretation of her theory. Finally, I am grateful to Tony Anderson for his collaboration on the commonsense inference experiment, and to Andrew Ortony for a provocative critique.

1 I originally directed this criticism at Gentner's theory; Holyoak (1985) makes a similar point. Gentner (personal communication) has pointed out that the criticism is misdirected. Her claim is correct, now that the first step in her theory is to establish structural relations and then to derive object mappings from them. Hence, the sun will be mapped onto the pendulum or clockwork that causes the hands to revolve; i.e., the causal relations establish the mapping. What remains to be explained is the origin of the more profound analogy of the two above.

2 Gentner has sometimes said that the process is syntactic, but it is clear that this label is misleading (personal communication). The mapping process in the program modeling the theory (see Gentner, this volume) works by taking into account the labels in semantic networks and the structural relations between them; i.e., if two relations have the same name, the program sets up a match between them provided their arguments are objects or functions of objects. It matches relations with the same meaning.

REFERENCES

Falkenhainer, B., Forbus, K. D., & Gentner, D. (1986). The structure-mapping engine. In *Proceedings of the American Association for Artificial Intelligence*. Los Altos, CA: Kaufmann.

Gentner, D. (1983). Structure-mapping: A theoretical framework for analogy. *Cognitive Science, 7*, 155–170.

Gick, M. L., & Holyoak, K. J. (1980). Analogical problem solving. *Cognitive Psychology, 12*, 306–355.

Gick, M. L., & Holyoak, K. J. (1983). Schema induction and analogical transfer. *Cognitive Psychology, 15*, 1–38.

✓ Goodman, N. (1955). *Fact, fiction, and forecast.* Cambridge, MA: Harvard University Press.

✓ Hesse, M. B. (1966). *Models and analogies in science.* Notre Dame, IN: Notre Dame University Press.

Holyoak, K. J. (1985). The pragmatics of analogical transfer. In G. H. Bower (Ed.), *The psychology of learning and motivation: Advances in research and theory* (Vol. 19, pp. 59–87). New York: Academic Press.

✓ Johnson-Laird, P. N. (1983). *Mental models: Towards a cognitive science of language, inference, and consciousness.* Cambridge, MA: Harvard University Press. Cambridge: Cambridge University Press.

✓ Johnson-Laird, P. N. (1988). Freedom and constraint in creativity. In R. J. Sternberg (Ed.), *Creativity.* Cambridge: Cambridge University Press.

Johnson-Laird, P. N., Herrmann, D. J., & Chaffin, R. (1984). Only connections: A critique of semantic networks. *Psychological Bulletin, 96*, 292–315.

Johnson-Laird, P. N., Legrenzi, P., & Legrenzi, M. S. (1972). Reasoning and a sense of reality. *British Journal of Psychology, 63*, 395–400.

Kirkpatrick, S., Gelatt, C. D., & Vecchi, M. P. (1983). Optimization by simulated annealing. *Science, 220*, 671–680.

Newell, A., & Simon, H. A. (1972). *Human problem solving.* Englewood Cliffs, NJ: Prentice-Hall.

Skinner, B. F. (1953). *Science and human behavior.* New York: Macmillan.

Thagard, P., & Holyoak, K. J. (1985). Discovering the wave theory of sound: Induction in the context of problem solving. *Proceedings of the Ninth International Joint Conference on Artificial Intelligence* (pp. 610–612). Los Altos, CA: Kaufmann.

Wason, P. C., & Johnson-Laird, P. N. (1972). *The psychology of deductive reasoning: Structure and content.* Cambridge, MA: Harvard University Press.

Winograd, T. (1972). *Understanding natural language.* New York: Academic Press.

12

Levels of description in information-processing theories of analogy

STEPHEN E. PALMER

The chapters by Dedre Gentner, Keith Holyoak and Paul Thagard, and David Rumelhart in this volume present a broad spectrum of approaches to understanding the nature of analogical thought processes. Gentner spends a good deal of effort on formulating just what an analogy is; Holyoak and Thagard use production systems and spreading activation to simulate analogical processing in a problem-solving task; and Rumelhart explores the potential importance of connectionism for understanding analogies in the context of other "higher mental processes." How are we to integrate this enormous diversity in tackling the same underlying problem? Is one right and the others wrong? Which proposals actually conflict, and which ones are compatible? What have we learned from each one about analogical thought?

I plan to approach these questions within a broad metatheoretical framework that spans the unique as well as the common aspects of the three presentations. The framework I have in mind is closely related to David Marr's (1982) well-known distinction among three levels of analysis of an information-processing (IP) system: the *computational* level, the *algorithmic* level, and the *implementational* level. My own view of the situation is slightly different from Marr's in that I see IP theories as spanning a single continuum of possible theoretical levels defined at the "upper" end of the spectrum by *informational (or task) constraints*, at the "lower" end by *hardware constraints*, and in between by *behavioral constraints*. In this view, all psychological IP theories are algorithmic in Marr's sense, but they can still differ dramatically from each other in terms of level of abstraction. Higher levels of IP theory are related to lower levels within this spectrum by successive applications of the "decomposition assumption," in which the "black boxes" of IP theories are recursively broken down into flow diagrams of more primitive black boxes (Palmer & Kimchi, 1985).

In my view the chapters by Gentner, Holyoak and Thagard, and

Rumelhart seem so different because they are directed primarily at different levels of analysis. Gentner aims, more than the others, at the highest level of the problem, trying to get clear on just what an analogy *is* and what operations *must* be part of understanding one. Rumelhart makes a brilliant stab at the lowest level, trying to see how neurologically plausible IP mechanisms might be able to accomplish analogical reasoning and related thought processes. Holyoak and Thagard worry less about either informational or hardware constraints and try to construct a working simulation model that conforms generally to existing behavioral evidence. Despite these differences in thrust, they all make some proposals in the middle of the spectrum and try to be faithful to important aspects of human behavior in at least some analogical tasks. It is primarily here that they conflict. My plan is to discuss the papers by levels, first at the upper, informational end, then in the middle where they overlap in content, and finally at the lower, hardware end where Rumelhart has the field to himself.

Informational constraints: What is an analogy?

At the highest level of analysis we are faced with what Gentner refers to as "competence" issues: What *is* an analogy and what *must* be true if a person can be said to understand one? These issues are at what Palmer and Kimchi (1975) call the "mapping level" because they concern informational constraints on what situations people would take to be analogous. In a sense, the objective at this level is to capture only the input–output mapping of people's analogical thought processes without regard to just *how* they might be accomplished in more specific terms.

Gentner's interest in this level of analysis is reflected in the kinds of questions she asks experimentally. Many of them are aimed at getting measures of the "goodness" or "soundness" of analogies and various types of near-analogies, just the sorts of studies one needs to figure out what kind of internal structure analogies have. Holyoak and Thagard are principally interested in how analogies can be used to help solve problems and in what sort of learning takes place when they are used. Rumelhart is interested in how people might come up with a potential analogy in the first place. Perhaps as a result, neither of the latter two chapters contains as many ideas about what constitutes an analogy as does Gentner's. Therefore, my comments at the highest level of IP theory will be directed at Gentner's structure-mapping theory (SMT).

Gentner's chapter itself suggests an analogy to me: that analogies are like representations. I will use this analogy to frame my discussion of informational issues because I think it illuminates some of the proposals she has made and brings them into sharper focus.

How are analogies like representations?

To begin, I should make clear what analogy I am proposing. At one point in her description of the structure-mapping theory (SMT) of analogy Gentner writes:

> The central idea in structure-mapping is that an analogy is a mapping of knowledge from one domain (the base) into another (the target), which conveys that a system of relations that holds among the base objects also holds among the target objects. Thus an analogy is a way of focusing on relational commonalities independently of the objects in which those relations are embedded.... Objects are placed in correspondence by virtue of their like roles in the common relational structure. [Gentner, this volume, p. 201].

What struck me was the remarkable similarity between this description of analogy and my own description of a representational system:

> The nature of representation is that there exists a correspondence (mapping) from objects in the represented world to objects in the representing world such that at least some relations in the represented world are structurally preserved in the representing world. [Palmer, 1978, p. 267]

There are clearly important differences between analogies and representations, but these two descriptions are so similar that one can scarcely help but see the resemblance in underlying conceptions. Simply replace *representation* with *analogy, represented world* with *base domain,* and *representing world* with *target domain,* and the resulting sentence from Palmer (1978) might well have appeared in Gentner's chapter as a description of analogy.

What does this mean? What inferences should we draw from this underlying similarity? No doubt many are possible, but the one I want to focus on is that analogies and representations are the same sort of beast. They are both *model systems* in which, loosely speaking, one thing is taken to "stand for" another thing. In the case of analogy, the source domain is taken to stand for the target domain so that the target can be understood in terms of the source to solve some problem or merely to emphasize a particular fact. Calling an analogy a model does not really *do* anything, of course, unless there is some interesting conception of a model that will help us to clarify what sort of model an analogy is. And in this case I think that Tarski's (1954) model theory might provide such a conception. At least, I will use it as such.

Model theory

Tarski formalized modeling relations in set theoretic terms. Roughly speaking, one set of objects is said to model another set of objects if there exists a function that maps the former to the latter so that corresponding relations are preserved. Formally, a model, M, is an ordered triple consisting of a homomorphic mapping function, F, from one relational system, S, to another, S',

$$M = < S, S', F >.$$

The relational system, S, is an ordered n-tuple consisting of a set of objects, O, and some number, m, of relations on O,

$$S = <O, R_1, R_2, \ldots R_m >.$$

The second relational system, S', is defined analogously,

$$S' = < O', R_1', R_2', \ldots R_m' >,$$

and the function, F, maps objects in S to objects in S'

$$F: o_i \rightarrow o_i'$$

such that corresponding relations are preserved. The n-ary relations in relational system S are formalized as subsets of all possible n-tuples consisting of objects in O (i.e., subsets of $O \times O \times \ldots \times O$) for which the given relation holds. Thus F is a map from O to O', such that

$$< o_i, o_j, \ldots o_n > \varepsilon\ R_m \Rightarrow <o_i', o_j', \ldots o_n'> \varepsilon\ R'_m$$

where o_i' is the image of o_i under F, and so forth.

This is a very spare – indeed, probably too spare – and very general characterization of a model, and that is precisely why I think that it will be a useful one for present purposes. We can now view analogy as a special case of a model and say precisely what further restrictions are required for a model to qualify as an analogy and how analogies differ from other sorts of models, such as representations.

Defining terms

The first thing that needs to be done is to ask for definitions of some theoretical terms. Clearly, the *analogy* is the whole modeling system, M, defined by the mapping, F, of objects in the source domain, S, to the objects of the target domain, S'. Beyond this, Gentner discusses a number of important concepts, some of which are easy to formulate in model theoretic terms and others of which are more difficult. In any case, it is informative to examine Gentner's concepts of structural consistency, transparency, target validity, systematicity, and the differences she proposes among attributes, first-order relations, and higher-order relations to see whether these can be understood in the model theoretic framework.

Structural consistency and *target validity* have straightforward interpretations within model theory. In fact, they both specify necessary conditions for model theory to apply. Structural consistency refers to the possibility that each object in the base (i.e., source) is assigned to one and only one object in the target. That is, in a consistent analogy a given object in the source domain always stands for the same object in the target domain; its interpretation does not hop around from one thing to another. In model theoretic terms, this condition is required for the mapping from one relational system to the other to qualify as a *function*: If it is not "structurally consistent" (in Gentner's sense), then it is not a function, and there is no globally specifiable "model" (in Tarski's sense).

Target validity refers to the property of an analogy that minimizes contradictions between relations in the source domain and the corresponding ones in the target domain. In model theoretic terms, a model is "valid" in the target domain by definition, because saying that a source relation preserves the truth of its corresponding target relation clearly implies that there are no contradictions. Thus contradictions have the effect of restricting just what relations are included in the two relational systems being mapped.

Gentner includes these concepts in her discussion because analogies, unlike Tarskian models, are very "fuzzy" things. Many idealized conditions – such as structural consistency and target validity – may be violated to some extent, and the result may still seem to be an analogy to some degree. Perhaps analogies could actually be formalized as "fuzzy models" in the mold of Zadeh's (1965) "fuzzy set theory" and "fuzzy logic," but the development of this conjecture is well beyond the scope of this chapter. For now, I only want to emphasize that the properties of structural consistency and target validity have somewhat different roles to play in a theory of analogies than in Tarskian model theory. In a theory of analogy, treated as a natural category à la Rosch (1977), they are properties of the categorical "ideal"; in a theory of models, treated as an artificial category, they are defining characteristics of the formal concept.

Transparency and *systematicity* are also easily understood in a model theoretic framework, although they are not actually part of the definition of a model. *Transparency* refers to a property of the mapping from base to target wherein base objects map onto target objects that are *similar* in some sense. As several of Gentner's experiments show, this property is particularly important for people to notice an analogy spontaneously. A corresponding concept does not arise in model theory, of course, because the whole point of model theory is that *any* homomorphic mapping that preserves the relational structure of the source relational system is equally good as a model in a mathematical sense, independent of how "similar" the corresponding objects might be in one or another target domain. The concept of similarity itself has proved to be difficult to pin down (e.g., Goodman, 1968; Tversky, 1977), and trying to formalize it within model theory would necessarily open this Pandora's box of thorny issues. Certainly these are all implicit in Gentner's concept of the transparency of a mapping (Gentner, this volume, pp. 221–226).

In Gentner's SMT, *systematicity* refers to the mapping of whole relational hierarchies in the base domain onto those in the target domain. There is a restricted sense in which this is included in model theory: namely, all the relations contained in Gentner's hierarchies are relations that would be specified within corresponding relational systems. In another sense, however, it is *not* included, because model theory does not contain any formal apparatus for specifying *hierarchies* among relations. Gentner's theory includes hierarchial structure because she chooses to represent complex relations as composed of simpler ones. For instance, she represents the binary relation HOTTER THAN as an abstract, "higher-order" relation, GREATER THAN, holding between the TEMPERATURE "attributes" of the two objects – that is, GREATER THAN [TEMPERATURE (object1), TEMPERATURE (object2)]. One might represent the same information with equal plausibility merely as a relation holding between two objects – that is, HOTTER THAN (object1, object2). Similarly, she represents causal relations hierarchically – for example, CAUSE [PUSH (object1, object2), COLLIDE (object1, object2)] – rather than merely as a binary relation – for example, CAUSE-TO-COLLIDE-BY-PUSHING (object1, object2). These are the kinds of hierarchies to which Gentner refers in her discussion of systematicity, and it is clear that they do not exist in Tarskian model theory, at least as applied to ordinary conceptions of what constitutes objects and relations.

The reason Gentner postulates such hierarchies, of course, is that they are part of her theory of mental representation. She feels that within the mental world complex ideas and relations are – or can be – psychologically decomposed into simpler ones that are structured hierarchically. For such hierarchical structure to be formally specified in model theory, the entities to which the relational systems refer must also be mental rather than physical. In other words, the "objects" of the relational system must be *conceptual entities*, including relations like CAUSE and GREATER THAN as well as concepts for standard objects like *table* and *dog*. In this case, it is straightforward to include Gentner's hierarchies in a model theoretic framework (although it is beyond the scope of this chapter to do so). However, it must be acknowledged that the objects and relations in question no longer refer directly to the physical world but refer to concepts inside people's heads which *then* refer to physical objects and relations. This is fine, but it clearly shows that at least part of Gentner's "conceptual"-level theory really does rest on her specific proposals about how to represent complex relations hierarchically.

The issues surrounding systematicity and relational hierarchies are closely related to what may be the most important problem in SMT: namely, the differences among "attributes," "first-order relations," and "higher-order relations." They are important because they are the key, according to Gentner, to understanding the differences among true analogies, mere-appearance matches, literal similarity, and anomaly. In particular, the claim is that "object attributes" in the two domains do not have to match, whereas "higher-order relations" (also called "relational structure" and "structural relations") *do* have to match. If so, we have to know how to distinguish the type that needs to match from the type that does not. I will refer to this as the *relation-sorting problem*.

Indeed, before we even get to this relation-sorting problem, we need to notice the even more fundamental distinction that is clearly implied by this claim: namely, that for at least some relations, the *same* relation must hold for corresponding objects in the source and target domains. Recall that basic model theory requires only that *corresponding* relations hold for corresponding objects. This is essentially the way things work in SMT for object attributes. In the heat/pressure analogy, for example, object temperatures can be modeled by water pressures; they do not have to be modeled by water temperatures. This is at the root of Gentner's claim that, in analogy, objects do not have to *resemble* their corresponding base objects; they do not have to have the *same* attributes, merely *corresponding* ones. Not so for other relations, apparently. The fact that differences in pressure *cause* water to flow so as to reduce those differences must be modeled by differences in temperature *causing* heat to flow in an analogous fashion. Whether or not this turns out to be necessary or even desirable for specifying the nature of analogy is another question. The answer hinges on several other important issues, including the relation-sorting problem.

Given that some relations among corresponding objects have to be the *same* and others merely *corresponding*, Gentner has proposed some criteria for classifying these two kinds of relations. In previous formulations, she suggested a clean, syntactic distinction between object attributes (as *one-place* predicates or *unary* relations) and all other relations (*two-or-more-place* predicates or *binary-or-greater* relations). This clearly will not do, as she herself admits. My problems with this neat "*n*-ary" formulation are twofold.

First, there are many binary (or greater) relations that presumably do *not* need to match, particularly those tied to attributes like size, color, weight, and so on. For instance, in the heat/pressure analogy, water EXERTS MORE PRESSURE on the beaker than on the vial, and the corresponding relation in the heat domain is that the coffee is HOTTER THAN the ice cube. To me, this seems to be an example of corresponding relations holding rather than identical relations holding. For Gentner, however, they are identical because she represents them both more abstractly as the same GREATER THAN relation holding between two attributes or functions. It is unclear which conception is correct or even how to decide the issue. It is similarly unclear whether DIFFERENCE-IN-PRESSURE-CAUSING something to happen is the *same* relation as DIFFERENCE-IN-HEAT-CAUSING something to happen, or whether they are merely *corresponding* relations. Gentner calls them the same because, as mentioned previously, she has chosen to represent complex relations by decomposing them into hierarchies of primitive (or at least more primitive) relations. In the standard application of set theoretic model theory, there is no provision for representing such differences. However, it could be incorporated, as previously suggested, by modeling conceptual entities rather than physical ones so that relations become "conceptual objects" whose interrelations can then be specified in the relational system.

This brings me to a second, related problem with the *n*-ary formulation. Whether a given relation is unary, binary, or whatever is hard to specify a priori; it depends at least somewhat on how one *chooses* to represent it. For example, the obvious way to represent the fact that a bear is bigger than a breadbox is a binary relation, BIGGER THAN (BEAR, BREADBOX) but one could also choose to use a more specific unary relation, BIGGER-THAN-A-BREADBOX (BEAR). In this manner, any *n*-ary relation can be reduced to a smaller number of arguments simply by binding one or more of them into the predicate itself – at the expense of proliferating the number of such relations, of course. The point is only that the order of a relation is not God-given or dictated by logic alone but something that results from representational choices made by a theorist. This may turn out to be an empirical question. If one could define a procedure for deciding how people actually represent such relations, then Gentner's n-ary formulation may turn out to be right after all.

Perhaps the goal of defining *crisp* boundaries between true analogy, mere-appearance matches, literal similarity, and anomaly is pointless. After all, Gentner herself presents a diagram showing a continuum among these cases. Rumelhart also implies unclear boundaries in his description of analogy as being at the end of a continuum from literal similarity to generalization to reminding to reasoning by example. But they both still require some sort of distinction (Gentner) or well-defined continuum (Rumelhart) between those aspects that can differ and those that cannot. In the final analysis, what *any* analogy theorist will have to do to make a convincing case is to tell us what the basis of this distinction is, and why.

Behavioral constraints: process models of analogical thought

Beyond the informational constraints implied by the task, analogy theorists must take into account people's observable behavior. Many of the most important constraints come from the problem-solving literature. Here we must consider empirical facts such as that one analogy may be more likely to be solved than another, that one will take longer to solve than another, and that one situation will spontaneously give rise to an analogy whereas another will not. The differences among such analogies occur not so much at the level of informational constraints as at the level of how people process them. That is, all such analogies may have the same high-level formal description and yet may differ substantially in the ways in which people actually process them. In Palmer and Kimchi's (1985) analysis, more specific process models are generated in information-processing theory by recursively decomposing the operations postulated at higher levels. It is at these lower levels that the assumptions of different models are likely to make differential predictions about behavioral observations.

Both Gentner and Holyoak and Thagard make proposals at the upper end of this middle level of processing models in what would seem to be the first application of recursive decomposition. Gentner divides analogy processing into roughly five stages, which she describes as: (a) accessing the base domain, (b) performing the mapping from base to target (which she divides further into two parts), (c) judging the soundness of the match, (d) storing inferences in the target domain, and (e) extracting the common principle. We can identify pretty much the same stages in Holyoak and Thagard's analysis, although they talk about them in slightly different terms: (a) accumulating activation in the source domain, (b) setting up a mapping, (c) extending the mapping, (d) performing analogous actions, and (e) generalizing from the results. Thus, at the upper level of process models there seems to be substantial agreement, at least among these theorists.

In the remainder of this section I will concentrate my comments on Holyoak and Thagard's proposals because their theory is directed most squarely at this middle level; that is, it offers the most complete account of what might be going on during analogical thought process. Gentner's proposal is less complete in the sense that she has nothing to say about the first stage (how the source domain is accessed) and little to say about the last (extracting the common principle), both of which are important components of Holyoak and Thagard's process model. Rumelhart's proposal is far less complete in that it is *only* about accessing the source domain.

Holyoak and Thagard specify the processing of analogies using two of the most popular "middle-level" processing constructs of IP psychology: production systems (Newell & Simon, 1972) and spreading activation (Collins & Loftus, 1975). Accessing the source domain is accomplished in their system by spreading activation through associative links, especially among subgoals. These associative links are presumably preexisting structures in the mind of the analogizer that encode prior experience with the relevant concepts. (For Gentner and Rumelhart, by contrast, accessing the source domain takes place by virtue of similarity rather than association.) The mapping from source to target is set up by tracing the activation back through prior associations to determine which concepts correspond to which. The mapping is then extended by mapping corresponding arguments of those concepts that have been established by the initial map based on associative activation. This complete mapping is then exploited in problem solving by performing actions in the target domain analogous to those that resulted in solution in the source domain. Thus analogical problem solving is ultimately accomplished by having the goals and subgoals in the source serve as a model for a plan consisting of the corresponding goals and subgoals in the target. Finally, if an analogy does lead to the solution of the new problem, the model generalizes from the two solutions to form a new abstract problem schema. Abstractions are made by comparing analogous concepts in the two solutions, and storing common higher-order concepts. All of these operations seem to be specified in enough detail to produce a working simulation model of analogical problem solving. (The reader is referred to their chapter for a more complete description.)

Even though I applaud the specificity of Holyoak and Thagard's proposals, I cannot help but worry that their theory will work only on the sort of "toy system" problems they have described in their chapter. I am particularly worried that, as the size of the data base grows, the number of associations and potential mappings will very quickly swamp the system and make it difficult or impossible to reason analogically in a sensible amount of time (see also Johnson-Laird, this volume). I also worry about the specificity of the knowledge that they need to include in their examples. Do we really need to suppose that people have a rule like "If x is an army and y is a road between x and some z, then x can move to z"?

Even if we grant this kind of knowledge representation, I worry about whether their proposal would still carry through if the situation were changed even slightly. For example, the rule just mentioned will not work if, say, there happened to be an open drawbridge between the army and the fortress. One could always add to the rule a condition that there *not* be an open drawbridge on the road between x and z. The trouble is that this is just one instance of which there are an infinite variety, any of which would cause the rule to fail. For instance, the road cannot be covered with land mines, or ablaze with burning oil, or submerged under 2 feet of mud, and so forth. Adding all of these conditions to the rule would lead, at *best*, to an extremely unwieldy representation of the condition–action pairs, and one that is not psychologically realistic. To be fair, many of these problems are not specific to Holyoak and Thagard's theory of analogy but are pervasive in the artificial intelligence literature. The question is whether these problems can be surmounted and, if so, whether the same type of theory Holyoak and Thagard have proposed will prove a viable account of analogical problem solving.

Hardware constraints: the microstructure of analogical thought

The only theorist who attempts to decompose information-processing operations "all the way down" to the level of hardware primitives is

Rumelhart. He presents a connectionist-style information-processing theory of analogy that almost exclusively concerns the stage we have called *accessing the source domain.*

One of the claims of connectionism is that the process of recursive decomposition in information-processing theories does not happen in small steps. Rather, it is claimed, one goes very quickly from some high-level description of a process to one in terms of quasi-neural primitives (Smolensky, 1986). Rumelhart's theory is a good example. In his view, the source domain is accessed by an almost unitary process in which units within a vast network pass activation and inhibition among each other, and the network settles into a minimum-energy configuration that ends up representing the source domain. Rumelhart's specific proposal about analogy concerns how such a connectionist network could come up with analogies by systematically relaxing low-level constraints on input feature values that represent the target domain. He suggests that if the lowest-level features of the input are allowed to vary freely, rather than being "clamped" by the input, such a system will perform analogical thought processes as a natural extension of the similarity-processing capabilities of such networks.

For me, Rumelhart's approach has enormous intuitive appeal. His idea that multiple constraints act in parallel through a fast automatic process that is conceptually continuous with similarity matching is an ingenious one. However, it is clearly just a conjecture with little to back it up. There is presently no working program that actually performs the operation and no behavioral evidence suggesting that this approach is preferable to others. Until substantial progress is made on both of these fronts, it would be premature to evaluate Rumelhart's idea by standard scientific criteria.

It is perhaps easy to see how Rumelhart's model might be a good way to access a potential source domain for an analogy. It is less clear, however, that connectionist networks could be used to implement some of the other, more sequential processing that seems to be implied by higher-level descriptions of analogical thought. For instance, how is the mapping from source to target carried out, evaluated, and exploited in problem solving? Some of Rumelhart's later proposals about simulation and mental models may be relevant here, but a lot more work is needed to make their implications clear for analogical reasoning. It is also worth mentioning that Rumelhart faces a problem similar to Gentner's relation-sorting problem in that he must come up with a principled description of which features to relax and in what order. Intuitively, the idea of relaxing the most superficial features is clear, but it is less than an adequate description of how to implement the process in a working model.

In most respects, Rumelhart's theory is much more different from Gentner's and Holyoak and Thagard's than they are from each other. Rumelhart's theory takes a dramatically different view of representation as being distributed rather than localized, and a different view of processing based on the parallel activation through dynamic associative networks rather than on the sequential following of logical rules. No doubt his theory would conflict more directly with the others if it were extended to encompass the further processes that seem to be involved in analogical thought.

Conclusion

I have discussed the three chapters in terms of a general description of information-processing models. According to this analysis, Gentner, Holyoak and Thagard, and Rumelhart differ strongly in the level at which they attack the problem of analogy. These levels are largely complementary and, as a result, I think we can learn a good deal from each one. From Gentner we learn about high-level informational constraints on analogy: what an analogy is and how it relates to other kinds of similarity-based comparisons. From Holyoak and Thagard we learn about middle-level processing models and their relation to behavioral data on problem solving collected in the laboratory. They have also done the most complete analysis of the entire process of analogical thought, using standard information-processing techniques like productions systems and spreading activation to construct a working simulation. From Rumelhart we learn about the lowest-level processes nearest to the system's hardware and how these may be important in constructing models of thought, even higher-level processes such as analogy.

My own conclusion from these three very interesting chapters is that there is more than one way to skin an analogy. All three contribute substantially to what we know about how people produce, understand, and make use of analogies in thought and reasoning. Perhaps we will someday soon be able to see how they all fit together in the complex processes we call "analogy."

REFERENCES

Collins, A. M., & Loftus, E. F. (1975). A spreading-activation theory of semantic processing. *Psychological Review, 82* 407–428.

Goodman, N. (1968). *The language of art.* Indianapolis, IN: Bobbs-Merrill.

Marr, D. (1982). *Vision.* San Francisco: Freeman.

Newell, A., & Simon, H. A. (1972). *Human problem solving.* Englewood Cliffs, NJ; Prentice-Hall.

Palmer, S. E. (1978). Fundamental aspects of cognitive representation. In E. Rosch & B. B. Lloyd (Eds.), *Cognition and categorization* (pp. 259–302). Hillsdale, NJ: Erlbaum.

Palmer, S. E., & Kimchi, R. (1985). The information processing approach to cognition. In T. Knapp & L. C. Robertson (Eds.), *Approaches to cognition: Contrasts and controversies* (pp. 37–77). Hillsdale, NJ: Erlbaum.

Rosch, E. H. (1977). Human categorization. In N. Warren (Ed.), *Advances in cross-cultural psychology* (pp. 1–49). London: Academic Press.

Smolensky, P. (1986). Neural and conceptual interpretations of PDP models. In J. L. McClelland, D. E. Rumelhart, & the PDP Research Group, *Parallel distributed processing: Explorations in the microstructure of cognition* (Vol. 2, pp. 370–431). Cambridge, MA: MIT Press (Bradford Books).

Tarski, A. (1954). Contributions to the theory of models. *Indigationes Mathematicae, 16,* 572–588.

Tversky, A. (1977). Features of similarity. *Psychological Review, 84,* 327–352.

Zadeh, L. A. (1965). Fuzzy sets. *Information and Control, 8,* 338–353.

13

The role of explanation in analogy; or, The curse of an alluring name

GERALD DEJONG

Introduction

Artificial intelligence has a long and continuing interest in analogy (Burstein, 1985; Carbonell, 1985; Evans 1968; Forbus & Gentner, 1983; Kedar-Cabelli, 1985; Winston, 1980). From a computational point of view, more controversy surrounds analogy than any other single topic in the cognitive arena. From the perspective of an outsider, researchers appear to be doing wildly different things, all under the rubric of analogy. Perhaps this is just the natural result of a healthy diversity of thought. On the other hand, it may be a manifestation of the seductive name *analogy*. Somehow, "analogy" and "intelligence" seem to go hand in hand. The notion of researching analogy conjures up the illusion, at least, that one is directly addressing the problems of thinking and reasoning. Why is this? One possible reason is that analogy truly is central to thought. Several researchers have advanced the claim that thought is primarily metaphorical or analogical. A more cynical view is that analogy is a fuzzy concept that means different things to different people. But so is intelligence. Though researchers do not agree on what either term means, they can concur with abstract claims like "analogical reasoning is a fundamental component of intelligence." It is perhaps this view that prompted Saul Amarel at the 1983 International Machine Learning Workshop to propose a moratorium on the term *analogy* in machine learning. Perhaps the field has fallen prey to a seductive term. Still, one gets an intuitive but compelling feeling while reading almost any of the chapters in this volume that, yes indeed, this research is on the right track; it may not be the full answer yet, but it is moving in the right direction. Only later does one question the validity of this universal feeling. In this chapter I offer a framework in which to fit some of the more computationally oriented of the previous chapters. Is it a complete, exhaustive account of the types of analogy? Perhaps not, but it too seems to be on the right track.

346

By limiting the focus to some of the "computationally oriented" theories I mean to include a subset of those theories that have been implemented or are sufficiently specific and processlike that it appears they could be implemented without much embellishment. In particular I will focus on the chapters by Ryszard Michalski, David Rumelhart, Dedre Gentner, John Anderson and Ross Thompson, and Keith Holyoak and Paul Thagard. I begin with a brief interpretation and evaluation of these chapters, followed by the outline of a framework that may help distinguish two important and different kinds of analogy.

Commentaries

In his chapter, Michalski advocates a representation scheme for concepts that involves two levels. The first (the *base concept representation*) captures the common, typical, and context-free components of a concept's meaning. The second (the *inferential concept interpretation*) relates observations to the concept's base representation. This level involves dynamically drawing conclusions about the concept's properties through the system's inference rules. The inferential interpretation, which can be sensitive to both context and background knowledge, extends the concept's meaning into "practically an open space of possibilities" without requiring an inordinate amount of storage. For Michalski, *analogy* is a combination of inductive and deductive inference and is one of a number of methods available at the inferential interpretation level. Thus, his use of analogy is as a tool in the attack of the broader issue of knowledge representation.

Intuitively, this seems like a very good idea. It could, for example, allow a system to tag the concept of *boat* directly with the characteristic "floats in water" but not explicitly represent that characteristic on the concept of *basketball* though all normal basketballs float, this characteristic is somehow less salient of *basketball* than of *boat*. The approach allows such less salient characterisstics to be accessible through the system's inferential mechanism without clogging the concept memory with nonuseful information. It also points to a direction by which some of the concept instability problems mentioned by Lawrence Barsalou (this volume) might be handled. He mentions a kind of context sensitivity for the definitions of concepts; the characteristic "eaten by humans" is not normally applied to the concept *frog* but can become active for *frog* in the context of a French restaurant. A suitable inferential mechanism could probably exhibit this behavior.

One problem is that no theoretical basis is offered to decide how to distribute a concept's characteristics between the levels. Many of the examples are quite compelling. However, it is only intuitively that the decision can be made. One would hope for a more formal motivation to distinguish the two levels. Of course, the correct level for a characteristic may simply require the human intuition of a programmer. A more pleasing possibility is that further research will yield a formal and theoretical definition of the distinction between "base" and "inferential" levels, which might lend itself to automation.

A potentially more severe problem with this approach can be seen by taking further advantage of Barsalou's concept of instability. Consider the concept of *inner tube* and its characteristic "floats in water." Should this characteristic be stored explicitly (level 1) or be inferred (level 2) as it is for *basketball*? For the particular automobile inner tube on a Lincoln Town Car speeding away from a gangland hit job, the characteristic "floats in water" seems irrelevant indeed. However, for the particular inner tube supporting little Joey in his family's swimming pool that characteristic is quite central. Though one could get by with the "floating" property at either the first or the second level, it seems much more natural for the first case to place it in the inferrably accessible level 2 and in the inner-tube-as-a-raft case to store the property directly at level 1. This is a problem. A single characteristic like "floats in water" should not be stored at both levels. Indeed, there is no reason to do this since once a characteristic is available at level 1 there is no benefit in making it also available via level 2. Indeed, duplication at both levels incurs a fair storage penalty.

An obvious way to fix the problem would be to treat the word *inner tube* as ambiguous. It can be viewed as a single lexical item that refers to two distinct concepts. The first meaning would be a large rubber thing used to help a car roll smoothly; the second meaning would be a large rubber thing used to support a person in a swimming pool. Upon reflection this is a bad idea. The problem is that we are now allowing a distinction between two concepts purely in terms of the *use* of the real-world referent and not based on any identifiable intrinsic property of the referent itself. This is dangerous because the number of concepts quickly explodes. We may need a third *inner tube* concept to represent the use of an inner tube as a sled on a snowy hill in the winter. The two-tiered representation makes no guarantee that this explosion is bounded. The function of an inner tube is slightly different on a 1967 Buick than it is on a 1973 Volkswagen – not in the characteristsic of "floating" but in others like "maximum pressure." We may be compelled to separate these as distinct concepts as well. This would quickly result in an unacceptable number of minutely different concepts. The cost in storage and in extra disambiguation processing would greatly outweigh the comparatively small storage advantage endemic to the two-tiered system. Intuitively, the approach seems promising. It needs more work and formalization, as is not uncommon with ongoing research.

Rumelhart presents a brief account of the parallel distributed processing (PDP) model that he and his colleagues have been researching (e.g. Rumelhart, Smolensky, McClelland, & Hinton, 1986). Rumelhart argues that a PDP model can naturally account for three types of reasoning that underlie processing novel situations. They are *reasoning by similarity, reasoning by mental simulation,* and *formal reasoning.* The first, reasoning by similarity, would seem to be the most important for our purposes. Memory retrieval in a PDP system is done almost as a content-addressable memory. One "clamps" whatever attributes one knows of the item to be retrieved, and the other attributes settle into appropriate corresponding values, thereby filling out the concept. Rumelhart advances a novel way of lookng at analogical access in which one gradually weakens the clamped inputs until an appropriate settling of the system occurs. Inputs representing concrete microfeatures are weakened in preference to those representing abstract microfeatures. Thus, the retrieved item shares abstractions with the original input but may have little surface similarity. The retrieved item is a candidate analogy to the input item.

There are several problems with Rumelhart's claims. First, the algorithm for analogy access is far from implemented. Indeed, it is really only hinted at. However, it seems to be a promising approach, and specificity will come with future work. Second, the chapter includes several sections that are only tenuously connected with analogy or similarity. This is not in itself bad, but it seems a pity not to devote more space to the chosen topic. Finally, it seems that the approach may suffer from the occlusion of interesting and productive analogies by surface similarities or mere-appearance matches. Because the clamped inputs are gradually weakened, a close match would seem to be found before a match at a more abstract level. Such a close match would likely have more the flavor of a pure "reminding" than of an analogy. Imagine trying to discover the analogy between sailing on stormy seas and a marriage. Initially we might clamp some of the inputs (microfeatures) from our last episode of sailing in stormy weather, hoping that, via weakening, an interesting analogy (like a marriage) will turn up. These inputs would, presumably, result in retrieval of the full memory of last Wednesday when I sailed in bad weather. This retrieval must be rejected as a candidate analogy and the inputs slightly weakened. Next, we might retrieve the time three weeks ago when I sailed in bad weather, which must also be rejected, followed by the time last month when I considered going sailing and decided not to because of a strong wind, followed, perhaps, by a vivid recall of the scene from *Mutiny on the Bounty* in which Marlon Brando almost falls overboard during a gale, and so on and on. What is wrong with this sort of hypothesis and test? There are often too many bad hypotheses. These hypotheses, though close to the clamped source concept, miss the deeper, more satisfying mappings so characteristic of interesting analogies. Furthermore, the test may be difficult. It seems to require standard serial reasoning to reject one hypothesis before going on to the next. Such an algorithm sacrifices the "settling" metaphor in exchange for the standard Von Neumann approach. Still, Rumelhart advances a truly different and interesting, if somewhat underdefined, approach to an important component of analogy processing.

Gentner's chapter is ostensibly about analogical learning. In fact, the implications for learning are only briefly and superficially treated at the end. What remains, however, is one of the most complete accounts of analogical mapping. Gentner gives five steps for analogical processing: (a) source access, (b) mapping, (c) match evaluation, (d) storing inferences, (e) extracting principles. Not surprisingly, a central notion is that of structure-mapping, which states that analogy is the mapping of a system of relations from the source domain to the target domain. It is important that the systems involve relations rather than attributes and that the relations' identities are unimportant; that is, goal and causal relations occupy no special place in structure-mapping.

The discussion is primarily centered on the first three of the five steps, which are, perhaps, the most crucial and specific to analogy processing. The second step is the only implemented one. The first and third are more speculative. The computer system that implements the second step is called SME, for structure-mapping engine.

The theory of structure-mapping and the SME implementation have implications for the other two steps. Structure-mapping is a purely syntactic manipulation. Since the identities of the relations do not affect the structure-mapping process their semantics are, and must be, ignored by SME. This means that no world knowledge is brought to bear on the mapping process, which, in turn, means that the process is a very efficient one. Thus, the access step need not be as discriminating as may be required by other theories. It costs little for SME to weed out incorrectly accessed source domains. On the other hand, the structure-mapping process may construct mappings that may be fine from a syntactic viewpoint but are precluded by semantic considerations (see Johnson-Laird, this volume). This places an added burden on the match evaluation process, which is not discussed in much detail.

The access process, though far from implemented, is duscussed in processing terms. The problem is: How can a system retrieve a relevant source if it does not already know the "correct" analogy mapping? One possibility is for the abstract plan or other conceptual features to be used to index the source. The source example, when originally processed, would be stored under these conceptual indexes. Then, when the target example is to be processed, the system would need to glean one or more of these conceptual indexes from the partially processed target example. The relevant source example can then be used to aid in the completion of the target processing. This approach is particularly popular in artificial intelligence (AI). Gentner argues against this approach on psychological grounds, citing a number of experiments that indicate that it is difficult for people to make use of abstract conceptual characteristics as retrieval cues. Instead, Gentner advances the possibility of repeated near-literal similarities as a mechanism by which abstract relational commonalities could be gradually made more accessible. As these commonalities become strengthened, the relevant source examples become more easily retrieved and access is less sensitive to irrelevant surface similarities.

Overall, Gentner's chapter is a pleasant combination of experimental results and reasonably precisely specified process theory. It is particularly heartening to see psychologists directly concerned with constraints imposed by computational considerations. One word of caution is needed in this regard. Often, computational trade-offs exist. Computational choices that make one subprocess easier to implement may impose an intolerable computational penalty elsewhere. There is no obvious reason to believe this is the case with the structure-mapping account of the mapping process. However, a full computational account of at least access and match evaluation are necessary to complete a validation of the theory on computational grounds. My own interpretation of structure-mapping is presented in Figure 13.1.

A second computational question arises concerning access. Many psychological works are cited which present evidence that access is best promoted by surface commonalities rather than by more abstract problem structure or causal model commonalities. These results seem undeniable. However, they cry out for some computational investigation or, at least, speculation. From a naive computational viewpoint, it seems far more desirable to access past examples based on their

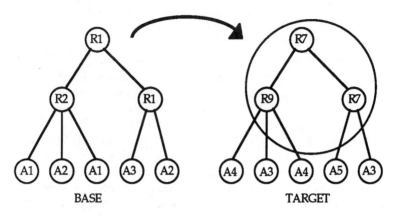

Figure 13.1. Structure-mapping.

underlying conceptual structure rather than on surface features. This is particularly true if the remembered source examples are to be used for analogical problem solving. That people do not use this sort of indexing indicates that we most probably do not yet fully understand the computational requirements for the accessing process. Some computationally motivated speculation about why people are the way they are would be desirable. Instead, Gentner simply accepts these results. Although there is nothing wrong with this, one cannot help mourning the missed opportunity for a computationally informed psychologist (a rare breed) to comment on her view of why the accessing process might be driven so strongly by surface features.

One very positive facet of Gentner's view of analogy is that it supports an analysis of what I will call *nonjustifiable* analogies. These are analogies in which the target is not entailed by the same abstract model illustrated by the source in such examples as "the sweet fruit of patience" or "Experience is the comb that nature gives us after we are bald." This point will be discussed later. The advantage is seldom apparent because the examples with which Gentner illustrates her process model are nearly always *justifiable* analogies.

Anderson and Thompson give a tentative but well-defined account of how a form of analogical reasoning might be implemented. An implementation exists in PUPS (Penultimate Production System), which is the successor to ACT* (Anderson, 1983). Interestingly, and honestly, the authors point out early in the chapter that "This new theory does not yet really exist." It is difficult to know what it means for the theory not to exist but yet to have an implementation of that theory. Perhaps it indicates that John Anderson has finally completed his transition from mainstream psychologist to mainstream AI researcher.

For Anderson and Thompson (as for Ross, this volume), solving a problem by analogy involves retrieving an example similar to the current problem. This is the access process, and, of course, it is done via spreading activation through the system's network memory. Next, a mapping function is generated between the problem and the example based on what is understood thus far about the problem.

The main domain used to illustrate the system is LISP programming. In PUPS, each LISP concept is a schema with three primary slots: isa, form, and function. The *form* specifies the LISP symbols for the concept. The *function* specifies in PUPS symbols what the concept does. The *isa* slot gives the category type of the concept.

The source concept has all slots filled; the target may be missing information. There are three types of analogical mappings: The first fills the missing form slot of a target concept having an existing function slot from a source form via a mapping defined by the two existing function slots. The second type fills the missing target function slot via a mapping defined by the existing form slots of the target and source concepts. The third, which is termed *refinement*, embellishes a target's function slot via a mapping defined by the existing target function and an already embellished source function slot.

Anderson and Thompson root their analogy processing in three principles: (a) no function in content, (b) sufficiency of functional specification, and (c) maximal functional elaboration.

Sadly, the first example, a simple one to illustrate the analogy steps, serves primarily to stultify the system's behavior. The example shows how the system infers the proper LISP expression to obtain the first element of the list *(a b c)* by analogy to the expression *(car '(p q r s))*, which is known to obtain the first element of the list *(p q r s)*. Even though the example quite clearly illustrates the underlying processing, it is a poor one. In my own pretheoretic intuition these match too well to qualify as a proper analogy. One might begin to question Anderson and Thompson's definition of what constitutes an analogy. Nonetheless, this appears only to be a problem with the choice of examples. A much more satisfying later example shows the system inferring the function of the unknown "summorial" concept by analogy to the known "factorial" concept. My own understanding of the first two types of analogies is illustrated by Figure 13.2.

Either the form or the function of the target is missing. The other target slot must be known. A mapping is defined between the known

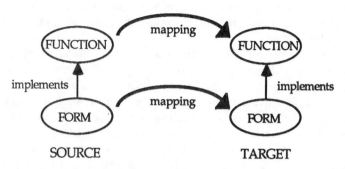

Figure 13.2. PUPS analogy (1 & 2).

target slot and the corresponding source slot. This mapping, when applied to the other source slot produces a filler for the unknown target slot. The third type of analogy (refinement) would be represented identically except that the forms would be replaced by unembellished function slots.

Holyoak and Thagard advance a system called PI (processes of induction) to model analogical problem solving through rule-directed spreading activation. The whole system has the flavor of a "general cognitive architecture" like ACT*, PUPS, or SOAR (Laird, Rosenbloom, & Newell, 1986). The propositionlike concepts are, somewhat counterintuitively, termed *messages*. Rules of the system relate these propositions in a standard condition–action framework. The entire structure forms a network memory. Propositions explicitly mentioned in the problem specification are initially active. Other propositions are activated via the rules. If all of the conditions of a rule become active, the propositions on the action side also become active. Rule importance is judged by three contributions: the rule's strength (past success), its degree of activation (calculated from its component's activations), and its relevance to the current goals (which enhances only rules that would directly achieve a current component goal). Activation proceeds "in parallel." A further addition allows "effector" rules to propose tentative "projections," which are designed to capture the notion of trying out a potential strategy. When the strategy succeeds or fails, the initiating rule strength is increased or decreased. There is a standard activation decay calculated for each proposition that does not participate in a time step. This is a standard forward-chaining mechanism with two exceptions: the parallelism and the projection notion. There is a backward-chaining mechanism, but it is not described in any detail.

The major example discussed is the classic analogy between the source of splitting up an attacking army to capture a fortress and the target of destroying a cancerous tumor with X-rays without destroying healthy tissue as well (Gick & Holyoak, 1980). The system possesses the knowledge of how the army can split up and each component can move separately to the fortress. The analogy's success depends on the source and target problem statements sharing the "betweenness" concept and on a known association linking the DESTROY concept with the CAPTURE concept.

There are some significant questions, if not problems, with the computational approach outlined by Holyoak and Thagard. The first concerns some technical questions about the implementation. How is the credit assignment problem handled? The outlined algorithm would seem to adjust correctly only the strength of effector rules. How is backward chaining accomplished? We are not told how the parallelism was simulated on a serial computer. Is there always a unique resolution to concurrent decisions? If so, in what sense is this a truly parallel algorithm? The second major problem is one of grain size and representations. The DESTROY-TUMOR problem specification is, in a sense, just the right one to spark the analogy and, perhaps, not as natural or objective as it might be. For example, the spatial relation of the tumor to the radiation uses the *between* predicate and explicitly mentions a third argument of flesh. This makes the analogy mapping much easier to discover but already biases the concept of the problem toward the notion of a roadlike conduit through the flesh. There is no mention of other intervening material (like the atmosphere) or what properties it must have (like being reasonably transparent to X-rays). The third, and to my mind, most severe problem is with Holyoak and Thagard's view of what constitutes an analogy. The problem here is that the ultimate solution to the target concept makes use of a known common abstraction between the source and the target. The abstraction can be thought of as "convergence" and is represented by two known predicates, *split* and *move-separately-to*. This is represented in Figure 13.3.

If the general notions of *split* and *move-separately-to* are already known, and they are known to be applicable to X-rays (which apparently is the case), then there seems to be no obstacle to solving the tumor problem with the system's standard forward inferencer. In that case there seems little need for analogical reasoning. This misgiving may just be the lack of a second clarifying example, which saved Anderson and Thompson from a similar criticism. On the other hand, even if the criticism is valid, Holyoak and Thagard are to be commended for being explicit about their representations, although one

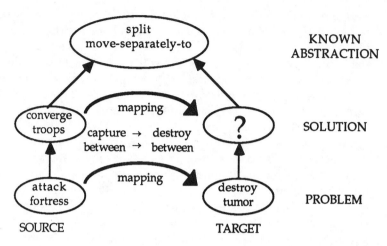

Figure 13.3. Fortress–tumor analogy.

might hope for a more concrete statement of the algorithm. The general problem of what might constitute an analogy is pursued further in the next section.

The PI system ultimately constructs a new problem schema, which supports reasoning about similar future convergencelike situations. This convergence schema is indexed by the problem predicates *between* and *overcome*, which, as it turns out, seems to be the association linking DESTROY and CAPTURE alluded to earlier. The new schema suggests that the action *split* may lead to a solution. Interestingly, the *move-separately-to* predicate is not mentioned. My own intuition is that *move-separately-to* would be a more convincing central notion than *split* in the convergence schema. The knowledge contained in a convergence schema is applicable to non-*split* kinds of situations and should be accessible from them. For example, in the real solution the X-ray beams do not typically start out as a single beam that is split; either they are generated by several independent beams, or a single beam is used within which the patient is rotated, thus changing the path. The notion of convergence is still a central one although there is no *split* action.

Note that while PI's newly formed concept is a generalization of the individual source and target examples, it is more specific than the system's original background knowledge; it requires the context of *between* and *overcome* to be present whereas *split* does not.

One possible problem is that the *split* and *move-separately-to* concepts were accessed from the source (fortress) problem specification. There is no indication that *split* or *move-separately-to* is any less accessible from the target (tumor) problem specification. Indeed, the analogy processing would seem to require this. Thus, the general knowledge that a *split* and a *move-separately-to* in combination can transfer an abstract object (whether it be X-radiation or an army) to an otherwise inaccessible location would seem to have been implicitly in the system all along. In this case there would seem to have been no inductive leap resulting in a nondeductive conclusion. Again, the system did not really need to perform the analogical reasoning; nonanalogical deductive reasoning would have worked as well.

General discussion

First, some words on specialized architectures are in order. Three of the chapters made claims based on specialized architectures: Rumelhart (PDP), Anderson and Thompson (PUPS), and Holyoak and Thagard (PI). All of these special architectures include some form of parallel processing.

Rumelhart is the most explicitly outspoken about the necessity for the non-Von Neumann architecture, saying (pp. 298–99) "we have (perhaps inadvertently) carried much of the baggage of the Von Neumann computer into the 'computer metaphor' and thence into our formal theories and into our intuitions." Interestingly, half of the remaining systems, those by Anderson and Thompson and by Holyoak and Thagard, both of which I discuss only because they represent computational (rather than parallel) approaches, also rely on non-Von Neumann architectures. Why is this? In all three cases the solution to "analogy access" can be traced to parallelism (though in a very different way for Rumelhart than for the others). For Rumelhart the PDP or "connectionist" model pervades his view of analogical processing. For the other two systems, the nonstandard architecture is of the production-system variety and seems more driven by a desire for a general cognitive architecture than by the needs of the analogy algorithms. Nevertheless, they are clearly not proponents of Von Neumann-type architectures.

Let us consider the remaining two models: Gentner's structure-mapping and Michalski's two-level concept representation. Here, one can make an interesting observation, which further questions Rumelhart's contention about computer metaphor baggage. These two systems are not particularly wedded to the Von Neumann fetch-execute-store cycle. Gentner's structure-mapping could be done largely in parallel if one were inclined to so implement it; Michalski's two-level representation system imposes no special constraints at all on the process model of how inferences are made. Rather, it comments on the structure of memory, and in this regard Michalski's view is perhaps more similar to the PDP model than to the other systems.

It seems that, at least in the field of computational analogy modeling, Rumelhart's fears are quite counterindicated. The Von Neumann computer metaphor has not severely limited our collective imagination, though it has certainly colored it.

A much more controversial point concerns local versus distributed concept representation – whether there is a bounded and identifiable area in memory corresponding to an individual concept or whether a concept is individuated only by a unique *pattern* that permeates all or much of memory. Even here, Rumelhart has, perhaps surprisingly, an ally in Michalski's two-level concept representation. For it, too, defies bounded locality of concepts. The second (inferential) level has no limit to its definition.

Some might object that *all* of the implementations were actually programmed on standard serial computers. However, this point, though true, is hardly fair since the shoehorning of the nonstandard systems into a Von Neumann machine extracts a huge performance penalty and even precludes the possibility of investigating large examples.

Next and finally, I wish to explore the original issue of diversity in the concept of analogy among researchers. Is the commonality only the attraction of the rubric *analogy*, or can we impose some order on the apparent chaos? As a secondary goal we would like to account for the intuitive dissatisfaction mentioned earlier with examples such as Anderson and Thompson's initial extract-the-first-element-of-the-list example and with Holyoak and Thagard's treatment of the fortress/tumor example. Unlike Anderson and Thompson's, this example "feels" like a proper analogy. Can we perhaps recast their treatment better to bring out this intuition?

I begin by introducing the distinction between *analogy* and *reinstantiation* and the distinction between *justified* and *nonjustified* analogies. For the moment I assume the reader's intuitive notion of analogy and define reinstantiation as shown in Figure 13.4.

The known example on the left in Figure 13.4 is very familiar. The example on the right is less familiar and is missing several important features. The left example "maps" to the first as indicated by the curved arrow connecting them. The "known abstraction" is general knowledge of the system, which applies in the same way to both examples, and one can think of it as the *explanation* of why the examples work.

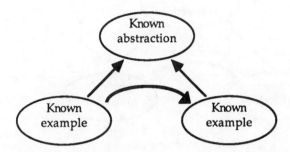

Figure 13.4. Reinstantiation.

To make this a bit more concrete, consider the problem of Janet, a neighbor, starting my automobile. Suppose that Janet has never started my car. This event will be identified with the lower-right bubble of Figure 13.4. That known event represents the problem specification of Janet getting my car started. The lower-left bubble is to be identified with the problem of Janet starting her own car. Janet's car is a blue 1981 Toyota Tercel sedan. She has started her own car thousands of times. The procedure is subject to minimal causal variation. This fact, also, is well known to her. Her faith in the start-the-car procedure is rooted in her general mental model of automobiles and their starting procedures, which is to be identified as the higher bubble of Figure 13.4 labeled "known abstraction."

As it happens, my car is also blue. It is also a Toyota Tercel and is a 1981 model. One difference is that mine is a hatchback. The mapping between the left and right lower bubbles is very strong. Note that is is a true *mapping* and not a *matching* as there is no identity at the level of the problem specification. My car is a different car. There is a correspondence between their parts. Her gas pedal is similar to mine but different; operating one does not operate the other, and so on.

It seems entirely unreasonable to believe that Janet should or would employ this mapping, no matter how strong, to solve the problem of starting my car. A far more reasonable, efficient, and believable way to solve the problem is for her simply to reinstantiate her general automobile-starting knowledge for my car. This would correctly and effortlessly dictate otherwise problematic constraints, such as the need for my particular key instead of hers.

When a problem is within the scope of a general and familiar abstraction it is always preferable to use the general mental model to

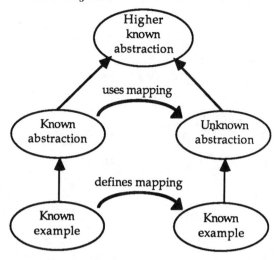

Figure 13.5. Reinstantiation.

draw inferences about the new situation rather than to attempt un-substantiated and often bizarre mappings.

This, it seems to me, is at the heart of my trouble with Anderson and Thompson's first example. I am no longer a naive subject for LISP programming examples. My general knowledge, though perhaps limited, has long since tightly connected the symbol *car* to its function. To my knowledge I have never typed the precise string "*(car ' (p q r s))*" to LISP. Yet, it is unthinkable to suppose that I would guess what would be returned by forming analogical mappings. The example might possibly be quite compelling to a sufficiently naive subject, but the subject would have to be phenomenally naive about programming languages not to guess the correct abstraction from a single instance.

Figure 13.5 represents a certain embellishment on Figure 13.4. In Figure 13.5 we separate the two constituents of the lower bubbles of Figure 13.4. In a problem-solving context the lower bubbles of Figure 13.5 are to be thought of as "problem specifications," and the next "known abstraction" bubbles represent the solutions to those problems. Note that the solution of the left problem is known but the right is unknown. Again, the higher common abstraction represents the system's general knowledge, which explains both solutions in the same terms.

Note the similarity between Figures 13.5 and 13.3, which represents the Holyoak and Thagard fortress/tumor "analogy." The "higher known abstraction" is an explanation of how *split* and *move-separately-*

to satisfy the abstract problem. We might term this abstraction *con-vergence*. For Holyoak and Thagard, the abstraction is known to the system (it must be since the system used this abstraction in its solution to the fortress problem). One possibility is that the abstract concepts are not accessible in the tumor case, although it is not clear why *split*, for example, should be connected to the event of soldiers taking different numbers of steps in different directions but not be connected to breaking an X-ray beam into smaller beams. Furthermore, it would appear that the system does indeed already know that the concept *split* can be applied to X-ray beams.

The problem I have with this example is that, to have the knowledge that the system appears to have, it makes little sense for it to form the mapping. In this criticism we should be more fair than to pick on only Holyoak and Thagard. They have the misfortune to have been more complete in their algorithm specification. Gentner's once-favorite analogy between the solar sysem and the atom suffers the same problem. To have understood either example entails that one already understand the abstraction of central force systems. If the abstraction already exists, there is no reason to form an analogical mapping. Any interesting causal inference is better made via the abstract explanation.

How could these examples make sense as analogies? One possibility is as illustrated in Figure 13.6. In this figure the "higher abstraction" is not known to the system. It is through analogy (and only through analogy) that the second example's abstraction is resolved. Once this is done the system might speculate about what a common higher abstraction might be.

In the fortress/tumor example, this would correspond to the system's not possessing general concepts for *split* or *move-separately-to*. There would instead be specializations of these concepts that apply only to the source example. The system would know about individual humans taking different numbers of steps in different directions and the implications of these actions for the humans' locations. The problem of achieving the "correct" analogical mapping under these circumstances is far more troublesome. This is particularly true if the system has a reasonable number of other facts that relate to the participating concepts but that turn out to be irrelevant to this analogy. Once both problems have been solved, the analogy might help guide the system to postulate a new causal abstraction via induction.

A better use for these difficult analogies is as a mechanism to convey such inarticulable higher abstractions. A teacher assures the student that an important common abstraction exists and then gives worked

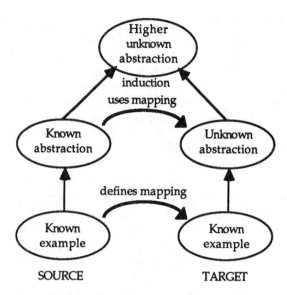

Figure 13.6. Justified analogy.

examples to illustrate it. The analogy mapping, perhaps constructed with the teacher's guidance, serves to aid the induction process of the student. The analogy is then not spontaneous on the part of the student but rather serves to convey difficult abstract concepts such as "central force system."

Analogies of the form of Figure 13.6 are termed *justified* because the mapping is a manifestation of an underlying common higher abstraction. Analogies in support of problem solving tend to be of this type. The higher abstraction is then the common abstract causal theory in which each problem solution is rooted. Not all analogies are of this type.

Figure 13.7 represents a *nonjustified* analogy. In this kind of analogy there is no common higher abstraction. An example of this type would be Gentner's "sweet fruit of patience." In one possible reading, the source is composed of the known example of "sweet fruit" together with its abstractions, among them that it can give pleasant sustenance to the body. The second (left) known example is "patience." The correct mapping might then be the inference that it gives pleasant sustenance to the mind.

In the "sweet fruit of patience" example there is no obvious abstraction of which the mapping is a manifestation. Rather, it is de-

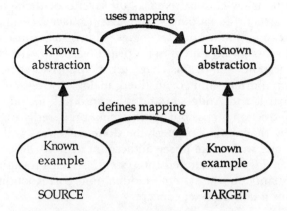

Figure 13.7. Nonjustified analogy.

signed to communicate an inference about "patience" without literally stating it.

Not all problem-solving analogies need be of the justified variety. Indeed, Anderson and Thompson's factorial/summorial analogy is nonjustified. There is no abstract causal theory that constrains the *function* of anything simply because it is named "summorial." For humans, the similarity between the names "summorial" and "factorial" might well help in accessing the source, but the actual mapping is not entailed or limited by any abstraction.

The distinction can be drawn between justified and nonjustified analogy research in artificial intelligence also. To some researchers (e.g., Carbonell, 1985; Falkenhainer, Forbus, & Gentner, 1986), analogy involves an unjustified mapping. Others (e.g., Davies & Russell, 1987; Kedar-Cabelli, 1985) have a distinctly justified if not outright deductive flavor. Still others (Falkenhainer, 1986) are in between.

Conclusion

I have offered a brief framework that distinguishes among some analogies and nonanalogies. The distinction hinges on whether or not there is a common abstraction or explanation possible between the source and target analogy components and whether that common abstraction is known to the analogizer. The framework captures some pretheoretic intuitions concerning a number of example analogies cited in the reviewed chapters. Beyond this intuitive appeal I am prepared to make no claims. From the perspective of this framework we can formulate a few closing remarks on several of the systems. First, Gentner's structure-mapping would seem to have a certain advantage in processing nonjustified analogies. This is so because mapping is defined syntactically and is not a priori biased toward causal accounts. On the other hand, this characteristic deprives structure-mapping of an important hint for justified analogies. Gentner, Holyoak and Thagard, and Anderson and Thompson all include generalization or induction steps, but none seems prepared to be too concrete on how that should properly be done. Likewise, with Rumelhart's PDP, one would like to see an account of how the process of drawing an analogy itself altered the system, perhaps resulting in a shift in the semantics of the system's hidden units corresponding to the acquisition of a new abstract concept.

NOTE

The preparation of this chapter was supported in part by the Office of Naval Research under Grant N–00014–86–K–0309. I am grateful to Andrew Ortony and Stella Vosniadou for helpful comments on an earlier draft.

REFERENCES

✓Anderson, J.R. (1983). *The architecture of cognition.* Cambridge, MA: Harvard University Press.

Burstein, M. H. (1985). *Learning by reasoning from multiple analogies.* Unpublished doctoral dissertation, Yale University, New Haven, CT.

Carbonell, J. G. (1985, March). *Derivational analogy: A theory of reconstructive problem solving and expertise acquisition* (Tech. Rep. CMU-CS-85-115). Pittsburgh: Carnegie-Mellon University, Department of Computer Science.

Davies, T., & Russell, S. (1987, August), A logical approach to reasoning by analogy, *Proceedings of the Tenth International Joint Conference on Artificial Intelligence* (pp. 264–270), Milan.

Evans, T. G. (1968). A program for the solution of geometric analogy intelligence test questions. In M. Minsky (Ed.), *Semantic information processing* (pp. 271–353). Cambridge, MA: MIT Press.

Falkenhainer, B. (1986). *An examination of the third stage in the analogy process: Verification-based analogical learning* (Tech. Rep. UIUCDCS-R86-1302). Urbana-Champaign: University of Illinois, Department of Computer Science.

Falkenhainer, B., Forbus, K., & Gentner, D. (1986, August). The structure-mapping engine. *Proceedings of the American Association for Artificial Intelligence* (pp. 272–277), Philadelphia.

Forbus, K. D., & Gentner, D. (1986). Learning physical domains: Towards a theoretical framework. In R. S. Michalski, J. G. Carbonell, & T. M. Mitchell (Eds.), *Machine learning: An artificial intelligence approach* (Vol. 2). Los Altos, CA: Kaufmann.

Gick, M. L., & Holyoak, K. J., (1980), Analogical problem solving, *Cognitive Psychology*, 12. 306–355.

Kedar-Cabelli, S., (1985, August). Purpose-directed analogy. *Proceedings of the Seventh Annual Conference of the Cognitive Science Society* (pp. 150–159), Irvine, CA.

Laird, J. E., Rosenbloom, P. S., & Newell, A. (1986). *Universal subgoaling and chunking: The automatic generation and learning of goal hierarchies.* Dordrecht, Holland: Kluwer.

✓Rumelhart, D. E., Smolensky, P., McClelland, J. L., & Hinton, G. E. (1986). Schemata and sequential thought processes in PDP models. In J. L. McClelland, D. E. Rumelhart, and the PDP Research Group, *Parallel distributed processing: Explorations in the microstructure of cognition:* Vol. 2. *Psychological and biological models* (pp. 7–57). Cambridge, MA: MIT Press (Bradford Books).

Winston, P. H. (1980). Learning and reasoning by analogy. *Communications of the Association for Computing Machinery, 23*, 689–703.

Similarity and analogy in development, learning, and instruction

The contributions included in Part III focus on developmental and instructional aspects of similarity and analogy. In her chapter, Ann Brown argues that young children can transfer knowledge across analogous domains and that findings that they can not are an artifact of the paradigms used to assess transfer. Stella Vosniadou also argues that children are capable of using analogical reasoning to acquire new knowledge and that what develops is not analogical reasoning per se but the content and organization of the knowledge base to which analogical reasoning is applied.

Brian Ross discusses the role that remindings play in acquiring knowledge about unfamiliar domains and suggests using surface similarity as a way to enhance analogical access. In their contribution, John Bransford, Jeffery Franks, Nancy Vye, and Robert Sherwood offer several proposals about how to make the knowledge base more flexible. They suggest teaching people in problem-oriented environments, rather than teaching facts, and they mention various instructional techniques for promoting the noticing of similarities and differences. Rand Spiro, Paul Feltovich, Richard Coulson, and Daniel Anderson discuss the advantages and disadvantages of using instructional analogies to acquire knowledge in ill-structured domains. Finally, William Brewer offers a commentary on the contributions to Part III, focusing on the role of analogical reasoning in knowledge acquisition.

14

Analogical learning and transfer: What develops?

ANN L. BROWN

Introduction

Inductive reasoning is ubiquitous in human thinking. Children, like adults, must constantly make inferences that are not deductively valid. Predictions, generalizations, and inductive projections from known instances are all examples of inductive reasoning; all involve the transfer of the known to the unknown.

Such flexible use of knowledge is often cited as a hallmark of human intelligence. At the same time, transfer is thought to be an elusive quality. Herein lies a conundrum. How can one simultaneously hold that the existing state of knowledge profoundly affects learning and that transfer of knowledge across situations is difficult to engineer without heroic effort? Taken at face value, there is an uneasy sense of contradiction in the juxtaposition of these two widely held beliefs.

Nowhere is this juxtaposition more apparent than in discussions of children's learning. One of the more ubiquitous claims concerning young children is that they tend to acquire knowledge in such a way that it is closely tied, restricted, or welded to habitual occasions of use. Flexible application of knowledge is not thought to characterize the reasoning processes of the young (Brown, 1974, 1982; Rozin, 1976). But, whereas theories of encapsulated knowledge are widely held, so too are theories that attribute many developmental differences solely to disparities in knowledge between children, "universal novices" (Brown & DeLoache, 1978), and adults, who are comparative experts in many domains. But how can young children be prisoners of a knowledge base that they cannot access? In this chapter, I will attempt to resolve this apparent paradox by considering what is known about analogical transfer in children.

Although the focus will be on analogy as a learning mechanism, I will argue that one cannot discuss the development of analogical reasoning in a vacuum. Rather, it is necessary to consider the role such

369

processes must play within a theory of learning and development in the wider sense. For example, what is the role of analogical transfer in knowledge acquisition? Does this role vary with the age of the child and the type of knowledge in question? Are there domains of knowledge that young children are predisposed to learn about early? If so, how do these biases guide future knowledge acquisition, and with what consequences for analogical processing? Does competence in analogical reasoning progress in a content-free manner, or is it highly dependent on specific domains? Any discussion of the development of analogical transfer must eventually be situated in the context of these wider issues of a theory of learning.

In this chapter, I will argue that analogy as a learning mechanism is a crucial factor in knowledge acquisition at all ages. What may look like recalcitrance in young children's ability to use what they know to solve new problems is an artifact of what they have been required to learn and the settings in which they have been required to learn it. In particular, I argue that all knowledge is not equal, and all conditions of learning are not equal.

Consider, first, knowledge. Imagine a hypothetical continuum of knowledge such as:

Theory	*Causal explanation*	*Meaningful solution*	*Arbitrary solution*

A *theory* would be defined as a coherent explanatory network of interrelated concepts. A *causal explanation* would refer to a principled understanding of part of a larger system, such as the fact that inanimate objects need to be pushed, pulled, or propelled into action. A *meaningful, isolated solution* would be one readily understood but not forming part of a larger system, such as Duncker's (1945) famous tumor problem currently popular in the work of Gick and Holyoak (1980); and an *arbitrary solution* would be something like "Red is correct," because the experimenter has randomly chosen that attribute. A great deal of the findings about transfer in children can be explained within this framework.

If that which is to be transferred consists of a coherent theory or a causal explanation that is understood, it is difficult to impede a flexible application of prior knowledge. It is when the application of a previously learned isolated rule or specific solution is required that observers decry a lack of transfer. It is common for fragmentary knowledge to be embedded in one context, a tendency that is an impediment when prior knowledge could be useful but also offers protection from massive interference. Transfer in young children is no exception. They rely on their emergent naive theories of persons, objects, and events to grant coherence to novel situations; but they are hesitant to apply fragmentary, unassimilated knowledge, which tends to remain embedded within specific contexts (Brown & Campione, 1981, 1984). In the first part of this chapter, I will address the issue of how children's knowledge of the world, and particularly their understanding of possible causal mechanisms, predicts the facility with which they learn and transfer.

Just as all knowledge is not equal, so too all conditions of learning are not equal. In the second part of the chapter, I will discuss the conditions of learning that facilitate flexible use of knowledge even in very young children. Whereas the first part is devoted to the place of analogical learning mechanisms in *conceptual development*, the second part is concerned with *engineering* transfer in situations where flexible access to knowledge is known to be difficult for both adults and children. In particular, I will consider both conditions that *impede* cognitive flexibility, such as negative learning sets, functional fixedness, and cognitive embeddedness, and those that *enhance* flexibility, such as positive learning sets, functional flexibility, and reflection.

Learning, transfer, and development

The predominant view

By far the majority of information concerning children's transfer has come from a classic laboratory transfer paradigm wherein a set of problems, which share some type of similarity in the experimenter's world view, are presented back to back to see if the subject *notices* the similarity and *applies* what was learned on the first task to subsequent tasks. I call this the "Now-for-something-completely-different approach," or the A B C paradigm, because a standard feature of this laboratory game is that no hint of the similarity among Tasks A, B, and C is leaked to the unsuspecting subject, who usually responds in kind, with no indication that the new is related to the old. Following this standard result, it is traditional to puzzle about the subjects' blindness in discussion sections; after all, the analogies are perfectly clear to the experimenter. We might step back for a minute, however, and ask: Why should anyone transfer under the standard A B C paradigm? If one were in the habit of noting similarities among all adjacent events, one would soon be overwhelmed by interference.

The current state of play in studies of laboratory transfer in children is that they show little evidence of spontaneous transfer in the classic A B C paradigm, 20% spontaneous transfer being the commonly reported figure for both adults and children when age-appropriate tasks are used (Brown, Kane, & Echols, 1986; Crisafi & Brown, 1986; Gick & Holyoak, 1980, 1983; Holyoak, Junn, & Billman, 1984). It has been claimed that below 5 years of age, transfer rarely occurs, and it is a widely held belief that the younger the learner the less likely is transfer. What explanations are offered for this?

Although there are some who hold to a simple deficit theory wherein below some magical age the child's ability to transfer, or reason by analogy, is thought to be weak to nonexistent, by far the most popular developmental explanation for the transfer reluctance of the young is a stagelike notion that implies a different basis of thinking in younger and older children. The most popular of these is the perceptually bound hypothesis.

The perceptually bound hypothesis. The claim that transfer is mediated by the degree of perceptual similarity among stimulus environments is a time-honored position, dating back at least to Thorndike's influential theory of *identical elements*. Thorndike and his colleagues (Thorndike, 1913; Thorndike & Woodworth, 1901) claimed that transfer occurred if and only if "identical elements" were shared between tasks. Although exactly what constituted "identical elements" was in considerable dispute, it was taken to mean identical at the level of surface features, such as color, shape, and size. Judd (1908), the leader of the opposition, argued that transfer is determined by the extent to which the learner is privy to underlying shared principles, through either discovery or instruction. Unfortunately, he was ignored, and it became generally assumed that transfer is a rarity and that when it occurs it is most often cued by some shared surface features of the stimulus environments. To cut a long battle short, Thorndike won, and psychology gained 60 years of identical elements in such guises as primary stimulus generalization, and Judd lost, taking with him the belief in underlying causal principles – even though Thorndike eventually capitulated, a change of heart that had little apparent effect on the continuing popularity of the original identical elements theory (Brown, 1986; Orata, 1945). This issue of surface features versus deep structure as mediators of transfer is again popular; witness the concentration in this volume on reminding, accessing, or noticing analogies or problem isomorphs.

The position with children below 5–7 years of age is that they are assumed to be *extreme Thorndikians*; that is, they are thought to be even more reluctant to transfer and even more reliant on perceptual similarity than are adults. They are called perceptually bound, meaning that they are unduly influenced by the appearance of things. This is another conundrum, for if, as we now know, even infants are sensitive to deep relational properties of, for example, mechanical causality (Baillargeon, Spelke, & Wasserman, 1985; Gibson & Spelke, 1983; Leslie, 1984a; Spelke, 1983) and learn about such deeper properties rather than more peripheral ones, why should older children have the opposite bias? At the very least, this seems like wasteful programming.

The question then is: Is it true? Are young children perceptually bound? There is an impressive stagelike data base showing a tendency to respond on the basis of perceptual similarity on a variety of tasks such as classification, free association, free recall, and word definitions (Mansfield, 1977), as well as analogy and metaphor (Gentner & Toupin, 1986; Vosniadou, 1987). In fact, no one denies that physical similarity is important in triggering access in young children, but it is for adults as well (Anderson, 1987; Ross, this volume). The question is whether they are *all-important* for young children; that is, can children transfer on any other basis? Consider three potential explanations of the seeming perceptual capture of young learners:

1. *The developmental-stage argument*: Children are perceptually bound initially but then, at a later stage, consider other bases for categorization. For example, Quine (1977) argues that children begin with an innate, perceptually bound similarity metric which is replaced over time by emergent theories. Children form their first concepts through perceptual similarity and only later import increasingly more complex theoretical knowledge into their conceptual systems.
2. *The developmental-preference argument*: Children can use a variety of bases for partitioning their world, but they prefer to rely on perceptually salient features. We know, for example, that they prefer to match on the basis of thematic relations even when taxonomic knowledge is readily available to them (Smiley & Brown, 1979). So too they often prefer perceptual matches even when alternative relational choices could be made (Brown, Ryan, Slattery, & Palincsar, work in progress). But, in both cases, it can be shown that minimal prompts are all that is needed to release the alternative level of analysis.
3. *The lack-of-knowledge argument*: Children rely on appearance as a fall-back option when there is no other basis on which to judge. Rather than there being a developmental shift from perceptually bound to theoretically based, all conceptual systems are integrated with theory from the earliest age, but children's theories are less well developed than adults'. In the absence of the requisite knowledge, it is difficult to imagine any other basis for partitioning than appearance, whether one is an adult or a child. For example, adults, asked to predict the likelihood that others in the domain *bird* have a disease if one bird has, based their predictions on the similarity of the in-

stances over which the projections must be made (Rips, 1975). Without an elaborated theory of avian disease, naive adults have no other
basis on which to constrain their inductive projections *but* perceptual
similarity. Reliance on surface similarity is indeed a typical finding
with novice learners. For example, Chi, Feltovich, and Glaser (1981)
found that novice physicists sorted physics problems in terms of
surface similarity, such as key words in the problem, or at best in
terms of the objects ("rotational things") mentioned. By contrast,
surface features did not influence the experts, who classified according to the major physics principles governing solutions; indeed,
the deep structure relations guiding their classifications could be
detected only by other expert physicists.

Young children, universal novices, with their impoverished and
sometimes radically different theories, find themselves dependent on
surface cues more often. They know little about many domains. What
else can they do but fall back on surface commonalities? Thus, what
may look like profound developmental differences in the basis of
conceptualization, or in the type of reasoning available to the child,
may actually be a reflection of the status of young children's core
theories (Carey, 1985a; Keil, 1986).

Of biological kinds and essences: of cabbages and kings. If this
position is true, then one would expect to find a radically different
picture of children's learning in domains for which they do have some
of the requisite knowledge. Consider one such domain, biological
knowledge (Carey, 1985b; R. Gelman, Spelke, & Meck, 1983; Keil,
1986). Biological knowledge evolves slowly. Initially, the child lacks
the superordinate concept *living thing*, differentiating plants and animals as separate categories. The young child appears to reason on
the basis of a naive psychology based on intention, regarding animals
as "behaving beings" that eat, breathe, sleep, and reproduce because
of intention. Older children see animals as functioning because of
their membership in biological categories. These differences in basic
core concepts, or "ontological commitments" (Carey, 1985b), have
profound effects on the child's transfer, whether measured by inductive projection (Carey, 1985b), judgments of category errors (Keil,
1983), or forced-choice method of triads matching (S. Gelman &
Markman, 1986). It is the state of theory, not age, that determines
judgment of category membership, "one's theories explicate the world
and differentiate it into kinds" (Murphy & Medin, 1985, p. 291).

As an example, Carey (1985b) has shown that even 4-years-olds are
capable of overcoming appearance matches to project biological properties to unknown species, within the constraints set by their immature

theories. Children of this age reason on the basis of similarity to the prototype of *person*, in contrast to adults, who use the concept *living thing* to constrain their inductive projections. Given this constraint, 4-year-olds' pattern of projections makes perfect sense. Told that people have a certain organ (spleen), they project the new organ in decreasing likelihood to mammals, birds, insects, and worms but not to inanimate objects. But when taught that a bee has the organ, they fall back on perceptual similarity (bee/bug) as the basis for transfer. Similarly 4-year-olds, told that a person has a spleen, believe that a worm is more likely to possess that property than is a mechanical monkey, even though they judge a mechanical monkey as more similar to a person than is a worm. They differentiate surface similarity from category membership, falling back on similarity when theory fails.

Similarly, S. Gelman and Markman (1986) pitted biological category membership *against* perceptual similarity. Four-year-olds were shown two pictures, for example, one that looked like an ostrich and one of a bat with outstretched wings. They were taught a new fact about each. In this example, they were told that "this bird [pointing to the ostrichlike picture] gives its baby mashed up food" and "this bat feeds its baby milk." They were then required to infer which of the facts applied to a third picture that looked very much like one of the preceding two but was given the same category label as the picture it did not physically resemble. For example, shown a picture of a bird with outstretched wings, perceptually very similar to the bat picture, they were asked, "What does this *bird* do – feed its baby milk or give it mashed up food?" No child responded consistently on the basis of perceptual matches, whereas 37% of 4-year-olds consistently relied on shared category to draw inductions, even though perceptual similarity would lead to a different conclusion. These data were replicated with 3-year-old children (S. Gelman & Markman, 1987).

Natural categories such as biological kinds encompass dense clusters of properties, some known to the layman, some known to the scientist, and some yet to be discovered (Kripke, 1971; Putman, 1970; Schwartz, 1979). Members of a kinds are expected to share properties – in the case of biological kinds, properties such as method of reproduction, internal organs, and even genetic structure if the predictor has the requisite scientific knowledge to appreciate this fact. These expectations can be made in the *absence of perceptual support*, for even if a member does not look like other members it will be expected to share common properties, many of which are unseen anyway (internal organs) or perhaps still unknown (DNA structure). Children honor this rule to the extent that they have the requisite knowledge.

It is claimed that there is something about natural kinds that is especially likely to support inductive inference. For example, assuming one knows that a human being, or a certain animal, has blood, bones, certain internal organs, produces live babies, and so on, one can make sensible projections to other objects, depending on what kind of thing they are (rabbit, whale, willow tree, chair, lump of gold, coffee pot, etc.). In contrast, assuming one knows that a certain animal mimics a skunk as a method of camouflage, it would be unreasonable to project this information broadly to other animals. Keil (1986) argues that from an early age we have a natural bias to go beyond characteristic features and seek underlying causal explanations. The rich underlying causal structure of natural kinds is thought to be particularly supportive of induction, even in the absence of perceptual support.

Thus, it would seem that young children do transfer their knowledge and can do so on deeper bases than mere appearance matches. What determines the extent of their knowledge projections is not some developmental constraint on the inductive process itself but a constraint on the type of knowledge to be transferred and its status within their emergent conceptual theories. It is not that children are incapable of inductive projections on the basis of underlying "essences"; it is just that their inchoate theories are often insufficient to warrant such inferences.

But just what is an essence? Medin and Ortony (this volume) describe a theory of psychological essentialism, arguing that knowledge representations embody "essence placeholders" that contain complex and often inchoate theories of what makes a thing the thing that it is (Murphy & Medin, 1985). As these theories are elaborated with time and experience, what the essence placeholder contains may change, but the function of the placeholder remains. Properties of things lie on a continuum of centrality ranging from the core concept (or essence) to superficial appearance. The more central, essential, core concepts "constrain or even generate" the surface properties that might be useful in identification, enabling two things with very different surface properties to be judged the same kind of thing. Medin and Ortony argue that:

First, people act as if their concepts contain essence placeholders that are filled with "theories" about what the corresponding entities are. Second, these theories often provide or embody causal linkages to more superficial properties. Our third tenet is that organisms have evolved in such a way that their perceptual (and conceptual) systems are sensitive to just those kinds of similarity that lead them toward the deeper and more central properties. Thus whales, as mammals that look more like fish than like other mammals, are the exception that proves the rule: Appearances are usually not deceiving.

This means that it is quite adaptive for an organism to be tuned to readily accessible, surface properties. Such an organism will not be led far astray because many of these surface properties are constrained by deeper properties. [Medin & Ortony, this volume, p. 186]

Developmental constraints on learning

Does psychological essentialism have the essence of a developmental theory of knowledge acquisition? Could it be that children come equipped with bundles of essence placeholders that help them sort the superficial properties of things into meaningful categories? In order to explain why young children learn and transfer certain properties rapidly but not others, something like this must be operating. But the trouble with this approach is that there would have to be a great many essence placeholders, and few believe that it is parsimonious to endow infants with too much prescience, or that infants come equipped with essence placeholders for whales, let alone unicorns! But what if we kept the idea of deep structure constraining perceptual pickup and limited the number and types of structures with which we must endow the child initially?

Such a developmental-constraints argument is currently gaining adherents among those who study learning in young children (Brown, 1982; Carey, 1985b; Keil, 1981; R. Gelman, 1986; R. Gelman & Brown, 1985a; R. Gelman & Gallistel, 1978; Gibson & Spelke, 1983; Spelke, 1983). They argue that in both the animal learning and language literatures, great strides were made once a basically associationist learning model was replaced by one grounded in the notion of species-specific biological constraints, predispositions, or biases to learn. By reason of the beast it is, an animal comes equipped to learn about certain privileged classes of information with particular survival value to that species (Hinde & Stevenson-Hinde, 1973; Seligman & Hager, 1972). It is argued that only by positing a system of constraints on human learning can one explain the puzzling disparity, from a strictly associationist point of view, between what infants can pick up perceptually and what they "choose" to learn about. For example, we know that infants are sensitive to the colors and forms of objects in that they dishabituate to changes along these dimensions (Cohen & Younger, 1983). Furthermore, infants categorically perceive color in much the same way that adults do; but this early sensitivity to color is *not* followed by rapid learning about, for example, color words (Bornstein, 1985). Indeed, color terms are learned late and with considerable difficulty. Linda Smith (this volume) demonstrates elegantly

that perceptual pickup of dimensional information and the understanding and use of dimensions of similarity are not the same thing.

So if infants do not "choose" to learn about color, what do they
learn about? There seems to be considerable agreement that they
learn rapidly about objects and people, not attributes of objects and
people but something much more akin to essences, such as what makes
them move. Infants from the earliest age seem to have different expectations for animate and inanimate things (R. Gelman, 1986; R.
Gelman & Spelke, 1981; R. Gelman, Spelke, & Meck, 1983). Young
children show early understanding that animate objects can move
themselves and hence obey what R. Gelman (1986) calls the "innards"
principle of mechanism. In contrast, inanimate objects obey the
external-agent principle; they cannot move themselves. If infants
come predisposed to differentiate animate and inanimate objects
(Trevarthen, 1977; Tronick, Adamson, Wise, Als, & Brazelton, 1975),
further differentiation into finer and finer distinctions could follow
as their knowledge of biology and physics increases. This progressive
differentiation would then form the basis of an understanding of
natural and material kinds.

It is also assumed that infants come predisposed to seek causal
explanations, but not just any cause, for they are particularly sensitive
to mechanical and personal causality (Brown, 1986; R. Gelman, 1986).
This initial cut on the world makes them learn rapidly that inanimate
objects need to be pushed, pulled, or propelled into motion, whereas
animate objects do not. Even 7-month-old babies are sensitive to this
need for point of contact in inanimate movement (Leslie, 1984a,
1984b). If we return to Medin and Ortony's point that deeper essences
constrain perceptual pickup, then one has an explanation for why
young babies differentiate between patterns of movement that represent human gait and biologically impossible movement in moving-
light displays. Furthermore, moving, dynamic light patterns are
needed to represent biological motions; successive static displays will
not do (Bertenthal, Profitt, & Cutting, 1984; Bertenthal, Profitt, Spetner, & Thomas, 1985; Fox & McDaniel, 1982).

It is also the initial need to separate things into animate and inanimate that explains why young children know so much about the
properties of objects (Baillargeon, et al., 1985; Gibson & Spelke, 1983;
Spelke, 1983). Object perception in infancy appears to be guided by
a coherent set of conceptions about the physical world: that objects
cannot act on each other at a distance; that one object cannot pass
through the space occupied by another; that movement must be ex-

ternally caused; that once set in motion, the path of motion has certain predictable properties, and so forth.

In brief, there are three essential interrelated parts to a structural constraints theory that have important implications for the study of learning and transfer. First, a core concept is the search for cause, for determinism and mechanism. Infants, just like adults (Reed, 1983), assume that events are caused, and it is their job to uncover potential mechanisms. Second, that which determines an event and delimits potential mechanisms is different for animate and inanimate objects. Thus, infants are guided by a naive theory of physical and personal causality; they come equipped to learn rapidly about this privileged class of mechanisms. Third, these core concepts determine, or at least constrain, what is selected from the range of available perceptual attributes to form the basis of emergent categories. Of the many sensations children are sensitive to, they learn most rapidly about those constrained by the core concept (see R. Gelman & Brown, 1985a, 1985b, for a more detailed discussion).

Causal structure and transfer

The foregoing steps toward a developmental theory of knowledge acquisition highlight the centrality of causal structure in understanding. On the basis of this theory, one would predict that, if there is *(a)* similarity at the level of *causal structure* and *(b)* the type of causal mechanism has been differentiated within the child's emergent theories of the world, then rapid transfer would be expected. Note that this is both a domain-specific and domain-general argument. Whereas a search for causal explanation (at least implicitly) may underlie children's knowledge-building in all domains, they cannot be responsive to causal mechanisms unless they have the domain-specific knowledge in question. As Bullock, R. Gelman, and Baillargeon (1982) point out, a child who does not know that sound waves exert force would most likely reject the notion that Ella Fitzgerald's voice could cause a glass to break. Similarly, the same child would surely be reluctant to claim that an "irredentist" was the cause unless he knew what an irredentist was, or at least what kind of thing it was. The state of children's theories about the world must have a profound influence on their learning and transfer.

How do these developmental constraints map onto current theories of analogical transfer? The most promising theory of analogical learning, because it gives causal structure preeminence, is Gentner's (1983) structure-mapping theory. This theory describes a set of implicit rules by which people are said to interpret analogy, which is seen as a mapping of knowledge from one domain (the base, or the source) to another (the target). Predicates are mapped from the base to the target according to the following rules: (a) The properties (attributes) of the objects in the base are discarded; (b) the relations among the objects in the base are preserved; and (c) higher-order relations (relations among relations) are preserved at the expense of lower-order relations. This last rule is the principle of *systematicity*, and it is within this principle that causal structure is emphasized. Connected systems of relations rather than isolated predicates are more likely to be transported. "The advantage of the predicate-structure approach is that it allows for mapping higher-order relational structure, such as causal relations" (Gentner, 1983, p. 14). So far, so good; it is the search for causal structure that facilitates broad understanding. But, in her developmental extensions, Gentner seems to favor a version of the perceptually bound hypothesis, when she argues that children rely on attributes rather than relations, and that systematicity "may make a somewhat later developmental appearance" (Gentner & Toupin, 1986). Thus there seems to be a conflict with the position I am advocating, which gives preeminence to systematicity at all ages, given that it involves the right kind of causal explanation.

The resolution lies in the argument that, just as all knowledge is not equal, all systematicities are not equal either. Let us consider two examples of systematicity used by Gentner. Her favorite example is the analogy between Rutherford's model of an atom and the solar system. In order to see the systematicity between these two examples, one would need a great deal of formal knowledge. Properties such as "revolves around," "attractive force," "more massive than," and "distance" are all causally interrelated if one understands the notion of a central force system. This is an example, par excellence, of the type of abstract knowledge acquired late, and as the result of schooling. The person on the street has seen neither the atom nor the solar system. Discovery of the systematicity in this comparison would indeed be late developing, if it develops at all, and would be highly dependent on formal education.

In contrast, consider the example (Gentner, this volume) of a simple causal chain form of systematicity:

$$\text{CAUSE [PUSH } (b_i, b_j), \text{ COLLIDE } (b_j, b_k)]$$

$$\text{CAUSE [PUSH } (t_i, t_j), \text{ COLLIDE } (t_j, t_k)]$$

Seeing the common causal structure of push/collide in two stories where different objects are doing the action is, presumably, a very simple case of systematicity. Now is this late developing? I think not. Given the evidence of children's early precocity concerning the nature of objects and what makes them move (Alpert, 1928; Baillargeon et al., 1985; Buhler, 1930; Gibson & Spelke, 1983; Leslie, 1984a, 1984b; Richardson, 1932a, 1932b; Spelke, 1983), this is where I would look for evidence of very early reliance on systematic relations and causal explanations. Indeed, whether children respond on the basis of attributes or lower-level relations, or are sensitive to higher-level causal relations among relations could be viewed as an indication of their depth of understanding within a domain, rather than their developmental status across domains.

We have some initial evidence that this is true (Brown, 1986; Brown & Slattery, work in progress). In order to study learning and transfer in very young children, we looked for a domain in which we knew that infants show early sensitivity to causal mechanisms, and where they choose to play with toys that exploit that knowledge. For these reasons, we decided to look at tools, particularly tools that afford certain relationships of point of contact, such as pulling and pushing.

We know that babies show early sensitivity to such causal mechanisms. Leslie (1984a, 1984b) showed 4–7-month-old babies moving film stimulus displays in which, for example, a moving block travels toward a stationary block and is clearly seen to propel the stationary block into motion. In a second film, the moving block stops short of contact. In another example, a hand approaches a stationary doll and either picks it up and moves away or moves away in tandem but without physical contact, the doll trailing behind as it were. Using a habituation technique, Leslie demonstrated that infants are highly sensitive to such spatiotemporal discontinuities. They see the hand or the block as an agent to cause movement in an inanimate object. But the no-contact, no-pickup scenarios are seen as anomalous events – a magical violation of causal principles.

This early sensitivity is reflected in studies of exploratory play, with 1-year-olds who work long and hard at mastering the functions of such tools as sticks and strings. By far the best descriptions of such self-motivated learning are Piaget's concerning his own children between the ages of 9 and 18 months. By 10 months of age, these children clearly understood the need for a point of contact to bring inanimate objects into range. For example, Jacqueline (9 months) discovers by chance that she can bring a toy within reach by pulling

382   ANN L. BROWN

a blanket (support) on which it is placed. After failing to reach a toy
duck she grasps the blanket which shakes the duck. "Seeing this, she
immediately grasps the coverlet again and pulls it again until she can
attain the objective directly – during the weeks that follow, she frequently utilizes this schema" (Piaget, 1952, p. 285). And Lucienne,
once she had experienced the action of a support, rapidly generalizes
the schema to sheets, handkerchiefs, tablecloths, pillows, boxes, books,
and so on. By 1 year of age, Lucienne cannot be fooled by elaborate
systems of overlapping pillows, drawing toward her only the particular
pillow that acts as a support for the desired object. Once the baby
understood the notion of the support, this knowledge transferred
rapidly to all potential supports. The same is true of sticklike things
(push schema) and stringlike objects (pull schema), as "means for
bringing" (Piaget, 1952, p. 295). Each new acquisition brings with it
its own penumbra of generalization:

Let us note that once the new schema is acquired, it is applied from the outset
to analogous situations. The behavior pattern of the string is without any
difficulty applied to the watch chain. Thus, at each acquisition we fall back
on the application of familiar means to new situations according to a rhythm
which will extend to the beginning of systematical intelligence. [Piaget, 1952,
p. 297]

Given this early sensitivity and spontaneous learning, I would predict that there would be ready transfer in laboratory situations if
pulling or pushing were the underlying causal mechanism. Is this
true? Apparently not; at least this did not seem to be the case in a
series of laboratory transfer studies where sticks and strings were used
(Alpert, 1928; Matheson, 1931; Sobel, 1939), where it was claimed
that insightful learning or transfer *does not exist* below 3–5 years of
age. How can this be? If infants are so fascinated by such tools, why
can't they learn to solve problems that exploit this knowledge? Yet
another conundrum to be explained is the contrast between the early
sensitivity and persistent self-motivated learning about tools reported
in the infant and naturalistic studies and the seemingly dramatic lack
of insight in laboratory transfer studies.

Let us look more closely then at these early laboratory studies. First,
they share a major drawback in that they were so closely modeled on
Kohler's (1925) classic work with problem solving in apes that they
could hardly be regarded as offering a hospitable environment for
young children. The toddlers were required to retrieve objects with
sticks, through the bars of cages (cribs). And it did not occur to anyone
that a set of boxes can be stacked and climbed to reach a desired
object more readily by apes than by less agile human 18-month-olds!

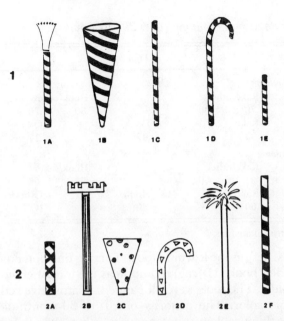

Figure 14.1. Representative learning and transfer tool sets from the "pull" condition used with 2-year-olds (from Brown & Slattery, work in progress).

Second, and more serious for my argument, is that the stimulus dimensions manipulated in these early studies were *not relevant to pulling or pushing.* Rather than varying relevant attributes such as length or rigidity of the means for bringing, influenced as they were by Thorndike, they varied perceptual similarity of the learning and transfer tools. And whereas all of these early studies claimed to find no evidence of insightful learning and transfer below 3 years of age, the claim is based on very little data. Below 30 months, the children are usually reported as nonresponsive, or as "finding the tools themselves more motivating than the incentives" (Sobel, 1939).

Not happy with the existing data base, we designed a tool-use transfer study where we manipulated perceptual similarity but also two variables relevant to the solution, length and the degree to which the instrument "affords pulling or pushing" (Brown & Slattery, work in progress). I will illustrate the main point by describing some data from the pull condition in 20–30-month-old children.

The child and the mother sat side by side, the child restrained by a "Sassy-Seat" that effectively prevented reaching beyond arm's length. A desired moving, noise-making toy (carousel) was out of reach. In front of the child was a set of tools. In Figure 14.1 are

Table 14.1. *Transfer data: pull condition (age: 20–30 months)*

Condition	Tool				
Conditions with no correct solution					
(1) 1 short tool	Rake/other			Hook/other	
	.70	.30		.80	.20
(2) 2 short tools	Rake		Hook		Other
	.35		.47		.17
Conditions with correct solution					
(3) 1 long tool	Rake/other			Hook/other	
	.91	.09		.93	.06
(4)ᵃ 2 long tools	Rake		Hook		Other
	.60		.40		0

ᵃInsufficient data for statistical analysis.

examples of the tools. Set 1 is the learning tools. There is one potential puller, a long, rounded hook (1D), agreed upon as the tool of choice by experts (3-year-olds). The tools were all painted an attractive red-and-white candy-cane color. The majority of 20- to 30-month-old children could solve this problem spontaneously. When they failed, the mother was urged to demonstrate the pulling solution. After three such demonstrations, the child was given a set of transfer tools. A representative example is also shown in Figure 14.1. In two conditions there was a correct choice, a tool long enough to reach and with an effective head. The transfer set shown in Figure 14.1 has a correct solution, as the rake (2B) is long enough. In two of the conditions no tool was "correct" because the ones with an effective pulling head were too short. We scored which tool the child chose, hastily giving a long enough tool after the trial on which the children were duped with too small tools.

The data from the four conditions are shown in Table 14.1. Children in all conditions transferred the pull solution, taking 23 seconds to choose an effective tool. They did not select the tool that was identical in color (i.e., tool 2F in Figure 14.1). And they showed no preference for the physically similar hook (2D) over the physically dissimilar rake (2B). If one potential puller is the right length, it predominates. They learned that what was needed were an effective pulling head and the correct length. They actively sought the appropriate tool; they were not distracted or influenced by physical similarity.

I conclude that young children do show rapid insightful transfer if they are familiar with the mechanism of causality that underlies the deep structural similarity between problems. If we are dealing with such privileged domains, transfer is not an issue; it can be assumed. Even 2-year-olds can override surface features of physical similarity and respond in terms of causal relations if they know what kind of thing it is that they are dealing with, if they understand the causal mechanism in question.

I would like to argue, then, that a search for causal explanation is the basis of broad understanding. Wide patterns of generalization, flexible transfer, and creative inferential projections are all indexes of deeper understanding. Causal knowledge works to make certain patterns of correlated properties more salient than others and provides a rationale for their interrelationship (Johnson-Laird, Herrmann, & Chaffin, 1984; Wattenmaker, Nakamura, & Medin, 1988).

To go back to the original argument, why do children act as if they were perceptually bound? The predilection to operate as if surface features were important is the result of three factors. First, in the real world they usually are important. As Medin and Ortony (this volume) point out, the surface features that we pick up are often constrained by deeper structural meanings; appearances are usually not deceiving; surface similarity is usually correlated with deep structural similarity; and organisms are sensitive to just these kinds of correlated similarities that lead to the deeper and central properties. Second, because of these correlated relations, sensitivity to surface features has a *high probability of paying off*; noting stable similarities among the surface properties might act as a crutch to new learning while the child is differentiating the core structures within his or her emergent theories. Third, for young children, and novices, who have not yet differentiated the deeper structure, appearance matches serve as a fallback option when theory fails.

Dependence on surface similarities is useful but fallible, however, as all surface similarities do not correlate with deep structure; appearances, as in the case of whales and fishes, can be misleading. If the child is captured by superficial features that are *not* rooted in a stable causal explanation, learning should be fleeting and fragile. The typical pattern of laboratory transfer suggests that it is just such momentary partial understandings that are being captured. Rapid, transitory judgments in the absence of causal explanation are not the basis for sustained learning or conceptual change.

In the next section, we turn to a series of studies on young children's transfer where the main focus was on engineering transfer in situations where it is difficult to obtain, where the situations are arbitrary and children are equated for knowledge by their lack of it, a typical ploy of developmental psychologists.

Factors that affect flexible access to knowledge

In this section, I will argue that, just as all knowledge is not equal, so too *all conditions of learning are not equal*. I will illustrate this point by describing a series of studies with preschool children, although there is no reason in principle to suggest that the crucial variables hold only for the young. We know that learners of all ages have difficulty accessing their knowledge in flexible ways; inert knowledge is not just a problem for the young (Bransford & Franks, this volume; Bereiter & Scardamalia, 1985; Brown & Campione, 1978, 1981).

The basic learning situation I use is the classic paradigm (A B C), where children are set a series of problems that differ in surface format but share similarity at a deeper level. Two classes of tasks were selected: (a) *tool-use* studies, where children, who understand the action of sticks, strings, and so on, must solve novel problems that involve creative uses of these instruments; and (b) *biological themes*, where children learn simple animal defense mechanisms by listening to short stories. Within both domains, the children would be asked to solve classic "arbitrary-solution" problems. However, in both domains, they would have enough sophistication to understand the solutions.

In the tool-use studies, children, who understand the action of sticks and strings, are required to apply this knowledge of basic mechanisms to creative but arbitrary solutions. In the Brown and Slattery work mentioned previously, the task was a natural use of tools; the child could not reach a desired toy, and in plain sight was an available reacher. In the studies to be described here, the tool-use solution is "unnatural," or a trick, as it were; the child must invent a novel solution to a deliberately ambiguous situation.

The biological domain was chosen as one for which children would not have any existing background knowledge and for which there is no readily available causal explanation; for example, there is no inherent reason why a crested rat should mimic a skunk as a method of defense. However, there are higher-order relations in the domain that can be learned. We also intend to look at a third domain, that of natural kinds (S. Gelman & Markman, 1986) and compare and contrast learning and transfer within the three types of knowledge. Here I consider the biological themes and tool-use studies only.

The major factors that affect flexible access in these situations are shown in Table 14.2. I consider three classes of variables. The first two deal with "meta"-level explanations of why children perform poorly. First, perhaps they simply do not know the *rules of the game* (Flavell, 1985). The second class has to do with another type of meta-

Table 14.2. *Factors that affect flexible access to knowledge*

I. Learning the game
A. Instructional analogies
    Using analogies as tools for communication and exposition
B. Learning to learn
    Forming a mind-set to look for analogies

II. Reflection
Concentrating attention on the underlying goal structure
A. By prompting
B. By asking the learner to teach
C. By discussion

III. Flexibility or encapsulation
A. Cognitive encapsulation

    Negative learning set
    Functional fixedness
    Cognitive embeddedness

B. Cognitive flexibility

    Positive learning set
    Functional flexibility: perceiving the solution as appropriate to many contexts
    Cognitive disembedding: via reflection on the deep structure

---

cognition, *reflection*; perhaps children have difficulty reflecting on their own thought processes.

The third set of variables has to do with the factors that promote cognitive encapsulation or cognitive flexibility. Here we borrow from the traditional problem-solving literature of the 1930s and 1940s. The Gestalt literature on problem solving included a great deal of discussion of three factors that impede flexible use of knowledge: (a) *Einstellung*, or *negative learning sets*, such as that of the famous water-jar problem described by Luchins (1942); (b) *functional fixedness* (Duncker, 1945), where a potential solution tool is "burdened" by its habitual use and is thereby rendered unavailable for a novel use; and (c) *cognitive embeddedness* (Scheerer & Huling, 1960), where a potential solution tool is not seen, although in plain sight, because it is embedded in a familiar context. However, little attempt was made to study the flip side of these issues: What are the conditions of learning that lead to "functional flexibility" or "cognitive disembedding," terms not even invented because of the focus on blocks to, rather than opportunities for, cognitive flexibility?

I argue that three mechanisms serve to enhance conceptual flexibility: (a) positive learning set; (b) *functional flexibility* – conditions that encourage the learner to perceive the solution as widely applicable; and (c) *cognitive disembedding*, whereby the learner is encouraged to reflect on the deep structure of the analogous problems. Each of these factors from Table 14.2 will be considered in turn.

Learning the game

Instructional analogies. If young children perform poorly because they do not understand the rules of novel laboratory games, how might one set about making things clearer? One possibility is simply to use analogies in a sensible fashion. In classic laboratory tests of transfer, the experimenter acts as a problem poser rather than a teacher. She presents Problem A, followed by Problem B, with no hint that the problems are similar in any way; no indication is given that Problem B is another token of the same type as Problem A. The whole trick is that children should notice the similarity on their own. In contrast, consider how analogies are actually used in instruction. Typically, Problem A, for example a simple fractions problem, is introduced. Next, Problem B is presented *explicitly* in order to illustrate Problem A. A classic example of an illustrative analogy for introducing fractions would be that of a pizza that must be divided into equal portions. The similarity of the illustrative pizza analogy to the fractions problem at hand is quite explicit and fully discussed by the teacher. In short, it is part of a communicative pact in instruction that analogies are introduced as explicit examples and transfer between them socially mediated. If analogies are presented in this informative way, will young children learn from them?

We examined this question in a series of studies with 3–5-year-old children (Brown, Kane, & Long, in press). All children were introduced to related problems requiring them to use tools to either pull, stack, or swing. Sample pairs of problems are given in Table 14.3. The children were assigned to one of three conditions: Instructional Analogy, Reminder, and Control. In the Instructional Analogy condition the children were given the first (stacking) problem (e.g., John, the garage-mechanic) and asked to solve it. When they could not, the experimenter put it aside and consoled the child.

Well, that's a really hard problem. Most kids don't get that right away. Keep thinking about how [the protagonist] might solve the problem because we will come back and help him later. But now we are going to work on an easier problem *which will help us solve the* [first protagonist] *problem.* Let's just tell [the first protagonist] that we won't forget, that we'll be back later after we have learned how to help him.

Table 14.3. *Tool-use problem pairs*

Problem Set 1: Stacking

A. John (Jean), the garage mechanic, has a problem. He needs to take all of the tires that have been delivered to his garage and put them up on a shelf. But the shelf is too high and he doesn't have a ladder, so he can't reach the shelf by himself. How can he solve his problem? *Solution*: Stack two tires and stand on top of them.

B. Bill (Brenda), the farmer, has a problem. He needs to put his bales of hay on top of his tractor so he can take them to the market. But Bill isn't tall enough to reach the top of the tractor by himself. How can he solve his problem? *Solution*: Stack two bales of hay and stand on top of them.

Problem Set 2: Pulling

A. Mrs. (Mr.) Smith is a lady who grows flowers. One day she is working in her garden, removing weeds (with a hoe) when she hears a little boy crying. She looks up and sees that the little boy has fallen down a big hole at the bottom of her garden. She can't reach him because the ground around the hole will give way. How can Mrs. Smith help? *Solution*: Mrs. Smith sticks out her hoe, the boy grabs it, and he is pulled up.

B. Linda (Steven), the girl guide, has a problem. She is fishing (with a pole) when suddenly she sees that a boat with a little girl in it has broken away from the dock and is floating downstream. She has to get the little girl and the boat back to shore. How can Linda solve her problem? *Solution*: Linda holds out her fishing pole and has the little girl grab it, and she pulls the boat to shore.

Problem Set 3: Swinging

A. Carolyn (Carl), the nurse, has a problem. Earlier in the day when the water wasn't deep she walked across the stream to go visit a sick lady in the house on the other side. But while she was there, the weather got very bad, there was a big flood, and now the water is too deep and fast for her to walk, jump, or swim across. She needs to get back to the other side before dark. How can she solve her problem? *Solution*: Grab onto a willow tree branch on the bank and swing across to the other side.

B. Mr. (Mrs.) Brown, the telephone repairperson, has a problem. He is up on a roof to connect the telephone wires to the two telephone poles. He has all of his tools up there. Suddenly, he notices that the house is on fire. He needs to get to the roof on the other house to save himself. How can he solve his problem? *Solution*: Grab onto the telephone wires and swing across.

The children then received the second (stacking) problem (e.g., Bill, the farmer), which they "solved" collaboratively with the experimenter. After this, the first unsolved problem, John was brought back and the children were told that because we now know how to help the second protagonist, "we can go back and help [the first protagonist], can't we?" The fact that the two problems were alike was stressed, but the actual point of similarity was not mentioned.

The same general procedure was followed for the Reminder group, except that after failure to solve the first problem, the link between it and the to-be-learned second problems was not made explicit. After solving the second problem, they received the minimal reminder, "Oh, now we can help the [first protagonist] can't we?" They received the same order of problems, however (A B A), as did the Control group, where no mention of problem similarity was made.

The experiment was repeated using simple biological themes material. Two of three problems were randomly selected; all involved illustrated stories about animals, including the critical information of how they defend themselves. In all cases, the defense mechanism was *mimicry*; further, all animals used visual mimicry in that they revealed markings to look like a more dangerous animal, "to make themselves more scary," in 3-year-old parlance. The first animal, the *crested rat*, parts its hair when threatened to reveal skunklike markings. The *hawkmoth caterpillar* turns over to reveal markings on its underside that resemble a poisonous snake; and the *capricorn beetle* reveals wasplike markings when under attack. In both sets of experiments, the patterns were the same. If the analogies were explicitly used for instructional purposes, most children transferred. These data are shown in Figure 14.2. Tool solutions were transferred less readily than defense mechanisms, but this difference was reliable only in the Reminder condition. Children needed only minimal prompts to transfer the mimicry solution, but in the tool-use scenarios, they needed to have it explicitly spelled out that Problem B was the same as Problem A. And, having seen the point in the A B A paradigm, they readily transferred (100%) to a totally novel Problem C. Using analogies in sensible ways, to instruct children to solve the unfamiliar by recourse to the familiar, results in ready transfer, even in children as young as 3 years of age.

Learning to learn: a mind-set to look for analogous solutions

In the following series of studies we set out to examine whether an abstract *positive learning set* to transfer could be established under conditions where there is no surface similarity in the *tool* or in *the action* that leads to solution and where the child would not be told that the problems were alike (Brown & Kane, 1988). Children would be set a series of problem pairs and required to use the information in the first problem of a pair to solve the second. Over a series of such tasks, would the child pick up the abstract rule, "transfer prior solutions," even when that solution is novel across pairs? Such a positive learning set would consist of something very abstract indeed, that is, the expectation to solve problems by analogy. In other words,

INSTRUCTIONAL ANALOGIES

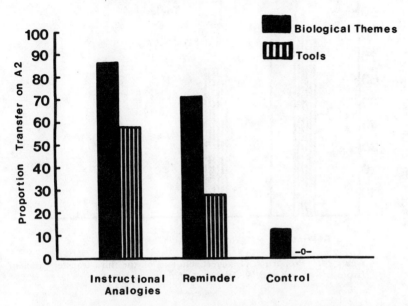

Figure 14.2. Proportion of correct solutions on the representation of the original unsolved problem (A^2) (from Brown, Kane, & Long, in press).

required to solve a series of isomorphic problem pairs, will the child develop a mind-set to look for analogous solutions within each pair even without verbal prompts to problem similarity?

To test this assumption, we again used two domains, the tool-use problem pairs illustrated in Table 14.3, and a set of biological theme stories. This time there were three sets of pairs. Two animals, the hawkmoth caterpillar (looks like a poisonous snake) and the porcupine fish (puffs itself up to twice its size and raises spikes), look like something *more dangerous* when under attack. Two animals, the arctic fox and the chameleon, *change color*, one by season and one on a momentary basis. The remaining two animals, the walkingstick insect and the pipefish, *change shape* as a means of camouflage. The mechanisms connecting the pairs are similar at a fairly high level of abstraction; the physical manifestation of the underlying mechanism is not at all similar. For each pair of problems (A B, & C), the solution to the first problem (A^1, B^1, C^1) was demonstrated by the experimenter; the analogous solution to the second problem (A^2, B^2, C^2) was the transfer probe.

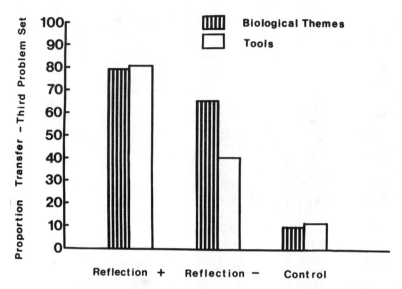

Figure 14.3. Proportion of correct solutions on the third transfer problem (from Brown & Kane, 1988).

Children 2 to 5 years old were assigned to one of three conditions. There were two learning-to-learn groups: Reflection and No-Reflection. In both, the children received the three pairs of problems in randomized order. The children in the Reflection condition received one of three kinds of aid designed to induce them to reflect on the solution of each problem: (a) *Hint*: after the A member of a pair, the experimenter told the child that the next problem was just the same. This explicit instruction proved effective in helping 2- to 5-year-olds transfer a simple physical solution across task boundaries (Crisafi & Brown, 1986); here it served as a base line against which other forms of reflection could be evaluated. (b) *Discussion*: after the B member of each pair, the experimenter prompted the child to discuss the similarity of the A and B problems. And (c) *Instruct*: after the B problem in a pair, the child is asked to instruct Kermit the frog puppet in the solution of the A and B problems, again a ploy that worked well with 3-year-olds in enhancing transfer of identical solutions across disparate tasks (Crisafi & Brown, 1986). No-Reflection children received the three sets of problems with no discussion. Control children received unrelated problems before tackling the problem pair that was the third of the series for the experimental subjects.

The data from the 3-year-olds are shown in Figure 14.3. The picture

Table 14.4. *Learning to learn: biological themes (examples of verbalization in discussion group)*

Aaron (3 years old)

1. E: Aaron, are this story about the fish [porcupine fish] and the story about the caterpillar [hawkmoth] the same kinds of stories?
2. A: Yes, they are the same.
3. E: Why are they the same?
4. A: Because these guys have a problem [*pointing to picture of fish*], and these guys [*pointing to picture of caterpillar*] have a problem too!
5. E: What is it that's the same? Tell me a little more.
6. A: Well, they both have the same kind of problem, I guess.
7. E: Which is what?
8. A: Both of them have a mean guy that wants to eat them all up. This guy [*pointing to caterpillar*] has a bird that wants to eat him. And the shark wants to eat him [*pointing to porcupine fish*].
9. E: So Aaron, what do they do? Is there any other way the two stories are the same?
10. A: Yes, they're the same all the way through the story [*said with great enthusiasm*].
11. E What do you mean "all the way through"? Could you tell me a little bit more what you mean?
12. A: When the bird wants to eat him [*pointing to caterpillar*] he gets really mean and changes himself into a snake. So the bird gets too scared and flies away.
13. E: So why is that the same then?
14. A: Because this one [*pointing to porcupine fish*] can look mean too! He gets mean and big and gets all his scary pointers [spikes] out and scares the shark away.
15. E: So is that why they are the same?
16. A: Yes. They both get mean and scary so they [predators] run away [*in an excited voice*].
17. E: They're pretty smart, huh?
18. A: Just like me!

---

is clear. By the third problem set both the children in the Reflection condition and those in the No-Reflection condition are showing significantly more transfer than is the Control group, a learning-to-learn effect. Again, biological themes are transferred more readily than tool solutions but only in conditions featuring minimal help.

The various help conditions all intensify the effect dramatically. Helping children reflect upon their solutions, through either discussing, hinting or having them teach others, forces attention to underlying deep structure and facilitates transfer to novel situations. Just what a discussion of similarity might look like in a 3-year-old is illustrated in the protocol shown in Table 14.4. Although Aaron appears reluctant to tell all he knows, persistence on the part of the experimenter pays off; in comments 12, 14, and 16, it is clear that Aaron has abstracted the essential principle that the two stories share.

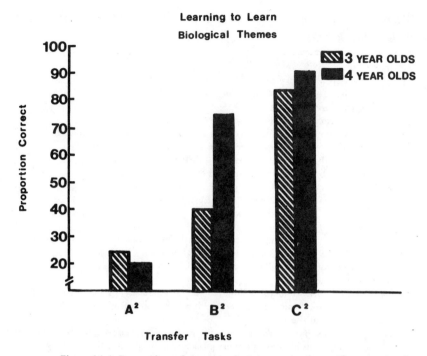

Figure 14.4. Proportion of correct solutions on the first (A^2), second (B^2), and third (C^2) transfer problem as a result of age (from Brown & Kane, 1988).

This experiment was essentially replicated using only the biological themes materials and the No-Reflection condition. Here children were in no way prompted to discuss or reflect on problem similarity. The data from this replication are shown in Figure 14.4, where it can been seen that both 3- and 4-year-olds show a dramatic learning-to-learn effect. The 4-year-olds have caught on to the rules of the game by the second problem pair; 3-year-olds need two examples before they show ready transfer across problem isomorphs. Young children readily develop a mind-set to look for analogies using the information provided in the first problem of a set (e.g., A^1, B^1) to solve the analogous second problem (e.g., B^2, C^2).

Reflection

An essential feature of the typical A B C paradigm is that the underlying structural similarity across problems is disguised by different relevant and irrelevant surface features. As described in the learning-to-learn studies above, we have found that manipulations that direct the child's attention to the underlying structure facilitate transfer. Asking the child to discuss problem similarity or teach each problem to a puppet leads to rapid transfer, because under such circumstances the child hones in on deep structure and disregards idiosyncratic surface features in his or her discussion or exposition. I will illustrate this point with just one example.

Brown, et al. (1986) considered transfer across "problem iso-morphs" based on the Genie problem introduced by Holyoak et al. (1984). The problems we used are shown in Table 14.5, and the common goal structure linking them is schematized in Table 14.6. Available on each problem is, among other potential tools, a large piece of paper that can be rolled into a tube. In the Genie story, the paper is called a magic carpet, and the Genie uses it to transport the jewels. The remaining two stories recruit the same solution. Children do not see this common goal structure and, as a result, fail to transfer. But in order to use the known solution of the source problem, the learner must retrieve it *in appropriate form*. The optimal level of rep-resentation is one that highlights the goal structure of the causal event sequence that is common across problems (Trabasso, Secco, & Van Den Broek, 1984). In noting the commonalities, the learner deletes the surface differences between problems and concentrates on the core similarities.

First, the problem that children experience is one of attention or retention; that is, do they notice and remember the source analog? Second, do children process the analogies at the most advantageous level of representation, concentrating on the causal goal structure (Black & Bower, 1980; Black & Wilensky, 1979)? If the stories are viewed as unrelated narratives, rather than as general problem paths, transfer is unlikely to occur.

Children from 3 to 5 years old were asked to solve the three anal-ogous problems illustrated in Table 14.5. They were assigned to one of three experimental conditions: Prompted Goal Structure, Recall, and Control. In the Prompted Goal Structure group, prompts were given in order to draw the child's attention to the common goal struc-ture of the three scenarios (see Table 14.6). After each scenario had been solved, the child was asked four questions to fill in the slots of a skeletal goal structure. First, the child was asked for the *protagonist*: Who has a problem (Genie, Rabbit, Farmer)? Then the child was asked for the *goal*: What did (the protagonist) want to do (transfer jewels, transfer eggs, transfer cherries)? Next the child was probed for the

Table 14.5. *The three analogous problems*

Problem 1. The Genie

A magic Genie lived for many years in a field behind a wall. His home was a very
   pretty bottle where he lived happily and collected a fine set of jewels. But one day
   an envious witch put a spell on the Genie. He was stuck to the spot, he couldn't
   move his feet, all his magic powers were gone. If he could move his home to the
   other side of the wall, he would be out of reach of the spell and his magic would
   come back. He had found an even prettier, larger bottle on the other side, but he
   has a problem. How can he get his jewels across the high wall into the new bottle
   without breaking them and without moving his feet? The Genie has all these
   treasures to help him [glue, string, tape, etc.]. Can you think of any way the
   Genie can get his jewels into the new bottle?

Problem 2. The Rabbit

Here is the Easter Bunny's problem. The Easter Bunny has to deliver all these
   Easter eggs to all the little children before Easter [tomorrow], but he has been
   working so hard all week, painting the eggs and hiding them for Easter egg hunts.
   He would really like to rest and to stay here with his friends and have a picnic. If
   he stays, he won't have time to finish delivering the eggs. The Easter Bunny has
   finished delivering all the eggs on this side of the river [*points to picnic side*], but he
   hasn't started on the other side. The Easter Bunny has a rabbit friend on the
   other side of the river who has offered to help him [*points to second rabbit waiting
   with an empty basket on the other side of the river*], but how can the Easter Bunny get
   the eggs across the river into his friend's basket? The river is big, there are no
   bridges or boats, and rabbits can't swim and don't like to get wet. What can he do?
   Can you think of anything he could use to get the eggs to the helpful bunny?

Problem 3. The Farmer

Farmer Jones is very happy. He has picked a whole bunch of cherries and is taking
   them to market. When he sells them, he will have enough money to go on
   vacation with his family. They will go to the seaside. He wants to deliver the load
   of cherries to the market. That morning there was a great storm, with rain,
   thunder, and lightning. But he cannot wait to take the cherries to market because
   the cherries are just ripe now and will go bad. On his way to market, he finds the
   road blocked by a very big fallen tree knocked over in the storm. What can he do?
   He must get his cherries to market quickly; otherwise, they will go bad. A friend
   has driven his tractor up to the other side of the tree and will lend it to Farmer
   Jones, but how will he get the cherries across the big, big tree? He can't reach
   over, and he mustn't damage the cherries.

---

obstacle: What is stopping (the protagonist)? And finally the *solution*
was requested: How did (the protagonist) get his (jewels, eggs, cherries) across? In the Recall condition, the children were simply asked
to tell all they could remember about the preceding story. In the
Control condition the children attempted the second problem with
no intervention, the typical procedure in the A B C paradigm. Note

Table 14.6. *Common goal structure of scenarios (from Brown, Kane, &*
Echols, 1986)

Scenario	Genie	Rabbit	Farmer
Progatonist	Genie	Easter Bunny	Farmer Jones
Goal	Transfer jewels across wall into bottle 2	Transfer eggs across river into basket 2	Transfer cherries across tree trunk into vehicle 2
Obstacle	Distance and wall	Distance and river	Distance and tree
Solution	Roll paper	Roll paper	Roll paper

that in all conditions no mention was made concerning problem similarity; the children had to notice this on their own.

About half of the students recalled what amounted to a perfect
synopsis of the goal structure. Therefore, the Recall students were
further divided into two groups: *(a)* Spontaneous Goal Structure,
where the child recalled all four elements of the goal structure (protagonist, goal, obstacle, and solution) and very little trivia; *(b)* Recall
Only, where the child recalled surface features of the story but omitted
critical structural elements. The resultant four groups then were the
Prompted Goal Structure, Spontaneous Goal Structure, Recall, and
Control. Of interest is whether these manipulations on the first problem in any way affect transfer to the second. In Figure 14.5, we can
see that children prompted to fill in the slots of the goal structure
significantly outperformed those in the Control condition. In addition, those children who spontaneously recalled the goal structure
transferred as well as those who were prompted on the critical
elements.

Children as young as 3 years of age can transfer a common solution
across analogous situations if they represent the source problem at
an appropriate level of analysis. Children who spontaneously represent stories in terms of an abstract situation (van Dijk & Kintsch, 1983)
or mental model (Gentner, 1983; Johnson-Laird, 1980) of the goal
structure underlying the critical event sequences also note the one-
to-one correspondences between the stories. In addition, mechanisms
that draw children's attention to the common deep structure of analogous problems facilitate transfer. Prompting the child to fill in the
slots representing the four key elements of the goal structure freed
or "disembedded" (Scheerer & Huling, 1960) the common abstract

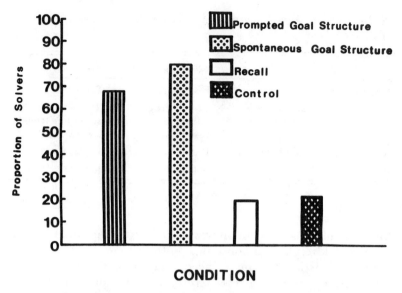

Figure 14.5. Proportion of correct solution to the first transfer problem as a result of recall conditions (from Brown, Kane, & Echols, 1986).

structure from its first specific context, thus permitting its flexible application.

Flexibility and encapsulation

So far we have shown that children as young as 3 years of age can transfer across tasks that differ in surface features but share an underlying goal structure. Furthermore, if their attention is drawn to the "game" of solving problems by analogy, they rapidly develop an abstract learning set to perform in this way. Finally, learning conditions that increase the likelihood that the child will reflect on the solution of each problem, via teaching or discussion, also result in flexible access to knowledge on subsequent problems. In this section we will consider the conditions of learning that lead to *more* rather than *less* flexible application of learned rules, borrowing from the Gestalt work on problem solving and creativity from the 1930s and 1940s.

As I pointed out earlier, the classic Gestalt literatures focused almost exclusively on factors that impede flexible problem solving such as *functional fixedness*, where a potential solution tool is overlooked because it is "burdened" by its habitual use, and *cognitive embeddedness*, where a potential solution object is not seen as such, although in plain sight, because it is embedded in a familiar context. Attempts to examine the corollary conditions that lead to "functional flexibility" or "cognitive disembedding" were not part of this literature. In this section I attempt to redress this omission, at the same time modifying the paradigms for use with young children.

Consider by way of example functional fixedness of an object (or more usually a tool) in problem-solving situations. Studies by Maier (1930, 1931, 1945), Duncker (1945), and others have shown that if a tool, A, has just been used for purpose x and the new task calls for purpose y, the availability of A for purpose y is reduced by its use in x. A is said to be "burdened" by its x function and therefore unavailable for use in a y function. This is particularly true if the x function is a natural one for A (A = hammer, x function = knocking in nails) and the y function is an invention (A = hammer, y function = using A as a weight on a pendulum). For example, Birch and Rabinowitz (1951) were able to show that the very same object can be fixed or available depending on prior experience. Adults were asked to complete an electrical circuit on a board by using either a switch or a relay. Next they were confronted with a variant of Maier's (1931) classic two-cord problem, where the subject is required to tie together the free ends of two cords that are suspended from the ceiling. The distance between the two cords is such that the subject cannot reach one cord if the other is held. The problem can be solved by tying a weight to the end of one of the strings, thus converting it into a pendulum, which can be set swinging and then be caught on the upswing while the stationary cord is held. The two cords can then be tied together. The solution is to use the switch or the relay as a weight. Although the Control group used the switch or relay with equal probability, all the Relay subjects used the switch, and 77% of the Switch subjects used the relay. When asked why they had used the switch (relay), the subjects gave plausible reasons why it was the *only* tool available. Would the same principles hold for children?

We began with a grade school sample and used the Genie, Rabbit, Farmer series of problems shown in Table 14.5. Kindergartners and second and fourth graders served as subjects. All children were shown the magic carpet (paper) solution to the Genie story and then attempted the two transfer tasks in counterbalanced order. The groups differed, however, in the experiences they had just *prior* to seeing the Genie solution. There were three conditions: Functional Fixedness, Flexibility, and Neutral. In the Functional Fixedness condition, children engaged in a pretest drawing session in which they used the (potential solution tool) paper, identical to that to be used in the problem sets. They completed three drawing tasks on three sheets of paper for future posting on the wall as artwork. As they had previously drawn on the paper, reinforcing the usual function of paper for children, its availability for potential tube solutions should be lessened. In the Flexibility condition, children performed three original tasks with the paper (drawing; making a house, tent, or plane; and playing a communication game), none of which involved a tube or conveyance function for the paper. It was hypothesized that this would encourage the children to regard the paper as a tool of many uses and enhance its availability for use as a solution tool. In the Neutral condition, children completed three irrelevant tasks before encountering the Genie series. The data for transfer to the first analogy (e.g., from Genie to Farmer) are presented in the top half of Figure 14.6. Prior experience with paper as a tool of many uses enhances transfer whereas experience with the tool in only one (habitual) function impedes transfer. The only difference between the younger and older children is how effective they are under neutral conditions. This effect is dramatic even though *the transfer part of the experiment was identical for all children*. The psychological availability of a common solution tool is determined not merely by its physical appearance but by its recent history of use (see Barsalou, this volume, on *recent context-dependent* information). Children whose recent experience involved using construction paper only as a medium for drawing did very poorly; using the paper exclusively for drawing fixes its function and makes it less available for creative solutions. In contrast, children whose prior experience involved using the paper in a variety of novel ways readily discovered tube solutions for the Rabbit/Farmer problems. Experimenting with a variety of uses for the paper frees it from a specific role, transforming it into a tool of many applications. The data in the second half of Figure 14.6 are from an essentially similar study with 3- to 5-year-olds solving simpler string-use tasks (see Brown & Kane, work in progress).

The generality of this finding and its potential educational significance are illustrated in a replication using exemplars from our biological themes domain, where 4-year-olds were asked to learn about mimicry-like defense mechanisms. In the Encapsulation or Fixedness conditions, the children learned three exemplars that are highly similar at the level of mechanism, all using visual mimicry: the *capricorn beetle*, which reveals wasplike markings when attacked; the *hawkmoth caterpillar* which has markings on its underside like a poisonous snake; and the *crested rat*, which when threatened parts its hair to reveal skunk-like markings. What the child learns is that animals defend

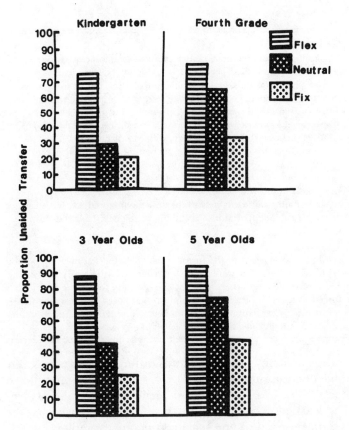

Figure 14.6. Proportion of correct solutions as a result of prior learning conditions: functional fixedness, cognitive flexibility, or neutral (from Brown & Kane, work in progress).

themselves by similar mechanisms, that is, by pretending to be something more dangerous than themselves. In contrast, the Flexibility group learned three exemplars that cover a range of possible mechanisms. For example, the hoverfly makes a sound like a bee (sound mimicry), the opossum freezes and plays dead, and the walkingstick insect changes its shape to look like a twig or a leaf. After learning their three examples, the children were introduced to a novel set of problems, Moths of Manchester and Pocket Mice, illustrated in Table 14.7, where a novel solution must be learned (natural selection based on color camouflage).

These data are shown in Figure 14.7. Of the Fixedness children, 76% transferred an old solution from the learning phase, compared

Table 14.7. *Transfer task*

Moths of Manchester

In an area of England called Manchester, before there were any factories, there was
a countryside and clean, clear air. There was no pollution [*explain with illustrative
picture of countryside prior to the Industrial Revolution*]. Peppered moths lived in the
area. They were mostly white in color, but some were gray and some were almost
black. Out of every 10 moths, 8 were white or off-white, and 2 were black.
[*Illustrate by placing eight Velcro-backed whitish moths on a white card with two blackish
moths.*] Over time Manchester became a big city, with lots of factories. The
factories put out smoke and pollution, and the air became darker and darker
[*illustration of factory stacks and pollution*]. What happened to the moths?
[*Two moths, one black and one white, are stuck on the factory habitat.*]
Hint 1: "Which moth would you rather be? Why?"
Hint 2: "The white moths can easily be seen against the polluted air; birds can
 catch them easily. Peppered moths still live in the city. How did this
 happen?"

Pocket Mice

Pocket mice lived in the sandy part of the forest. Most of the pocket mice were light
 brown (sandy) in color, but a few were reddish in color. But the sandy part of the
 forest became overcrowded, and there was not enough food for all the mice.
Some were forced to move to other parts of the forest where the soil was reddish-
 brown or dark brown. What happened? [*Repeat hinting procedure with Velcro-backed,
 sandy, red, and dark brown mice and three forest habitats as necessary.*]

---

with 23% of the Flexibility group. And this difference was not merely
one of numbers because those who did refer back to training did so
in different ways. The Fixedness children mentioned the general principle they had learned to encompass all three exemplars, whereas the
Flexibility group referred to one specific concrete exemplar. For example, the children in the Fixedness condition who learned three
exemplars of *become dangerous* suggested that the Moths defend themselves by "looking more scary," exactly as they had been taught. Sometimes their responses took some interpretation; we presume that the
child who suggested the moth turn into a big gorilla had in mind the
"more dangerous" theme even if he lacked somewhat an understanding of the constraints set on such mechanisms! If told the dark ones
survived, they suggest that dark ones are more scary. This group
came up with an average of 1.7 solutions. Satisfied with their learned
generalization (*look scary*), they did not seek a novel solution. In contrast, the Flexibility group mentioned several possible solutions, averaging 5.3 per child, and as a result, 82% invented the color change
as a potential solution. These data, on inventing the color solution,
are also shown in Figure 14.7.

To characterize the children's performance, it seemed as if the

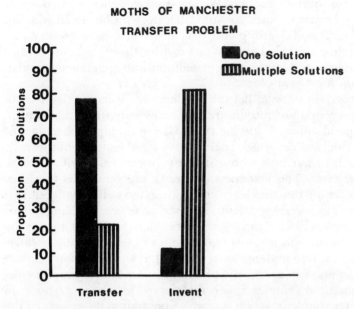

MOTHS OF MANCHESTER
TRANSFER PROBLEM

Figure 14.7. Proportion of transfer and invention solutions to the Moths of Manchester problem as a function of prior learning conditions (from Brown & Kane, work in progress).

Fixedness group had learned a general rule that they attempted to apply and this blocked them to alternative possibilities, an example of *negative transfer*. The Flexibility group had learned that there are a variety of solutions to problems of defense, leaving them more open to the novel *color-change* solution. Note, however, that none of these very young children really understood the actual mechanism of selection that underlies the Moth solution. Even those suggesting the efficacy of color change saw it as an immediate solution for these particular moths, in the fashion of a chameleon, rather than natural selection over time.

They could, however, transfer the color-change principle. When presented with the analogous Pocket Mice problem, 33% of the Flexible children immediately suggested the color change before the experimenter had finished describing the scenario, snatching up red and brown Velcro mice and placing them in appropriate habitats with great enthusiasm. After the problem was posed, 56% more of the Flexible children were successful (total = 89%) as were 73% of the Fixedness group, so there were no differences between groups on the transfer problem. Having learned Moths of Manchester, Pocket Mice were easy for these 4-year-olds. We saw scant evidence of the transfer reluctance shown on typical tool-use laboratory problems. In addition 30% of the Flexibility group and 16% of the Fixedness group spontaneously gave a detailed explanation of why Moths and Pocket Mice were the same problem, a rare expedition into spontaneous verbal justification for 4-year-olds.

It is important to note that the conditions of learning that lead to higher-order rule abstraction are not necessarily those that lead to broad generalization of specific rules. Giving multiple exemplars of the same rule, *look dangerous*, leads to very rapid learning of this rule, and indeed, to attempts to transfer it to the novel Moths of Manchester scenario. The Fixedness children's problem is *not* that they don't transfer but that they learn and transfer too well. Having learned one solution in several problems, they see no reason to change; their previous success *blinds* them to the novel color-change solution to the Moths problem. This result is reminiscent of Luchins's (1942) water-jar problem, where students were reluctant to set aside a well-learned complex solution to arithmetic problems in favor of a simpler rule. The automatized complex rule is transferred to new problems even though a far simpler solution is readily apparent to those without the prior experience with the difficult rule. So too, the Fixedness children were reluctant to abandon their successful *look dangerous* rule.

In contrast, the children in the Flexibility group learned that there are several potential solutions to an animal's defense needs. This prior training prepared them to look for novel solutions suitable to each animal's needs. Embedded in each story were clues to the animal's mechanism of defense. Forewarned that animals solve the problem in different ways, the children readily noted the emphasis on color in the Moths story and invented the color-camouflage solution. Conditions that breed creative flexibility, and even invention, are not necessarily the same as those that promote learning of a specific rule. Although we have known for a long time that "training in multiple contexts" facilitates transfer (Adams, 1954; Brown, 1978; Brown & Campione, 1978, 1981, 1984; Grether & Wolfle, 1936; Morrisett & Hovland, 1959), *not all contexts are equal*. Examples that exploit a range of potential applications, and thereby demonstrate flexible usage, are those that promote discovery of higher-level commonalities.

What develops?

Common across all these laboratory studies of transfer is the undoubted fact that the older children assigned to unassisted conditions transfer more readily than the younger ones. If it is true that what develops in analogical reasoning is not some fundamental difference at the level of representational format (Carey, 1985a), that children are not fundamentally different kinds of thinkers but rather, like adults, seek a causal explanation to grant coherence to the world around them, then we must look elsewhere for an explanation of their typically poor performance on transfer tasks. The most commonly proffered explanations are: (a) a lack of *knowledge*, particularly coherent causal explanations (theories if you will) of the domain in question; (b) differences in basic *mental capacity*, a moot point at this time (Brown, Bransford, Ferrara, & Campione, 1983); and (c) ineffective general processing, or *learning strategies*, of which we know little. All of these explanations are themselves desperately in need of explanation. Many factors could affect performance. For example, in studies of judgment of analogical appropriateness, do children know the rules of the game; do they know that they should judge relevance, goodness of fit, attempt an exhaustive match, and so on? As such tasks recruit metalinguistic judgments, is the ability to reflect on language as an object of thought in its own right a developmental problem? Many have argued that it is (Brown et al., 1983; Carey, 1985a; Flavell, 1982; R. Gelman, 1983). All these factors – knowledge, capacity, strategies, and metaconceptual factors, that is, the ability to think about one's mental representations and inferential processes – form a residual class affecting performance that can mask competence in the analogical transfer process itself.

What have we learned about age differences? First, they exist even when care is taken that neither the young nor the old have the requisite specific knowledge to solve the problems and the tasks are especially tailored to be suitable for the narrow age ranges under consideration in each study. With minimal prompts, even the youngest children could proceed merrily through a series of problems after experiencing the first solution, so it is difficult to imagine that the tasks were differentially overloading the information-processing capacity of the young. If it is not knowledge, because all were equated for their lack of it, or overloaded capacity, then what is responsible for the greater efficiency of the relatively older group in each study?

We have no ready explanation for this consistent developmental trend, but we do know that such findings are ubiquitous (Brown & Campione, 1984). Once one has ruled out knowledge and capacity, one is left with learning strategies and metaconceptual competence; and perhaps it is advances in these general factors that underlie the improvements we see. One explanation of the age difference is that

ANN L. BROWN

the greater efficiency of the older children reflects the fact that they can provide for themselves the type of help that we provide to enhance performance. They are more capable of reflecting on their problem solutions; they expect to extract a general rule; they look for the rules of the game; in short, they have learned more about learning. Efficient learners possess a repertoire of general strategies; they know more about learning; they apportion attention and effort appropriately; they monitor progress; they know when and how to seek advice. One aspect of their greater sophistication as learners is that they are better able to prepare for transfer; they engage in reasoning processes aimed at accessing and using knowledge. With experience, they develop a set to regard new problems not as isolated examples but as instances of a general class; they come to expect what they learn to be relevant elsewhere. Good learners perform thought experiments, seek appropriate analogies, and understand some of the principles involved in learning and reasoning. They have a greater metaconceptual grasp of the domain *learning* (Brown et al., 1983). Such general learning strategies are surprisingly difficult to define and even more difficult to study; but we will not get a clear picture of the development of learning unless we include this aspect of the child's performance.

Conclusion

It has been claimed that preschool children have particular difficulty transferring knowledge across analogous problems. In this chapter, I have argued that this is an artifact of the paradigm typically used to assess transfer and the type of knowledge that the child is required to apply.

All conditions of learning are not equal. Some promote and some impede cognitive flexibility. Some mechanisms that enhance flexibility are (a) positive learning set; (b) functional flexibility, perceiving the solution tool as one of many uses; and (c) cognitive disembedding, for example, via reflection on the deep structure of the analogous problems. Some mechanisms that serve to fix or encapsulate knowledge are (a) negative learning set; (b) functional fixedness; and (c) cognitive embeddedness.

Maximum flexibility is found under conditions where the basic transfer paradigm is modified to promote rather than test knowledge and/or where what is being acquired is a principled body of knowledge rather than an isolated rule. Exposure to multiple exemplars that exploit a range of potential applications is most likely to promote flexible learning.

Broad application of knowledge is particularly likely if there is similarity across problems at the level of causal structure and the type of causal mechanism has been differentiated within the child's emergent theories of the world. Children come endowed with predispositions to learn about certain privileged classes of information. These biases serve to constrain attention and guide learning (R. Gelman, 1986). The child is sensitive to and actively seeks out just those environments that feed these biases. This tendency makes learning and transfer easier, even possible. But note that this is still a *learning theory*. Children may come fortuitously endowed with predispositions to learn about certain things and not others. But they still have to learn about them. And we should not forget that human beings are efficient general-purpose machines, too. With experience, children will be able to learn almost anything by brute force, that is, will, effort, skill, and strategies. It just so happens (luckily) that they do not have to work so hard to acquire the fundamentals.

NOTE

The preparation of this manuscript was supported by grants from the National Institute of Child Health and Human Development, HD–06864 and HD–05951. Funds from the Spencer Foundation supported the author's fellowship at the Center for Advanced Study in the Behavioral Sciences at Stanford University in 1984–85. The author would like to thank Anne Slattery who collaborated on the infant tool-use studies and Mary Jo Kane for her collaboration on the biological themes and preschool tool-use studies. Special thanks are due to Joseph Campione, Rochel Gelman, Dedre Gentner, Doug Medin, Andrew Ortony, Bob Reeve, and Stella Vosniadou for their helpful comments on the manuscript during its various stages of development.

The development of the discussion in the first half of this chapter was greatly influenced by the author's year at the Center for Advanced Study in the Behavioral Sciences at Stanford in 1984–85. There, a group consisting of Ann Brown, Susan Carey, Rochel Gelman, and Frank Keil met regularly to discuss the topic of developmental constraints on learning. The author is especially indebted to Rochel Gelman for her consistent encouragement and advice on the development of this argument.

REFERENCES

Adams, J. A. (1954). Multiple versus single problem-solving. *Journal of Experimenal Psychology, 58*, 52–55.
Alpert, A. (1928). *The solving of problem situations by preschool children: An analysis*, (Rep. No. 323). New York: Teachers College, Columbia University.

408   ANN L. BROWN

Anderson, J. R. (1987). Skill acquisition: Compilation of weak-method problem solutions. *Psychological Review, 94*, 192–210.

Baillargeon, R., Spelke, E. S., & Wasserman, S. (1985). Object permanence in five-month-old infants. *Cognition, 20*, 191–208.

Bereiter, C., & Scardamalia, M. (1985). Cognitive coping strategies and the problem of "inert knowledge." In S. S. F. Chipman, J. W. Segal, & R. Glaser (Eds.), *Thinking and learning skills: Current research and open questions* (Vol. 2, pp. 65–80). Hillsdale, NJ: Erlbaum.

Bertenthal, B. I., Profitt, D. R. , & Cutting, J. E. (1984). Infant sensitivity to figural coherence in biomedical motion. *Journal of Experimental Child Psychology, 37*, 213–230.

Bertenthal, B. I., Profitt, D. R., Spetner, N., & Thomas, M. A. (1985). The development of infant sensitivity to biomechanical motions. *Child Development, 56*, 531–543.

Birch, H. G., & Rabinowitz, H. S. (1951). The negative effect of previous experience on productive thinking. *Journal of Experimental Psychology, 41*, 121–125.

Black, J. B., & Bower, G. H. (1980). Story understanding as problem-solving. *Poetics, 9*, 223–250.

Black, J. B., & Wilensky, R. (1979). An evaluation of story grammars. *Cognitive Science, 3*, 213–230.

Bornstein, M. H. (1985). Infant into adult: Unity to diversity in the development of visual categorization. In J. Mehler & R. Fox (Eds.), *Neonate cognition: Beyond the blooming, buzzing confusion* (pp. 115–138). Hillsdale, NJ: Erlbaum.

Brown, A. L. (1974). The role of strategic behavior in retardate memory. In N. R. Ellis (Ed.), *International review of research in mental retardation* (Vol. 7, pp. 55–111). New York: Academic Press.

Brown, A. L. (1978). Knowing when, where, and how to remember: A problem of metacognition. In R. Glaser (Ed.), *Advances in instructional psychology* (Vol. 1, pp. 77–165). Hillsdale, NJ: Erlbaum.

Brown, A. L. (1982). Learning and development: The problem of compatibility, access, and induction. *Human Development, 25*, 89–115.

Brown, A. L. (1986, November). *Domain-specific competence and general learning mechanisms: The problem of transfer.* Paper presented at the meeting of the Psychonomic Society, New Orleans.

Brown, A. L., Bransford, J. D., Ferrara, R. A., Campione, J. C. (1983). Learning, remembering, and understanding. In J. H. Flavell & E. M. Markman (Eds.), *Handbook of child psychology* (4th ed.): *Cognitive development* (Vol. 3, pp. 77–166). New York: Wiley.

Brown, A. L., & Campione, J. C. (1978). Permissible inferences from the outcome of training studies in cognitive development research. *Quarterly Newsletter of the Institute for Comparative Human Development, 2*, 46–53.

Brown, A. L., & Campione, J. C. (1981). Inducing flexible thinking: A problem of access. In M. Friedman, J. P. Das, & N. O'Connor (Eds.), *Intelligence and learning* (pp. 515–530). New York: Plenum Press.

Brown, A. L., & Campione, J. C. (1984). Three faces of transfer: Implications for early competence, individual differences, and instruction. In M. Lamb, A. Brown, & B. Rogoff (Eds.), *Advances in developmental psychology* (Vol. 3, pp. 143–192). Hillside, NJ: Erlbaum.

Brown, A. L.,& DeLoache, J. S. (1978). Skills, plans, and self-regulation. In

R. Siegler (Ed.), Children's thinking: What develops? (pp. 3–35). Hillsdale, NJ: Erlbaum.

Brown, A. L., & Kane, M. J. (1988). Preschool children can learn to transfer: Learning to learn and learning from example. *Cognitive Psychology, 20*, 493–523.

Brown, A. L., Kane, M. J., & Echols, K. (1986). Young children's mental models determine analogical transfer across problems with a common goal structure. *Cognitive Development, 1*, 103–122.

Brown, A. L., Kane, M. J., & Long, C. (in press). Analogical transfer in young children: Analogies as tools for communication and exposition. *Applied Cognitive Psychology*.

Brown, A. L., & Reeve, R. (1987). Bandwidths of competence: The role of supportive context in learning and development. In L. S. Liben (Ed.), *Development and learning: Conflict or congruence?* (pp. 173–223). Hillsdale, NJ: Erlbaum.

Buhler, K. (1930). *The mental development of the child*. London: Harcourt Brace.

Bullock, M., Gelman, R., & Baillargeon, R. (1982). Development of causal reasoning. In J. W. Friedman (Ed.), *Psychology of time*. New York: Academic Press.

Carey, S. (1985a). Are children fundamentally different kinds of thinkers and learners than adults? In S. F. Chipman, J. W. Segal, & R. Glaser (Eds.), *Thinking and learning skills* (Vol. 2, pp. 485–517). Hillsdale, NJ: Erlbaum.

✓ Carey, S. (1985b). *Conceptual change in childhood*. Cambridge, MA: MIT Press (Bradford Books).

Chi, M.T.H., Feltovich, P. J. & Glaser, R. (1981). Categorization and representation of physics problems by experts and novices. *Cognitive Science, 5*, 121–152.

Cohen, L. B., & Younger, B. A. (1983). Perceptual categorization in the infant. In G. K. Scholnick (Ed.), *New trends in conceptual representation: Challenge to Piaget's theory* (pp. 197–220). Hillsdale, NJ: Erlbaum.

Crisafi, M.A., & Brown, A. L. (1986). Analogical transfer in very young children: Combining two separately learned solutions to reach a goal. *Child Development, 57*, 953–968.

DeLoache, J. S., Brown, A. L., Kane, M. J. (1985, April). *Young children's error correction procedures in manipulative play*. Paper presented at the meeting of the Society for Research in Child Development, Toronto.

DeLoache, J. S., Sugarman, S., & Brown, A. L. (1985). The development of error correction strategies in young children's manipulative play. *Child Development, 56*, 928–939.

Duncker, K. (1945). On problem solving. *Psychological Monographs, 58* (Whole No. 270).

Flavell, J. H. (1982). On cognitive development. *Child Development, 53*, 1–10.

✓ Flavell, J. H. (1985). *Cognitive Development* (2nd ed.). Englewood Cliffs, NJ: Prentice-Hall.

Fox, R., & McDaniel, C. (1982). The perception of biological motion by human infants. *Science, 218*, 486–487.

Gelman, R. (1983). Recent trends in cognitive development. In J. Schierer & A. Rogers (Eds.), *The G. Stanley Hall lecture series* (Vol. 3). Washington,DC: American Psychological Association.

Gelman, R. (1986, August). *First principles for structuring acquisition*. Presidential

410   ANN L. BROWN

Address to Division 7 of the American Psychological Association, Washington, DC.

Gelman, R., & Brown, A. L. (1985a). Early foundations of cognitive development. *The 1985 Annual Report for the Center for Advanced Study in the Behavioral Sciences.* Stanford, CA.

Gelman, R., & Brown, A. L. (1985b). Changing views of cognitive competence in the young. In N. J. Smelser & D. R. Gerstein (Eds.), *Knowledge in the social and behavioral sciences: Discovery and trends over fifty years.* Proceedings of a Commemorative Symposium on the Fiftieth Anniversary of the Ogburn Report, *Recent social trends in the United States.* New York: Academic Press.

Gelman, R., & Gallistel, C. R. (1978). *The child's understanding of number.* Cambridge, MA: Harvard University Press.

✓ Gelman, R., & Spelke, E. (1981). The development of thoughts about animate and inanimate objects: Implications for research on social cognition. In J. H. Flavell & L. Ross (Eds.), *Social cognitive development: Frontiers and possible futures* (p. 43–66). Cambridge: Cambridge University Press.

Gelman, R., Spelke, E., & Meck, E. (1983). What preschoolers know about animate and inanimate objects. In D. Rogers & J. Sloboda (Eds.), *The acquisition of symbolic skills* (pp. 297–326). New York: Plenum Press.

Gelman, S., & Markman, E. (1986). Categories and induction in young children. *Cognition, 23,* 183–209.

Gelman, S., & Markman, E. M. (1987). Young children's inductions from natural kinds: The role of categories and appearances. *Child Development.*

Gentner, D. (1983). Structure-mapping: A theoretical framework for analogy. *Cognitive Science, 7,* 155–170.

Gentner, E., & Toupin, C. (1986). Systematicity and surface similarity in the development of analogy. *Cognitive Science, 10,* 277–300.

✓ Gibson, E. J., & Spelke, E. S. (1983). The development of perception. In P. H. Mussen, J. H. Flavell, & E. M. Markman (Eds.), *Handbook of child psychology* (4th ed.) Vol. 3, *Cognitive development* (pp. 1–76). New York: Wiley.

Gick, M. L., & Holyoak, K. J. (1980). Analogical problem solving. *Cognitive Psychology, 12,* 306–355.

Gick, M. L., & Holyoak, K. J. (1983). Schema induction and analogical transfer. *Cognitive Psychology, 15,* 1–38.

Grether, W. F., & Wolfle, D. L. (1936), The relative efficiency of constant and varied stimulation during learning. *Journal of Comparative and Physiological Psychology, 22,* 365–374.

Hinde, R. A., & Stevenson-Hinde, J. (1973). *Constraints on learning: Limitations and predispositions.* New York: Academic Press.

Holyoak, K. J., Junn, E. N., & Billman, D. O. (1984). Development of analogical problem-solving skills. *Child Development, 55,* 2042–2055.

Johnson-Laird, P. N. (1980). Mental models in cognitive science. *Cognitive Science, 4,* 71–115.

Johnson-Laird, P. N., Herrmann, D. J., & Chaffin, R. (1984). Only connections: A critique of semantic networks. *Psychological Bulletin, 96,* 292–315.

Judd, C. H. (1908). The relation of special training to general intelligence. *Educational Review, 36,* 28–42.

Keil, F. C. (1981). Constraints of knowledge and cognitive development. *Psychological Review, 88,* 197–227.

Keil, F. C. (1983). On the emergence of semantic and conceptual distinctions. *Journal of Experimental Psychology: General, 112,* 357–389.

Keil. F. C. 1986. The acquisition of natural kind and artifact terms. In W. Demopoulos & A. Marras (Eds.), *Language, learning, and concept acquisition* (pp. 133–153). Norwood, NJ: Ablex.

✓ Kohler, W. (1925). *The mentality of apes.* New York: Harcourt Brace.

Kripke, S. (1971). Identity and necessity. In M. Munitz (Ed.), *Identity and individuation.* New York: New York University Press.

Leslie, A.M. (1984a). Infant peception of a manual pick-up event. *British Journal of Psychology, 2,* 19–32.

Leslie, A. M. (1984b). Spatiotemporal continuity and the perception of causality in infants. *Perception, 13,* 287–305.

Luchins, A. S. (1942). Mechanization in problem-solving. *Psychological Monographs, 54* (Whole No. 6).

Maier, N. R. F. (1930). Reasoning in humans: 1. On direction. *Journal of Comparative Psychology, 11,* 115–143.

Maier, N. R. F. (1931). Reasoning in humans: 2. The solution of a problem and its appearance in consciousness. *Journal of Comparative Psychology, 12,* 181–194.

Maier, N. R. F. (1945). Reasoning in humans. 3. The mechanisms of equivalent stimuli and of reasoning. *Journal of Experimental Psychology, 35,* 349–360.

Mansfield, A. (1977). Semantic organization in the young child: Evidence for the development of semantic feature systems. *Journal of Experimental Child Psychology, 23,* 57–77.

Matheson, E. (1931). A study of problem-solving in preschool children. *Child Development, 2,* 242–262.

Morrisett, L., & Hovland, C. I. (1959). A comparison of three varieties of training in human problem solving. *Journal of Experimental Psychology, 58,* 52–55.

Murphy, G. L., & Medin, D. L. (1985). The role of theories in conceptual coherence. *Psychological Review, 92,* 289–316.

Orata, P. T. (1945). Transfer of training and educational psuedo-science. *Mathematics Teacher, 28,* 265–289.

✓ Piaget, J. (1952). *The origins of intelligence.* New York: International University Press.

Putman, H. (1970). Is semantics possible? In H. E. Kaifer & M. K. Munitz (Eds.), *Language beliefs and metaphysics.* New York: State University of New York Press.

Quine, W. V. O. (1977). Natural kinds. In S. P. Schwartz (Ed.), *Naming, necessity, and natural kinds* (pp. 155–175). Ithaca, NY: Cornell University Press.

Reed, S. K. (1983). Once is enough: Causal reasoning from a single instance. *Journal of Personality and Social Psychology, 45,* 323–334.

Richardson, H. M. (1932a). The growth of adaptive behavior in infants: An experimental study of seven age levels. *Genetic Psychology Monographs, 12,* 195–359.

Richardson, H. M. (1932b). Adaptive behavior of infants in the utilization of the lever as a tool. *Journal of Genetic Psychology, 44,* 352–377.

Rips. L. (1975). Inductive judgments about natural categories. *Journal of Verbal Learning and Verbal Behavior, 14,* 665–681.

Rozin, P. (1976). The evolution of intelligence and access to the cognitive unconscious. *Progression in Psychobiology and Physiological Psychology, 6,* 245–280.

Scheerer, M., & Huling, M. D. (1960). Cognitive embeddedness in problem solving. In B. Kaplan & S. Wepner (Eds.), *Perspectives in psychological theory: Essays in honor of Heinz Werner.* New York: International University Press.

Schwartz, S. (1979). Natural kind terms. *Cognition, 7,* 301–315.

Seligman, M. E., & Hager J. L. (1972). *Biological boundaries of learning.* New York: Appleton-Century-Crofts.

Smiley, S. S., & Brown, A. L. (1979). Conceptual preference for thematic and taxonomic relations: A nonmonotonic age trend from preschool to old age. *Journal of Experimental Child Psychology, 28* 249–257.

Sobel, B. (1939). The study of the development of insight in preschool children. *Journal of Genetic Psychology, 55,* 381–388.

Spelke, E. S. (1983, June). *Cognition in infancy* (Occasional Paper No. 23). Cambridge, MA: MIT.

Thorndike, E. L. (1913). *Educational psychology* (Vol. 2). New York: Columbia University Press.

Thorndike. E. L., & Woodworth, R. S. (1901). The influence of improvement in one mental function upon the efficiency of other functions. *Psychological Review, 8,* 247–261, 384–395, 553–564.

Trabasso, T., Secco, T., & Van Den Broek, P. (1984). Causal cohesion and story coherence. In H. Mandl, N. L. Stein, & T. Trabasso (Eds.), *Learning and comprehension of text.* Hillside, NJ: Erlbaum.

Trevarthen, C. (1977). Descriptive analyses of infant communicative behavior. In H. R. Schaffer (Ed.), *Studies in mother–infant interaction.* London: Academic Press.

Tronick. E., Adamson, L., Wise, S., Als, H., & Brazelton, T. B. (1975, March). *The infant's response to entrapment between contradictory messages in face to face interaction.* Paper presented at the meeting of the Society for Research in Child Development, Denver, CO.

van Dijk, T. A., & Kintsch, W. (1983). *Strategies of discourse comprehension.* New York: Academic Press.

Vosniadou, S. (1987). Children and metaphors. *Child Development, 58* 870–885.

Wattenmaker, W.D., Nakamura, G. V., & Medin, D. L. (1988). Relationships between similarity based and explanation based categorisation. In D. Hilton (Ed.), *Contemporary science and natural explanation: Common sense conception of causality.* Brighton: Harvester Press.

15

Analogical reasoning as a mechanism in knowledge acquisition: a developmental perspective

STELLA VOSNIADOU

Whether or not we talk of discovery or of invention, analogy's inevitable in human thought, because we come to new things in science with what equipment we have, which is how we have learned to think, and above all how we have learned to think about the relatedness of things. We cannot, coming into something new, deal with it except on the basis of the familiar and the old-fashioned. The conservation of scientific enquiry is not an arbitrary thing; it is the freight with which we operate; it is the only equipment we have. We cannot learn to be surprised or astonished at something unless we have a view of how it ought to be; and that view is almost certainly an analogy.

[Robert Oppenheimer, September 1955]

Interest in analogy has been generated to a large extent by a recognition of the role that analogy can play in the acquisition of new knowledge. Although our models of learning have stressed the importance of prior knowledge in thinking, remembering, and learning, they have remained mainly silent on the processes whereby new knowledge is acquired. One mechanism that has been recognized by scientists, philosophers, and psychologists alike as having the potential of bringing prior knowledge to bear on the acquisition of, sometimes, radically new information is analogy.

My purpose in this chapter is to examine analogical reasoning, paying particular attention to the role it plays in knowledge acquisition. This question will be approached from a developmental point of view. I will discuss how analogical reasoning is used by adults as well as by children, and I will speculate about how analogical reasoning may develop. The developmental questions are often ignored in our treatment of analogy. Yet they are critical both in order to understand the psychological processes involved in analogical reasoning (see also Gentner, this volume) and in terms of their implications for learning and instruction. For it is only if we understand how analogical rea-

413

soning develops with age and with the acquisition of expertise that we will be able to influence its development.

The first section of this chapter deals with the problem of what analogical reasoning is. It is argued that analogical reasoning involves the identification and transfer of structural information from a known system (the source) to a new and relatively unknown system (the target). Two different types of reasoning are discussed, and some of the psychological processes involved in their identification are examined. It is concluded that the *productive* use of analogy, the use of analogy to produce *new* knowledge about the explanatory structure of the target system, is often based on the recognition of some similarity in properties of the two systems and not on their explanatory structure, because the relevant structure of the target system is not known.

In the second section, a distinction is drawn between uses of analogical reasoning that require the relevant structure to be part of one's representation of the target and cases where analogical reasoning can produce this knowledge. With respect to the developmental question, the main thesis of this chapter is that analogical reasoning is available to children. Like adults, children can identify the similarity in the structure between two analogs when this structure is part of their representation of the source and target systems. Moreover, it appears that children can use similarity in salient properties between two systems as a vehicle for discovering structural similarities between them, just like adults do. It is concluded that what develops is *not* the analogical mechanism itself but the conceptual system upon which this mechanism operates.

Analogical reasoning: definitional issues

Mapping a relational structure

Two types of analogical reasoning. It is by now generally accepted that the process of reasoning by analogy involves transfer of structural information from a source to a target system. This transfer of knowledge is accomplished by mapping or matching processes, which consist of finding the correspondences between the two systems.

In most cases, an analogy is said to exist between two systems (concepts. theories, stories, etc.), which belong to fundamentally different or remote conceptual domains but which share a similar explanatory structure (hereafter, *between-domain* analogies). For example, the analogy between the atom and the solar system is based on the similarity in the structure of the two systems. The particular properties involved (e.g., sun–nucleus, electrons–planets) are very different. Similarly, in the analogy between the "radiation problem" (Duncker, 1945) and the "fortress problem" (Gick & Holyoak, 1980, 1983; Holyoak & Thagard, this volume), the particular properties involved (e.g., army and rays, fortress and tumor) are very different. However, the goals, resources, and constraints of the two problems (i.e., structural aspects) are similar and hence can be transferred from one problem to the other.

In other cases, analogical reasoning involves items that belong to the same or at least very close conceptual domains, as in the case of a Styrofoam cup that is used as an example from which to reason analogically about a ceramic mug, described by Kedar-Cabelli (1985; hereafter, *within-domain* analogies). The types of analogical reasoning described by Anderson and Thompson (this volume) and Ross (this volume) involve mainly within-domain analogies.

The distinction between within-domain and between-domain analogical reasoning is not a dichotomous one. Rather, it represents a continuum from comparisons involving items that are clear examples of the same concept to items that belong to different and remote domains. In that respect, the distinction between the two types of reasoning is similar to the distinction between literal comparisons and metaphorical comparisons (Ortony, 1979; Vosniadou, 1987a). The important point for the purposes of this discussion is that analogical reasoning can be employed between items that belong anywhere in the continuum from literal similarity to nonliteral similarity.

Can within-domain comparisons be analogies? Some theories of analogy consider within-domain comparisons as literal similarities rather than as analogies. For example, Gentner (this volume) argues that within-domain comparisons are not analogies because they involve items that are similar in many simple, descriptive, nonrelational properties. Gentner draws a distinction between object attributes (descriptive properties of objects, roughly expressed as one-place predicates) and relations (roughly two-or-more-place predicates) and argues that an analogy is defined by the presence of similarity in relations and the absence of similarity in object attributes. According to this view, in an analogy only relational predicates are shared, whereas in literal similarity both relational predicates and object attributes are shared.

Gentner is primarily concerned with characterizing static similarity statements of the sort "The solar system is like an atom," rather than the process of reasoning by analogy. But when it comes to characterizing such similarity statements the distinction between a within-domain and a between-domain comparison carries certain definitional implications. For instance, certain within-domain similarity statements (such as "Puppies are like kittens") *cannot* be considered analogies (although an analogy could be made out of them, as in "Puppies are to dogs as kittens are to cats"). When it comes to characterizing the process of reasoning by analogy, however, the distinction between within-domain and between-domain comparisons does not have any definitional implications. Analogical reasoning can be employed between any two items that belong to the same fundamental category if it involves transferring an explanatory structure from one item to the other.

In the system described by Kedar-Cabelli (1985), for example, an analogy exists between a ceramic mug and a Styrofoam cup to the extent that the example of a ceramic mug can be used as a source from which to determine whether the target satisfies a given goal (e.g., that of drinking hot liquids). Very briefly, the analogy mechanism operates as follows:

1. The system retrieves a familiar source example (e.g., a ceramic mug) together with an explanation of how this source example satisfies some goal (e.g., drinking hot liquids).
2. The system maps the explanation derived from the source onto the target and attempts to find out if this explanation is justified by the target example.
3. If the target example justifies the explanation, then it is concluded that it satisfies the goal (i.e., it can be used to drink hot liquids).

Although the base and target systems in this case share many similar simple properties, the reasoning process is analogical in nature because it rests on the mapping of an explanatory structure from the source system to the target system.

Consider another example: Suppose we want to find out if there is a day/night cycle on the moon. If we do not know the answer to this question directly, one way to answer it is to reason by analogy to the earth. We know that the day/night cycle on the earth is determined by the earth's rotation around its axis. If we know that the moon also rotates around its axis (or assume that it does on the basis of the other existing similarities between the moon and the earth), then we can come to the conclusion that there must be a day/night cycle on the moon.

Thus, although the statement "The earth is like the moon" can hardly be thought of as an analogy, the earth can nevertheless be used as a source from which to reason analogically about the moon. And, despite the many simple properties that the earth and the moon share (solid, spherical, suspended, rotating, etc.), it is only the *causal relation* between axis rotation and the existence of a day/night cycle that is mapped from the source to the target.

To conclude, we have argued that domain incongruence (belonging to different conceptual domains) is *not* a defining characteristic of analogical reasoning. The defining characteristic of analogical reasoning is similarity in underlying structure. Structural similarity can be found between items that belong to different conceptual domains as well as between items that belong to the same or similar domains. Domain incongruence is, however, a defining characteristic of non-literal (i.e., metaphorical) similarity (see Ortony, 1979; Tourangeau & Sternberg, 1982; Vosniadou, 1987a, for a more detailed discussion of this issue). The items juxtaposed in a metaphor must belong to different conceptual domains. This can be shown by the fact that between-domain analogies can be turned into metaphors (e.g., "Atoms are solar systems," "Inflation is disease," "Illiteracy is prison," and the like), but within-domain analogies (e.g., "A puppy is to a dog as a kitten is to a cat") cannot. "A puppy is a kitten" is just nonsense.[1]

Identifying similarity in relational structure

The role of "surface" similarity. The definition of analogical reasoning that I have offered focuses on the mapping of an explanatory structure from a source to a target system, ignoring the question of whether these two systems are similar in "surface" (simple, descriptive, non-analogy-related) properties as well. Similarity in surface properties may be relevant, however, in determining how a source analog is accessed in the first place. It could be argued, for example, that within-domain analogs can be identified on the basis of their similarity in simple, descriptive (and therefore easily accessible) properties, which may not have anything to do with the analogy in the first place. Since between-domain analogs do not share similarity in such non-analogy-related surface properties, they can be accessed only by noticing the similarity in their explanatory structure. This could be interpreted to mean that different psychological processes operate in accessing a between-domain analog than in accessing a within-domain analog. The argument I will advance in this chapter is that whereas different psychological processes can operate in accessing a between-domain analog than in accessing a within-domain analog, access to a *productive* between-domain analog (i.e., a between-domain analog that provides new knowledge about the explanatory structure of the target system) is often based on the same psychological process as access to a within-domain analog.

In support of the different-psychological-processes argument come the results of a number of experiments, which show that surface similarity (i.e., non-analogy-related similarity in simple, descriptive properties of objects like shape, color, size, names, profession, workplace of story characters, kinds of animals, etc.) is likely to be noticed more easily than similarity in underlying structure (e.g., Gentner & Landers, 1985; Holyoak & Koh, 1986; Vosniadou, Brown, & Bernstein, in preparation). The easy accessibility of surface similarity sometimes becomes the motivating force for selecting the wrong between-domain source analog (e.g., Ross, 1987).

Such experiments have served an important purpose in showing that people are more sensitive to similarity in descriptive properties than to similarity in structural aspects. They have erred only in allowing the inference that such a characteristic of the human reasoning system is an impediment to analogical reasoning. Contrary to commonsense expectations, similarity in descriptive properties of objects is often analogy-related. As Medin and Ortony (this volume) note, in our conceptual system, descriptive properties of objects are usually related to deeper, less easily accessible properties in a complex causal/relational network. In such a system, the easily accessible, descriptive properties that are analogy-related can become the vehicle for discovering the similarity in the underlying structure between two analogs. In fact, one of the reasons why people pay attention to "surface" similarities may be that such similarities can lead to the discovery of an analogy in a nonaccidental way (see also Brown, this volume; Ross, this volume). Being attentive to similarity in descriptive properties is thus one of the characteristics that an efficient analogy mechanism should have.

Accessing a productive between-domain analog. It could be objected here that the possibility of arriving at an analogy via similarity in the descriptive properties of two analogs can operate *only* in the case of within-domain analogical reasoning. The absence of descriptive properties in between-domain analogies necessitates that the identification of a between-domain analog must be based on some recognition of the structural similarity between the source and target domains.

Obviously, between-domain analogies can be accessed by recognizing the similarity in their underlying structure. The problem with this account of access is that it fails to explain how between-domain analogies can ever be used *productively*. As Hesse (1966) correctly observes, in order for an analogy to be used productively – that is, for it to lead to the discovery of new knowledge – it cannot be based on the realization that the two systems have a similar explanatory structure. Understanding that two systems have the same explanatory structure presupposes that one has a theory about both analogs. If a theory about the target is not available, as must be the case for an analogy to be used productively, then one is *not* likely to understand that the two systems have a similar structure.

In such cases the access problem can be solved if we assume that the between-domain analog is identified on the basis of some similarity in easily accessible properties of the two systems, just as in the case of many within-domain analogies. This argument rests on the presupposition that easily accessible similarity does not need to be similarity in descriptive properties. Rather, it can be similarity in relational, abstract, or conceptual properties, as long as these properties are salient with respect to people's underlying representations. This is why I shall use the term *salient similarity* to distinguish it from *surface similarity* (the differences between these two kinds of similarity will be discussed further in the next section). Such salient similarity can become the vehicle for discovering the presence of other, less easily accessible similarities and eventually the crucial structural correspondences between the two systems.[2]

An access process of this sort can be traced in the discovery of a number of scientific analogies, like the analogy between elastic balls and the behavior of gases, which apparently suggested itself because of the similarity in the behavior of bouncing balls and balloons and the effects of pressure on a surface due to expanding gas. Another example is the analogy between light and particles made by Newton. This analogy appears to be based on the observation that light is reflected when it hits a surface the same way that particles bounce back when they hit a surface. Properties such as the behavior of particles and the behavior of light may appear to the layman to be remote and inaccessible. Yet to the physicist working in the context of a certain theory they appear to be as real and easily observable as the solid nature and spherical shape of the earth and the moon are to us.

Surface similarity versus salient similarity

The access process for the productive use of between-domain analogies that I have proposed requires some modification of currently accepted notions regarding easily accessible similarity. It has been assumed that what is easy to access is surface similarity and that surface

similarity is either perceptual similarity (Rips, this volume) or similarity in object attributes (Gentner, this volume). In this section I shall
argue that similarity that is easy to access (i.e., salient similarity) can
be of a perceptual or conceptual nature, similarity in descriptive or
relational properties. What matters is only the status that these properties have with respect to people's underlying representations.

Similarity in object attributes. In her work, Gentner has drawn
a distinction between object attributes (simple, descriptive properties
of objects) and relations (complex, relational properties of objects)
and has argued that the latter are more difficult to access than the
former. However, although descriptive properties of objects are often
easy to access, this is not always the case. Take, for instance, the
analogy between the earth and the moon discussed earlier. One may
think that the similarity in object attributes like *solid* and *spherical* which
the earth and the moon share should be easily accessible. Using the
earth as a source analog from which to reason about the moon may
thus be considered rather trivial. Yet most children in our studies of
knowledge acquisition in astronomy (Vosniadou, 1987b; Vosniadou
& Brewer, 1987a) would never use the earth as a source analog from
which to reason about the moon, although adults would. The reason
is that until the end of the elementary school years many children do
not really believe that the earth is a sphere. Children's phenomenal
experience that the earth is flat is so strong that information coming
from adult sources regarding the shape of the earth is consistently
misinterpreted. Furthermore, many children do not know that the
moon is spherical either. Many believe that the moon is shaped like
a crescent or that it is circular but flat, like a disc. It is apparent from
the above that the characterization of "spherical" as an object attribute
of the earth and the moon carries no implications as to whether this
is an easily accessible property of the objects in question or not.

The argument that descriptive properties of objects are more easily
accessible than relational properties fails to take into consideration
the status that this information has in people's underlying representations. Since similarity judgments can be made only with respect to
people's underlying representations, it would be impossible to see
similarity between analogs whose representations do not include these
similar properties, or in which these properties are not salient. The
fact that a property is described as an object attribute does not necessarily mean that it is present in people's representation of that object
or that it is an easily accessible property. Similarly, describing a prop-

erty as relational does not imply that it is *not* included in people's representations or that it is not salient.

In fact, some developmental research indicates that relational properties of objects may be particularly salient even for young children. For instance, metaphor comprehension studies indicate that children find it easier to see similarity between moving objects belonging to different conceptual domains (like a ballerina dancing and a top spinning) than between stationary objects with similar object properties like a curvy river and a curvy snake (see Calhoun, 1984; Dent, 1984). Our studies of children's knowledge about the sun and the moon also show that children are very sensitive to the movement of these objects across the sky and their relation to the day/night cycle.

Perceptual similarity. Defining easily accessible similarity as perceptual similarity is also problematic. As Linda Smith (this volume) argues, the perception of similarity is not something static and well defined but something that changes with development (see also Piaget, 1969). What we perceive as similar at the time of birth is presumably determined by constraints on our perceptual apparatus. However, this "perceptual" similarity develops and changes with age and the acquisition of expertise. Moreover, to go beyond what may be considered as perceptual, developments in people's representations of concepts allow them to have easy access to information that may not be of a perceptual nature at all.

The above observations suggest that easily accessible similarity does not have to be perceptual similarity or similarity in object attributes. Rather, both descriptive and relational properties of objects can be easy or difficult to access depending on how salient these properties are with respect to people's underlying representations.

Finally, it appears that what constitutes salient similarity may change in the process of knowledge acquisition. The results of a number of developmental and expert/novice studies show that older children's similarity judgments are different from those of younger children (e.g., Carey, 1985b; Keil, 1987) or that experts categorize problems differently from novices (Chi, Feltovich, & Glaser, 1981). As Chi et al. (1981) have argued, there are fundamental differences in the representations of physics problems employed by experts and novices. Because of such differences, "experts are able to *see* the underlying similarities in a great number of problems, whereas novices *see* a variety of problems that they consider to be dissimilar because the surface features are different" (Chi et al., 1981, p. 130).

Conclusions

The analogy mechanism I have described can be characterized as a mechanism whereby a problem about a target system (*X*) is solved by:

1. retrieving a source system (*Y*), which is similar to *X* in some way
2. mapping a relational structure from *Y* to *X*
3. evaluating the applicability of this relational structure for *X*.

A distinction was made between the situation where *X* and *Y* represent examples of the same fundamental concept and the situation where *X* and *Y* belong to different conceptual domains. Although it is the latter type of analogy that has often been identified as the "true" case of analogical reasoning, it is important to notice that the same mapping process operates in both cases. In both cases an explanatory structure is mapped from the source to the target, and its applicability is evaluated on the basis of what is known about the target concept.

Although in many instances a between-domain analogy is identified on the basis of the structural similarity between the analogs, the productive use of a between-domain analogy (i.e., its use for the purpose of acquiring knowledge about the explanatory structure of the target system) requires an access process similar to the one used to access a within-domain analogy. In both cases, access to a productive analog must be based on similarity in some salient, easily accessible properties of the two systems.

Using analogical reasoning

In this section I will try to show how an analogy mechanism like the one described in the previous section is used and, particularly, how it is used to acquire new knowledge. Examples will be drawn from research describing adults' and children's abilities to reason analogically, and emphasis will be placed on how analogical reasoning develops with age and expertise. Finally, a distinction will be drawn between two cases where analogical reasoning can be used. The first is the situation where the employment of analogical reasoning requires that the underlying structure shared between two analogs is present in the subject's representation of both the source and the target systems at the time when the analogy problem is solved. The other is the situation where the underlying structure needs to be present only in one's representation of the source. Analogical reasoning can contribute most to the acquisition of new knowledge in this latter case. Instructional uses of analogy, where the source analog is given, and cases where similarity in explanatory structure is discovered on the basis of similarity in the salient properties of two systems are some instances where analogical reasoning can lead to the acquisition of new knowledge.

The ability to identify similarity in relational structure

In most experimental investigations of analogical reasoning (e.g., the solution of four-term verbal or pictorial analogies, the comprehension of analogies, the transfer of a solution from Story A to Story B), the application of analogical reasoning is based on the identification of the structural similarity of the two systems in the absence of any known similarity in easily accessible properties between them.

Take, for example, the situation where Story A is presented, followed by an analogous Story B, and where A contains some information that can be used to solve a problem about B (e.g., Brown, Kane, & Echols, 1986; Gentner, this volume; Gick & Holyoak, 1980, 1983; Holyoak, Junn, & Billman, 1984; Ross, 1987). In these situations one must identify the similarity in the structure between the two stories and, on the basis of this similarity, transfer the problem solution from Story A to Story B.

The results of a number of experiments employing this paradigm have shown that often the similarity in the structure of two analogs is not identified, with the corresponding result that Story A is not used as a source analog for Story B. However, in order to identify this structural similarity, the relevant structure must be present in the subject's representation of Stories A and B at the time when the analogy problem needs to be solved. It has now become apparent that analogous stories (problems, concepts, etc.) are not always represented at a level at which the underlying structural similarity is preserved, and as a result analogical reasoning cannot be applied to them.

Sometimes these appropriate representations are not achieved because of lack of the relevant knowledge in the knowledge base. This is often the case with children. At other times, the relevant relational structure could be inferred from what exists in the knowledge base, but it is not.[3] This creates the problem of "inert" knowledge discussed by Bransford, Franks, Vye, and Sherwood (this volume) and Brown (this volume). In general, it appears that when familiarity with the target and source domains is high then the likelihood of achieving an appropriate representation of the source and target system is increased (thus the observed differences in analogical reasoning between adults and children and experts and novices; e.g., Novick,

1988). When familiarity with the source and target domains is not very high but appropriate representations could be achieved by inference to what is already known, then certain experimental manipulations (e.g., presenting *two* instead of *one* source analog, giving subjects various hints indicating that the two systems are similar, increasing the similarity in descriptive properties of the two analogs, etc.) can bring about appropriate representations and thus facilitate analogical reasoning.

It becomes apparent from the above discussion that failure to reason by analogy in the cases where an appropriate representation has not been achieved carries few implications with respect to the ability to reason analogically per se (i.e., to identify and map a relational structure). The problem lies not in the analogical mechanism itself (the "analogy engine," as Gentner calls it) but in the representational structures on which this mechanism operates.

Lack of concern for children's knowledge about the source and target systems is a common problem in developmental research on analogical reasoning. When this problem is corrected, the possibility of discovering that children can reason analogically increases. There is now considerable evidence that suggests that when children represent the target concepts at the appropriate level of generality they can solve four-term analogy problems (Gentner, 1977), understand relational metaphors (Vosniadou, Ortony, Reynolds, & Wilson, 1984), and solve a problem after listening to a story in which an analogous problem is solved (Brown et al., 1986).

The shift from attributes to relations. Recently, Gentner (1987; Gentner & Toupin, 1986) has advanced the argument that, although children do not lack the fundamental competence to make relational mappings, they do not have the propensity to do so. According to Gentner, "there is evidence for a developmental shift from attributional focus to relational focus in production, choice, and rating of analogy interpretations" (Gentner, this volume, p. 223). This could be due either to lack of knowledge or to lack of some cognitive ability to observe relational similarity systematically.

Gentner (this volume) cites the results of two experiments (Gentner, 1988; Gentner & Toupin, 1986) to support the attribute to relations shift hypothesis. In Gentner (1988) children and adults were asked to interpret figurative comparisons of the sort "Clouds are like a sponge." Results showed that the children produced mainly attributional interpretations (e.g., "Both are round and fluffy"), whereas adults produced mainly relational interpretations (e.g., "Both can hold water and later give it back").

As I have argued elsewhere (Vosniadou, 1987a), there is a confounding of relational interpretation with lack of necessary knowledge in this experiment. In other words, the information that clouds are round and fluffy is usually part of children's knowledge about clouds, but the information that clouds hold water may not be. This criticism applies in general to the materials used. Consider another of Gentner's examples: "Plant stems are like drinking straws." Again, it is highly debatable whether one should expect a 5-year-old to know that plant stems have liquids running through them, whereas the knowledge that plant stems are relatively tall and thin is readily available. In order to test the hypothesis that children do not have the propensity to map relational information one must first insure that this information is part of children's knowledge base.

In the second experiment (Gentner & Toupin, 1986), children were asked to act out a story plot twice using different story characters. One of the variables manipulated was the degree to which the target objects resembled the source objects. Results showed a strong effect of the transparency of the character correspondences on transfer accuracy. Transfer accuracy was nearly perfect when highly similar characters were used and lower when the characters were quite different. Gentner (this volume) concludes that these results provide a striking demonstration of young children's reliance on surface similarities in transferring knowledge. However, reliance on surface similarity is not a developmental phenomenon. Surface similarity enhances analogical access and mapping both in children and in adults (Gentner & Landers, 1985; Ross, this volume).

The ability to map a relational structure

It could be argued that in an analogy comprehension task like Gentner's (1988) the relational structure does not need to be included in the subject's knowledge of the source. In an analogy comprehension task the source analog is given *explicitly* and does not need to be identified (as in four-term verbal analogies, or even in the case where two analogous stories or problems are provided). All that needs to be done in this case is to map the relevant *relational* structure from the source to the target. In other words, the children in Gentner's (1988) experiment could infer that plant stems have liquids running through them by transferring this information from the source to the target.

I can think of two responses to this argument. First, similarity statements of the sort "X is like Y" are ambiguous with respect to whether they should be interpreted as comparisons (in which case the *existing* representations of X and Y are compared) or as invitations to transfer information from the more familiar Y to the less familiar X. Second, even in the case where a mapping is considered, the mapping may fail for lack of adequate knowledge about which properties of the source could be safely mapped onto the target. Consider again the statement "Plant stems are like drinking straws." It is possible that there is so much discrepancy between what children think about plant stems and the possibility that they have liquids running through them that the mapping of the relevant property of "drinking straws" is not even considered. A similar mapping difficulty could be experienced by adults, as in the situation where a physics-naive individual is faced with statements such as "Heat is like water," "Particles are like light," and "Electrons are like a spinning top." Mapping an underlying structure may not necessarily require the presence of this structure in one's current representation of the target, but it certainly requires that enough is known about the target domain to make such a mapping from the source feasible.

This argument holds even when the information to be mapped is a simple, descriptive property rather than structural information. The case of transfer failure discussed earlier, regarding children's understanding of the statement "The earth is round like a ball," is a good example. The reason why children have problems with this statement is that their knowledge of the shape of the earth is incompatible with their knowledge of the shape of a ball. When children (or adults) try to make sense of such similarity statements, they often end up with gross misconceptions. For example, many children interpret the "earth is round like a ball" statement to mean that the earth is circular but flat, like a disc; others believe that the earth is like a truncated sphere and that people live on its flat top, or that people live inside the flat top of a sphere. Finally, some children think that there are two earths: a round one, which is a planet up in the sky, and a flat one on which the people live (Vosniadou & Brewer, 1987a, 1987b).

If the mapping operation were obstructed by difficulties in mapping *relations* as opposed to *object attributes* the children in our experiments should not have any difficulty understanding that the "earth is round like a ball." The mapping operation is limited because the knowledge of the target concept does not allow an easy mapping of the relevant information from the source. When what is known about the target is consistent with the direction and nature of the required mapping, then the mapping can take place regardless of whether what is mapped is a descriptive property, a relational property, or an explanatory structure.

Our own studies of analogy comprehension (Vosniadou & Ortony, 1983; Vosniadou & Schommer, 1988) show that children readily map an explanatory structure from a source analog to a target domain when this structure is available in their knowledge of the source and is also consistent with what they already know about the target domain. In these studies children read texts introducing them to relatively unfamiliar concepts (e.g., an infection) using an explanatory analogy from a more familiar domain (e.g., war). Children are asked to recall the texts, to describe the information contained in them to another child, and to answer various inferential questions about them. Results show that kindergartners and second grade children are perfectly capable of mapping the relevant structural information from the source to the target. In other words, they are capable of understanding that in an infection germs attack the body just as in a war enemy soldiers attack a country.

Most revealing in this experiment are children's inferences. Children often go beyond the information given to make correct or incorrect inferences about the target domain based on their knowledge of the source. If children did not have the propensity to make relational mappings, we should expect most of these inferences to involve the transfer of descriptive properties. Contrary to this prediction, our results show that descriptive properties are rarely transferred, but relational properties often are. Children do not infer, for example, that white blood cells look like people, wear uniforms, or carry guns when they are told that white blood cells are like soldiers. On the contrary, they often say that white blood cells can die from an infection, that they feel sorry when they hurt the germs, that they think that the germs are bad, and so on. Although many of these mappings are clearly inappropriate, they do demonstrate children's propensity to transfer relational information from the source when this information does not contradict what is already known about the target concept.

In fact, if there is something children could be accused of, this should be not the lack of relational transfer but overgeneralization and inappropriate transfer caused by lack of relevant constraints in their immature knowledge base. The phenomenon of overgeneralization and inappropriate transfer, common also to adults when using analogies in unfamilar domains (Halasz & Moran, 1982; Spiro, Fel-

tovich, Coulson, & Anderson, this volume), is particularly characteristic of the thought of the preschool child, as Chukovsky's (1968) often
hilarious examples amply demonstrate.

Finally, the claim that children may have the capacity to make relational mappings but not the propensity to do so is difficult to accept
because the perceptual information for events, for linguistic structure,
and for coordinated action that young children use to make sense of
the world around them is primarily relational. Brown (this volume)
reviews much of the relevant literature on cognitive development and
makes a persuasive argument for the claim that young children not
only can transfer their knowledge on "deeper bases than mere-
appearance matches" but also for the primacy of relational information. The view that infants come predisposed to seek causal explanations and to uncover potential mechanisms is also a point
discussed by Keil (1987).

In conclusion, it appears that both children and adults can see the
similarity in the underlying structure between two systems, concepts,
or stories that are not similar in descriptive properties if their current
representations of these systems already include the relevant structures. Both children and adults can also map an explanatory structure
from a source to a target system if their knowledge of the target is
not inconsistent with such a mapping.[4] What develops is not so much
the ability to engage in analogical reasoning per se but, rather, the
conceptual system upon which analogical reasoning must operate.

The ability to create a productive analogy

So far I have emphasized the importance of prior knowledge in analogical access and mapping. Obviously, it is not possible to identify
the structural similarity in two systems if the relevant structure is not
already present in one's representation of these systems. Instructional
uses of analogy can augment and modify one's knowledge about the
target system, but in these cases the source analog is given, not discovered. How can an analogy be discovered and also lead to the
acquisition of new knowledge, particularly knowledge about the explanatory structure of a system?

As was argued before, accessing a *productive* analog cannot be based
on the identification of the similarity in the explanatory structure of
two systems. Rather, it must be based on some similarity in easily
accessible properties between the two systems. Once access to a possible analogy has been achieved, the structure of the source can then
be mapped onto the target to solve a problem, answer a generative

question, provide a missing explanatory framework, or restructure the target concept. In the pages that follow some of these productive uses of analogical reasoning will be explored.

Transferring a structure from a within-domain example. The evidence that adults engage in analogical reasoning based on surface similarity to a within-domain example is abundant (e.g., see Anderson & Thompson, this volume; Ross, this volume). This is particularly the case when people reason in unfamiliar domains where they lack general rules. Universal novices as they are, children lack general rules and powerful domain-free problem-solving heuristics. As a result, they should be likely to use similarity-based analogical reasoning to solve problems and deal with everyday situations. Is there any evidence that children employ this kind of analogical reasoning?

According to Piaget (1962), reasoning on the basis of similarity to particular examples is the main form of reasoning for young children (2–7 year-olds). Here is an example of the kind of reasoning Piaget observed in his daughter Jacqueline at the age of 2 years and 10 months.

Obs 111(6) at 2:10(8). J. had a temperature and wanted oranges. It was too early in the season for oranges to be in the shops and we tried to explain to her that they were not yet ripe. "They are still green. We can't eat them. They haven't yet got their lovely yellow color." J. seemed to accept this, but a moment later, as she was drinking her camomile tea, she said, *Camomile isn't green, it's yellow already....Give me some oranges.* [Piaget, 1962, p. 231]

In this example the child uses the camomile as a base from which to reason about oranges. The reasoning is clear. The child takes camomile as the source from which to reason about oranges, possibly based on some easily accessible similarity between them (e.g., that they can both be yellow). The child then maps the explanatory structure of "when you make camomile tea" to solve the problem of "when you can eat oranges" (see Table 15.1). Based on the similarities in this relational structure the child arrives at the inference that "if camomile has turned yellow, then oranges must have turned yellow too." And if oranges are yellow, it means that they are ripe and ready to eat, since there is a particular causal relationship between "yellowness" and "ripeness."

According to Piaget (1962), this type of reasoning based on similarity to particular "images" is characteristic of the preconceptual child and is inferior to both deductive reasoning and analogical reasoning proper, which depend on a stable conceptual system and which develop at the stage of concrete operations. We now know that this view is not correct. Developmental research has shown that children are capable of forming consistent and stable classes from an early age and

Table 15.1. *Reasoning about oranges on the basis of their similarity to camomile*

Camomile (properties)		Oranges (properties)
You can make camomile tea out of it	→	You can eat them
↓		↓
When it is ripe	→	When they are ripe
↓		↓
When it is ripe it is yellow	→	When they are ripe they are yellow
↓		↓
It becomes yellow at a certain time of the year	→	They become yellow at a certain time of the year
It is yellow now		They must be yellow now

that they can reason deductively when the necessary knowledge is available (Carey, 1985a; Gelman & Baillargeon, 1983; Rosch, Mervis, Gay, Boyes-Braem, & Johnson, 1976; Smith, 1979; Sugarman, 1979). Alternatively, unlike Piaget's (1962) claims, adults often reason on the basis of similarity to particular cases, as suggested in such sources as Tversky and Kahneman (1982), Rumelhart and Norman (1981), and Rumelhart (this volume). In fact, the type of reasoning just described is similar to the kind of analogical reasoning described by Anderson and Thompson (this volume), Ross (this volume), Kedar-Cabelli (1985), and Carbonell (1986).

The analogical type of reasoning based on similarity discussed here is different from the probabilistic type of reasoning based on similarity identified by Carey (1985b). In her experiments, Carey asked children to decide whether certain animals had unknown properties like "spleens." Children below 10 answered this question by identifying the known spleen owner most similar to the object being probed and by deciding whether that object had a spleen or not on the basis of its similarity to the retrieved exemplar. In the absence of a known causal relation between the existence of spleens and a particular property or properties of the source, the children in Carey's (1985b) experiments determined the probability that the target had the property in question (e.g., a spleen) on the basis of the number of shared similar properties between it and the source exemplar. This type of similarity-based probabilistic reasoning is similar to the reasoning discussed by Brooks (1978) and E. Smith and Osherson (this volume). It differs from the similarity-based analogical reasoning discussed here, which involves the mapping of an explanatory structure. It appears that when there is no explanatory structure to be mapped, children (and adults) resort to similarity matches and apply some probabilistic reasoning on them.

Transferring an explanatory structure from a different domain. Adults often borrow an explanatory framework from a familiar domain in order to reason about a target system where an appropriate explanatory framework is missing. Presumably, this is done on the basis of some similarity in easily accessible properties of the two systems. It has been shown, for instance, that people borrow a "sand and grain" model to reason about the behavior of molecules in water (Collins & Gentner, 1987), or describe the workings of a home thermostat in terms of an analogy to a car accelerator (Kempton, 1987). Our investigations of knowledge acquisition in the domain of observational astronomy (Vosniadou & Brewer, 1987a; Vosniadou, 1987b) have shown that not only adults but children are capable of transferring an explanatory framework from a familiar to an unfamiliar domain. One such example is the use of people as a source analog from which to reason about the movement of the sun and the moon.

Preschool children have certain observational knowledge of the sun and the moon, but this knowledge cannot provide an explanatory framework for answering questions like "Where is the sun during the night?" "Where is the moon during the day?" "How does this happen?" "Why does the sun move?" and so on. In order to answer such "generative" questions, children need to borrow an explanatory framework from a different domain. Very young children (2–3-year-olds) usually transfer an explanatory framework from the domain of people. The reason seems to be the sun's and moon's appearance of self-initiated movement. Because self-initiated movement is a characteristic of animate rather than inanimate objects, children feel compelled to explain it in ways appropriate to an animate object. They thus provide psychological explanations of the sun's movement (e.g., the sun hides behind the mountain, the sun went home to sleep, the sun plays with the moon, etc.) and attribute to the sun (and moon) certain humanlike qualities related to the ability to move independently (i.e., intentionality, playfulness, fatigue, etc.).

It could be objected here that rather than thinking analogically, young children may simply fail to make a distinction between animate and inanimate objects. They thus attribute to the sun all the qualities that an animate object should have (e.g., see Piaget, 1962). This view is not consistent with research showing that children can observe the animate/inanimate distinction from very early on (Gelman, Spelke, & Meck, 1983; Carey, 1985a). It also does not agree with our findings that children attribute to the sun *only* those human qualities that are associated with self-initiated movement and no more. For example, the same children who say that the sun hides or sleeps to explain the day/night cycle do *not* think that the sun can eat or drink, that it can read newspapers, or that it knows what people do during the day. Finally, additional evidence for the analogical nature of children's thinking comes from the fact that some children borrow an explanatory framework from the domain of inanimate objects rather than the domain of animate objects. These children explain the sun's or the moon's movement as being caused by the push of the clouds or by the push of the air.

The type of analogical reasoning just discussed is not qualitatively different from the kind of analogical reasoning employed by adults when they borrow an explanatory framework from a different domain, such as the one found in the work of Collins and his colleagues (e.g., Collins & Stevens, 1984; Collins & Gentner, 1987).

Restructuring the knowledge base

One of the most significant roles that analogy can play in knowledge acquisition is as a vehicle for theory change. Analogies have often been cited as mechanisms for theory change in science. This is particularly the case when dissatisfaction with an existing theory is high and its replacement with a new theory is actively sought.

It is sometimes difficult to determine whether it is the analogy itself that caused the restructuring or whether some restructuring of the knowledge base occurred independently and made it possible for the analogy to be accessed in the first place. One such case is found in Rutherford's planetary analogy of the atom. The accepted model of the atom before the time of Rutherford was known as the "plum pudding" model. As the name suggests, according to the plum pudding model, the atom consisted of a positively charged sphere (the pudding) in which the negatively charged electrons (the plums) were embedded; see Figure 15.1(A). Rutherford's experiments showed that instead of being spread throughout the atom the positive charge is concentrated in a very small region, or nucleus, at the center of the atom; see Figure

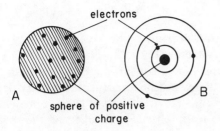

Figure 15.1. Models of the atom.

15.1(B). Once one starts thinking of the positive charge of the atom as concentrated in a small mass in the center of the atom and the electrons as being in the periphery, the similarity of the atom to the planetary system becomes quite salient. Once accessed, however, the adoption of the planetary analogy suggested possibilities about the structure of the atom that might not have been thought of otherwise, thus further aiding the process of theory change.

In other cases, access to an analogy that can lead to restructuring may be more fortuitous. Sometimes the perceived similarity in the formal equations used to describe two systems can become the vehicle for accessing a scientific analogy. In physics, identical equations can be used to describe fundamentally dissimilar systems. Scientists sometimes come across such similarities accidentally, and it often requires quite a lot of courage to follow the implications of these similarities to their logical conclusions. One such example is that of de Broglie's theory of matter waves. De Broglie noticed that Bohr's equations describing the orbits of electrons in an atom were the same equations used to describe the waves of a violin string. Taking this analogy seriously, he proposed a wave theory of matter that revolutionized atomic physics and became the foundation of quantum mechanics. Other examples include the well-known similarity in the formal descriptions of electromagnetism and hydraulics as well as that between a spinning top and the behavior of an electron (spin).

It is possible that children use analogical reasoning to restructure their knowledge base in ways similar to those of adults. We know that the spontaneous restructuring of the knowledge base does occur in children (Carey, 1985b; Chi, 1987; Keil, 1987; Vosniadou, 1987b). But we still do not know how such restructurings occur and the role that analogical reasoning may play in them. This is an interesting area for future research.

Conclusions

The ability to identify within-domain or between-domain analogies and to use them to solve problems about an unfamiliar target system is present both in adults and in children. It appears that both adults and children are capable of seeing the structural similarity between two systems when the relevant structue is part of their representation of these systems. They also seem to be capable of using the similarity in salient properties between two systems to discover a productive analog. Both adults and children are knowledgeable about the network of causal relationships that exist between "surface" and "deep" properties of a system (such as the relationship between *yellowness* and *ripeness*, or the relationship between *self-initiated movement* and *intentionality*) and capable of using the similarity in some of these properties as a vehicle for discovering an analogy. What develops is not, it would seem, the ability to engage in analogical reasoning per se but the content and organization of the knowledge base on which analogical reasoning is applied. The richer and more tightly structured one's representation of a system is, the easier it becomes to see the structural similarities between it and other systems and the greater the possibility of identifying productive analogs. The developments of the knowledge base make it possible to access more and more remote analogs, to see the structural relationships between superficially unrelated systems, and to map increasingly complex structures. Thus, although critically limited by the information included in the knowledge base, analogical reasoning can act as a mechanism for enriching, modifying, and radically restructuring the knowledge base itself.

NOTES

The writing of this paper was supported by Contract no. 400–81–0030 of the National Institute of Education and by a grant from the National Science Foundation, BNS–8510254. I wish to thank Costas Papanicolas for many insightful discussions on scientific analogies, and Bill Nagy, Usha Goswami, and Andrew Ortony for helpful comments on earlier drafts.

1 It could be argued that there is a way of turning some seemingly within-category comparisons into metaphors. For example, the statement "Chicago is the New York of the Midwest" appears to be metaphorica', although it juxtaposes two items (Chicago and New York) that do not belong to different conventional categories (both are cities). What is really juxtaposed in this metaphor, however, is *not* "Chicago versus New York" but "cities of the Midwest versus cities of the East." This becomes evident if we consider that the statement "Chicago is New York" is unacceptable. In order to make

a metaphor, the speaker must provide information to the listener about the relevant category that is being violated – in this case "Chicago as a city of the Midwest" versus "New York as a city of the East."

2 The access process for the discovery of *productive* between-domains analogs will be described in greater detail in future work. It is based on the assumption that in people's conceptual representations easily accessible properties (which can be either descriptive or relational in nature) are linked to less accessible ones in complex, causal, explanatory networks, such that the identification of similarity in one property can lead to the discovery of similarity in other properties and eventually to the discovery of structural correspondences between the two systems.

3 See Michalski (this volume) and Barsalou (this volume) on which aspects of people's conceptual knowledge may be profitable to represent at the "base" level of conceptual representations and which at the "inferential" level.

4 I do not mean to argue here that instructional analogies cannot be helpful in restructuring the knowledge base (see Vosniadou & Brewer, 1987a). I think they can, but they cannot do the job of restructuring on their own. Additional help is required by a teacher who understands the discrepancies between the two inconsistent representations of the same concept and guides the student through the restructuring.

REFERENCES

✓ Brooks, L. (1978). Nonanalytic concept formation and memory for instances. In E. Rosch & B. B. Lloyd (Eds.), *Cognition and categorization* (pp. 169–211). Hillsdale, NJ: Erlbaum.

Brown, A. L., Kane, M. J., & Echols, K. (1986). Young children's mental models determine analogical transfer across problems with a common goal structure. *Cognitive Development, 1*, 103–122.

Calhoun, A. W. (1984). *The effects of perceptual, functional, and action-based grounds on children's comprehension of metaphors* (Research Bulletin No. 7). Greensboro: University of North Carolina, Language Research Group, Department of Psychology.

Carbonell, J. G. (1986). Derivational analogy in problem solving and knowledge acquisition. In R. S. Michalski, J. B. Carbonell, & M. T. Mitchell (Eds.), *Machine learning: An artificial intelligence approach* (Vol. 2. pp. 371–392). Los Altos, CA: Kaufmann.

Carey, S. (1985a). Are children fundamentally different kinds of thinkers and learners than adults? In S. F. Chipman, J. W. Segal, & R. Glaser (Eds.), *Thinking and learning skills* (Vol. 2, pp. 485–517). Hillsdale, NJ: Erlbaum.

✓ Carey, S. (1985b). *Conceptual change in childhood*. Cambridge, MA: MIT Press (Bradford Books).

Chi, M. T. H. (1987, April). *Possible types and processes of knowledge reorganization*. Paper presented at the biennial meeting of the Society for Research in Child Development, Baltimore.

Chi, M. T. H., Feltovich, P. J., & Glaser, R. (1981). Categorization and representation of physics problems by experts and novices. *Cognitive Science, 5*, 121–152.

Chukovsky, K. (1968). *From two to five*. Berkeley: University of California Press.

✓ Collins, A., & Gentner, D. (1987). How people construct mental models. In D. Holland & N. Quinn (Eds.), *Cultural models in language and thought* (pp. 243–265). Cambridge: Cambridge University Press.

Collins, A., & Stevens, A. L. (1984). *Mental models of complex systems: Project summary* (Rep. no. 5788). Cambridge, MA: Bolt, Beranek & Newman.

Dent, C. H. (1984). The developmental importance of motion information in perceiving and describing metaphoric similarity. *Child Development, 55*, 1607–1613.

Duncker, K. (1945). On problem solving. *Psychological Monographs, 58* (Whole No 270).

✓ Gelman, R., & Baillargeon, R. (1983). A review of some Piagetian concepts. In J. H. Flavell & E. M. Markman (Eds.), *Handbook of child psychology: Cognitive development* (Vol 3, pp. 167–230). New York: Wiley.

Gelman, R., Spelke, E., & Meck, E. (1983). What preschoolers know about animate and inanimate objects. In D. Rogers & J. Sloboda (Eds.), *The Acquisition of symbolic skills* (pp. 297–326). New York: Plenum Press.

Gentner, D. (1977). Children's performance on a spatial analogies tasks. *Child Development, 48*, 1034–1039.

Gentner, D. (1988). Metaphor as structure-mapping: The relational shift. *Child Development, 59*, 47–59.

Gentner, D., & Landers, R. (1985, November). Analogical reminding: A good match is hard to find. In *Proceedings of the International Conference on Systems, Man, and Cybernetics*. Tucson, AZ.

Gentner, D., & Toupin, C. (1986). Systematicity and surface similarity in the development of analogy. *Cognitive Science, 10*, 227–300.

Gick, M. L., & Holyoak, K. J. (1980). Analogical problem solving. *Cognitive Psychology, 12*, 306–355.

Gick, M. L., & Holyoak, K. J. (1983). Schema induction and analogical transfer. *Cognitive Psychology, 15*, 1–38.

Halasz, F., & Moran, T. P. (1982). Analogy considered harmful. *Proceedings of the Human Factors in Computer Systems Conference*, Gaithersburg, MD.

✓ Hesse, M. B. (1966). *Models and analogies in science*. Notre Dame, IN: University of Notre Dame Press.

Holyoak, K. J., Junn, E. N., & Billman, D. O. (1984). Development of analogical problem-solving skill. *Child Development, 55*, 2042–2055.

Holyoak, K. J., & Koh, K. (1986). *Analogical problem solving: Effects of surface and structural similarity*. Paper presented at the annual meeting of the Midwestern Psychological Association, Chicago.

✓ Inhelder, B., & Piaget, J. (1958). *The growth of logical thinking from childhood to adolescence*. New York: Basic Books.

Kedar-Cabelli, S. (1985, August). Purpose-directed analogy. *Proceedings of the Seventh Annual Conference of the Cognitive Science Society*, Irvine, CA

Keil, F. C. (1986). The acquisition of natural kind and artifact terms. In W. Demopoulos & A. Marras (Eds.), *Language learning and concept acquisition* (pp. 133–153). Norwood, NJ: Ablex.

✓ Keil, F. C. (1987). Conceptual development and category structure. In U. Neisser (Ed.), *Concepts and conceptual development: Ecological and intellectual factors in categorization*. Cambridge: Cambridge University Press.

✓ Kempton, W. (1987). Two theories used for home heat control. In D. Holland & N Quinn (Eds), *Cultural models in language and thought.* Cambridge: Cambridge University Press.

Novick, L. R. (1988). Analogical transfer, problem similarity, and expertise. *Journal of Experimental Psychology: Learning, Memory, and Cognitiion, 14,* 510–520.

Oppenheimer, R. (1956). Analogy in science. *American Psychologist, 11,* 127–135.

Ortony, A. (1979). Beyond literal similarity. *Psychological Review, 86,* 161–180.

✓ Piaget, J. (1962), *Play, dreams, and imitation in childhood.* New York: Norton.

Piaget, J. (1969). *The mechanisms of perception.* London: Routledge.

Rosch, E., Mervis, C. B., Gay, W. D., Boyes-Braem, P., & Johnson, D.N. (1976). Basic objects in natural categories. *Cognitive Psychology, 8,* 382–439.

Ross, B. H. (1987). This is like that: The use of earlier problems and the separation of similarity effects. *Journal of Experimental Psychology: Learning, Memory, and Cognition, 13,* 629–639.

Rumelhart, D. E., & Norman, D. A. (1981). Analogical processes in learning. In J. R. Anderson (Ed.), *Cognitive skills and their acquisition,* (pp. 335–339). Hillsdale, NJ: Erlbaum.

Smith, C. (1979). Children's understanding of natural language hierarchies. *Journal of Experimental Child Psychology, 27,* 437–458.

Sugarman, S. (1979), *Scheme, order, and outcome: The development of classification in children's early block play.* Unpublished doctoral dissertation, University of California at Berkeley.

Tourangeau, R., & Sternberg, R. J. (1982). Understanding and appreciating metaphors. *Cognition, 11,* 203–244.

✓ Tversky, A., & Kahneman, D. (1982). Judgments of and by representativeness. In D. Kahneman, P. Slovic, & A. Tversky (Eds.), *Judgment under uncertainty: Heuristics and biases* (pp. 84–98). Cambridge: Cambridge University Press.

Vosniadou, S. (1987a). Children and metaphors. *Child Development, 58,* 870 – 885.

Vosniadou, S. (1987b, April). *Children's acquisition and restructuring of science knowledge.* Paper presented at the annual meeting of the American Educational Research Association, Washington, DC

Vosniadou, S., & Brewer, W. F. (1987a). Theories of knowledge restructuring in development. *Review of Educational Research, 57,* 51–67.

Vosniadou, S., & Brewer, W. F. (1987b, April). *Knowledge reorganization in the domain of observational astronomy.* Paper presented at the biennial meeting of the Society for Research in Child Development, Baltimore.

Vosniadou, S., & Ortony, A. (1983). The influence of analogy in children's acquisition of new information from text: An exploratory study. In P. A. Niles & L. A. Harris (Ed.), *Searches for meaning, in reading: Language Processing and instruction* (pp. 71–79). Clemson, SC: National Reading Conference.

Vosniadou, S., Ortony, A., Reynolds, R. E., & Wilson, P. T. (1984). Sources of difficulty in children's comprehension of metaphorical language. *Child Development, 55,* 1588–1606.

Vosniadou, S., & Schommer, M. (1988). Explanatory analogies can help children acquire information from expository text. *Journal of Educational Psychology, 80,* 524–536.

16

Remindings in learning and instruction

BRIAN H. ROSS

In learning a new cognitive skill, novices usually are required to solve many instructional examples. Under these circumstances, people often think back to an earlier example that the current problem reminds them of and use that earlier example and its solution to help them solve the current problem (e.g., Anderson, Farrell, & Sauers, 1984; Novick, 1986; Reed, Dempster, & Ettinger, 1985; Ross, 1984). This use of earlier examples has been suggested as a useful problem-solving heuristic (e.g., Polya, 1945; Wickelgren, 1974), and making analogies from earlier problems is considered by many researchers to be an important part of learning (e.g., Anderson, Farrell, & Sauers, 1984; Carbonell, 1983; Dellarosa, 1985; Gentner, 1980; Pirolli & Anderson, 1985; Reed et al., 1985; Ross, 1984; Winston, 1980).

My research in this area has focused on these remindings, their occurrence, their use, and their effects. Besides the effects that these remindings and their use may have on solving the current problem, they may be of interest for two additional reasons. First, as I will argue in more detail later, these remindings may affect performance not only on the current problem but on later problems as well. That is, remindings may affect what is learned. Second, the study of these relatively simple cases may provide particularly useful information about a number of important basic processes. Remindings may be useful not only because they occur and affect performance but also because they help us to examine similarity-based retrieval of relevant information, reconstruction, analogy, and generalization. We may learn much about processes that also operate on generalized knowledge by studying them at work on a restricted and relatively simple type of information.

In this chapter, I try to accomplish two goals. The first is to provide a framework for understanding the occurrence, use, and effects of remindings. The second goal is to consider how remindings might be a useful tool for aiding instruction. The main focus will be an examination of remindings during the early learning of a cognitive skill. I will present a framework I have been using to direct my investigation of remindings. The motivations that I have mentioned require a detailed examination of how these remindings are noticed, used to solve the current problem, and used to learn. Because of these motivations, the primary aim of my research has been to understand these processes in remindings. The major part of this chapter presents this framework with elaborations from recent research. Following this examination, I will consider some of the general characteristics of early learning that emerge from this work, some differences with other proposals, and how remindings might be used in studying other aspects of learning. Finally, there will be a speculative discussion of how remindings might be used in instruction. This chapter is principally concerned with remindings in the learning process, since the use in instruction needs to follow an understanding of the learning.

Remindings in learning

Introduction

Novices use various means to solve problems. When are remindings used? Although remindings could occur even when other means are available, they are probably more likely to occur and be made use of when the novices do not have other means available to solve the problems. Thus we may expect to see greater reliance on the use of earlier examples when learners are faced with novel or difficult tasks, such as early in learning (Pirolli & Anderson, 1985; Ross, 1984). However, it is important to realize that though remindings may be more likely to occur and be used in novel or difficult tasks the effects of these remindings may persist throughout learning.

Why might remindings be particularly useful in these situations? First, they may help the learner to remember the details of the method. As opposed to the largely independent parts of an abstract rule, the memory for what was done last time is highly interconnected and redundant, allowing the learner to piece it together without remembering separately each part and its position in the sequence. Second, even if the rule is well remembered, the novice may not be able to apply it to the current problem. Because this is a new domain, the concepts used in the rule may not be well understood, or they may be misinterpreted. Also, many remembered rules do not contain all the relevant information needed but, rather, assume some basic level of domain knowledge. Third, the learner may not have extracted all the relevant information at the time of the earlier episode and may now do so from the memory of it. Langley and Simon (1981) argue that one of the general conditions needed for learning is hindsight, the ability to reevaluate past performance in terms of subsequent knowledge of results and causal attributions.

Previous work and framework

My initial experiments in this area were demonstrations that remindings do occur in the learning of cognitive skills and can have large, predictable effects on performance (Ross, 1984). In one experiment, subjects learned to use a computer text editor. For each operation, two methods were taught, each using a different type of text. For example, the operation to "move words" was taught using one method that appended words and another that inserted words. One of these methods would be illustrated using text from a restaurant review, and the other would be illustrated using a poem. At a test requiring this editing operation, subjects would be asked to move words in another restaurant review or another poem. When subjects were reminded, there was a strong tendency (84% of the time) to use the method illustrated with similar text. (An example of these remindings is "Do it the way we did 'molasses,' " where the subject had replaced letters in *molasses* earlier.)

In another experiment, subjects learned each of six probability theory principles (see Table 16.2) by studying abstract information and the solution to a word problem (see Table 16.3) that illustrated the use of the principle. Each of these word problems had a particular irrelevant story line (e.g., IBM motor pool, airport merchants, golfers, and prizes). At test, subjects had to solve some word problems requiring these principles. The test-problem story line was either the same as the study-example story line for that principle (appropriate), a story line not shown before (unrelated), or a story line studied with one of the other principles (inappropriate). The appropriate condition led to highest performance, and the inappropriate condition led to lowest performance, as predicted by the use of remindings. These effects were not only reliable but very large, with proportions correct of .77, .43, and .22 in the appropriate, unrelated, and inappropriate conditions, respectively.

As a guideline for research, I proposed a general framework for remindings in the learning process (Ross, 1984), which is shown in Table 16.1. The basic idea is that to solve a problem learners probe their memory for relevant information. What is retrieved depends

Table 16.1. *A general framework for remindings*

Noticing of an earlier problem (reminding)
Reconstruction of that problem and its solution
Analogy from that problem and solution to the current problem
Generalization from the analogical process

---

upon the match between this probe and the information the learner has in memory. Novices are likely to include superficial aspects of the task in their probes (and their memory), so both structural and superficial aspects of the task may influence what is retrieved. A case in which the learner retrieves some matching information about an earlier example, that is, notices an earlier example, constitutes a reminding. However, noticing an earlier example is not sufficient for aiding performance. The example must be used. This use consists of remembering part of the earlier example and its solution by a reconstructive process. In addition, learners must map aspects of the earlier example to the current problem in order to extend the solution from the earlier example to the current one, that is, in order to make an analogy. This analogical mapping forces a small amount of generalization. This generalized knowledge from the mapping will probably not be nearly as general as the principle; rather, it will be a partially decontextualized episode or combination of episodes. This incremental generalization is one means by which learners may develop schemata and by which earlier examples may influence later performance.

Methodology

Before describing recent work and its implications for this framework, I need to provide a little more detail on the general method used and the logic underlying the main manipulations. Many of the experiments elaborating this framework have used the instruction of elementary probability theory, though some work has used text editors and a variety of less complex tasks. In the teaching of these probability principles, subjects are given study sheets with a principle, its associated formula, and an explanation of the principle. This is followed by a word problem that requires the use of the principle. The four principles that I have used most often are given in Table 16.2 along with their formulas and a brief explanation. Examples of the word problems for each principle are given in Table 16.3. The remaining

Table 16.2. *Principles used in many of the experiments*

Principle	Formula
Permutations of r from n^a	$1/[n\,(n-1)\ldots(n-r+1)]$
Combinations of h from j^a	$[h!\,(j-h)!/j!]$
Waiting time[b]	$q^{k-1}p$
At least once[c]	$1-[1-c]^t$

[a]Permutations and combinations are the probability of a particular one.
[b]Probability that an event, with probability p of occurring (and probability $q = 1 - p$ of not occurring) on each independent trial, occurs for the first time on trial k.
[c]Probability that a specified event (that has a probability c of occurring on each trial) occurs at least once in t independent trials.

part of the study sheet is set up like a workbook, in which the subjects, by answering simple questions about the problem, end up with a worked-out problem. The main reason for this format is to insure that the subjects are attending to the information. The answers to these questions are provided, and subjects are given time to review the sheet with these answers. (When the subjects are tested individually, the experimenter reviews the principle and answers any questions.)

This study phase is followed by a test phase in which subjects are asked to solve word problems requiring the taught principles. Depending upon the experiment, subjects either are given the appropriate formula or are not, the number of tests may range from 4 to 10, and additional dependent measures may be collected, such as latency and confidence. In many of these experiments, the superficial similarity between the study examples and test problems is manipulated. For instance, as in the experiment mentioned earlier, the word problems at study and test may have similar story lines (such as being about airports, golfers, IBM) or may have different story lines. In the experiments to be discussed, all the manipulations are made within subjects. With this general explanation of the method, we may now consider some recent findings and their implications for the framework.

An updated framework for remindings

The main goal of my research program has been to understand better the occurrence, use, and effects of remindings. As mentioned earlier, this work will not only help in understanding how novices solve prob-

Table 16.3. *Sample of the problems used in the experiments*

Permutations

The Mahomet Marathon attracts 44 entrants, but on the day of the race, only 31 runners are present, exactly the same 31 as the year before. If each year the runners present are randomly given a number from 1 to 31 to wear, what is the probability that the first 8 runners each wear the same number they did the year before?

Combinations

A drug dealer bought 50 pills, but when he was arrested he had 22 pills on him. Of the pills, 14 were amphetamines and 8 were placebos. He only had enough time to swallow 8 pills. He didn't have time to look, so these 8 pills were chosen randomly. What is the probability that the 8 pills he swallowed were all placebos?

Waiting time

To promote a hotel in Hawaii, the owners have imported thousands of oysters, 1/9 of them with pearls inside and 8/9 with no pearl inside. When guests check in they are each given an oyster to open. What is the probability that the 5th guest finds the first pearl?

At least once

On the local ballot are 10 offices. Each office has 3 candidates running for it: a Democrat, a Republican, and an Independent. If a voter randomly chose a candidate for each office (with each candidate having an equal 1/3 chance of being selected and a 2/3 chance of not being selected), what is the probability that the voter would vote for one or more Independents?

lems but also provide information on later effects of remindings on performance and allow a detailed examination of the basic processes shown in Table 16.1. The major part of this chapter, then, is a current view of these remindings. These ideas will be presented in terms of elaborations of the earlier framework. These additional details have resulted from recent experimental work in my laboratory (Ross, 1987, 1988; Ross & Sofka, 1986) and elsewhere (e.g., Gentner, this volume; Holyoak & Thagard, this volume). For clarity, the different processes will be examined separately, though it should become clear that they interact to a great extent.

Before proceeding to a consideration of the different processes, a comment is needed on a distinction that will be used throughout the chapter, that of superficial versus structural aspects of the problems (and the similarities between the problems). This distinction can be drawn in various ways (e.g., Gentner, this volume; Gentner & Landers, 1985; Holyoak, 1985; Holyoak & Thagard, this volume). For the purposes of the probability-principle word problems used in the research to be discussed here, I will adopt the following distinction. If changing the problem aspect would not result in a different means of solution, then it is superficial. If changing it would result in a different means of solution, then it is structural. Thus, numbers, story lines (e.g., IBM motor pool, airport desk assignment), and objects (e.g., mechanics and cars, airlines and desks) are superficial aspects of the problems. Structural aspects depend upon the principle underlying the word problem solution. To illustrate this distinction with the permutation principle, the structural aspects include the idea of assignment and that the ordering is important. If this latter aspect were changed so that order was not important, the solution would be changed as well (in this case, to a combinations solution). Clearly, because these are word problems being considered, the structural aspects will be included as part of the word problem. In the first example in Table 16.3, the fact that the first eight runners each have the same number that they had the year before is a structural aspect even though the runners and numbers are superficial aspects. Whatever the superficial aspects, the same idea of a particular, ordered assignment must hold for it to be solvable by the permutations formula.

Noticing. Much evidence now exists supporting the idea that the noticing of an earlier example is affected by the superficial similarity between this earlier example and the test problem (e.g., Gentner & Landers, 1985; Holyoak, 1985; Rosss, 1984). This evidence has led to the suggestion that overall similarity (i.e., all superficial and structural similarities) is determining reminding (Anderson, 1986; Gentner & Landers, 1985; Ross, 1984), but this suggestion needs to be amended due to the results of Ross (1987). Overall similarity is an incomplete description in that it does not make clear that this similarity is a relative similarity measure. I will elaborate on this point and the supporting evidence after describing the relevant experimental design.

In the experiments of Ross (1987), the superficial similarity between word problems was varied both in terms of story line and in terms of object correspondence (i.e., whether the correspondence between objects and variables was similar, reversed, or unrelated to the earlier study problem). The design, with the various conditions used across all the experiments, is given in Table 16.4. A sample word problem illustrating each of these conditions for the permutations principle is provided in Table 16.5 (see Ross, 1987, for more examples). As can be seen in the study example, the IBM mechanics are choosing what company car to work on. In the same/same condition test, the IBM mechanics are again choosing what company car to work on, though

Table 16.4. *Conditions from Ross (1987)*

Condition	Study–test relation		
	Story line	Objects	Correspondence
same/same	same	same	same
same/reversed	same	same	reversed
same/unrelated	same	unrelated	unrelated
unrelated/unrelated	unrelated	unrelated	unrelated

Note: Columns refer to the relation between the various aspects of the study example and test problem.

there have been some minor superficial changes between the problems. In the same/reversed condition test, it is now the cars (via the IBM salespeople who use them) that are choosing the mechanics, so the variable n (see Table 16.2) is the number of mechanics, not the number of cars. In the same/unrelated condition test, though the word problem is still about IBM (which is enough to remind people of the earlier example, as will be discussed later), the objects are computers and offices, which do not seem to have any natural correspondence to cars and mechanics.[1] Finally, in the unrelated/unrelated test condition, the story line (high school athletic team ticket sales), the objects (teams and teachers) and the object correspondences are unrelated to those in the study example.

A needed amendment to the idea that overall similarity determines reminding is that this similarity is a relative measure. Although this claim is not inconsistent with most accounts, the nature of the similarity is often not detailed. In Experiments 2a and 2b of Ross (1987), conditions same/unrelated and unrelated/unrelated were used to assess the influence of story-line similarity on noticing. Across the two experiments, the confusability of the principles was varied. As can be seen in Table 16.2, the principles often used in these experiments form two pairs of confusable principles. Permutations and combinations are very similar, the only difference being whether the order of assignment matters. The other two principles both involve multiple independent trials with the probability reflecting a particular outcome. For waiting time, the outcome is that the event occurs for the first time on the specific trial. For the final principle (which I will refer to as "at least once"), the outcome is that the event occurs at least once in the specified number of trials. They also both include exponents and subtracting an event probability from one to get the probability that an event does not occur. In Experiment 2a, these confusable

Table 16.5. *Sample permutations problems from Ross (1987)*

Study example

The IBM motor pool has to make sure the company cars are serviced. On a
particular day there are 11 cars and 8 mechanics. The IBM mechanics randomly
choose which car they will work on, but the choice is done by seniority. What is
the probability that the three most senior mechanics, Al, Bud, and Carl, will
choose the cars of the Chairman, President, and Vice-president, respectively?

Same/same test problem

The motor pool at IBM repairs the cars the company salespeople use. The IBM
mechanics randomly choose which car to repair, with the best mechanic choosing
first, etc. There are 16 salespeople who have cars and 5 mechanics. What is the
probability that the best mechanic gets to work on the car of the best salesperson
and the second-best mechanic gets to work on the car of the second-best
salesperson?

Same/reversed test problem

The motor pool at IBM repairs the cars the company salespeople use. The IBM
salespeople randomly choose which mechanic repairs their cars, with the best
salesperson choosing first, etc. There are 14 salespeople who have cars and 16
mechanics. What is the probability that the best mechanic gets to work on the car
of the best salesperson and the second-best mechanic gets to work on the car of
the second-best salesperson?

Same/unrelated test problem

The IBM offices need to be equipped with computers. Each IBM office randomly
chooses the computer it will get, but they choose in the order that they request the
computer. The supervisor of the supply department has 16 computers (each a
different size) and 5 offices request computers. What is the probability that the
first office to request a computer gets the largest computer and the next office
gets the second largest?

Unrelated/unrelated test problem

Valley Forge High School has 16 teachers that are willing to help with ticket sales
for the 12 athletic teams. Each team randomly chooses a teacher to help with its
sales, with the basketball team choosing first and soccer team second. What is the
probability that the algebra teacher sells tickets for the basketball team and the
geometry teacher sells tickets for the soccer team?

Note: The test conditions are explained in Table 16.4 and the text. Each subject who
received this study example would receive only one of these test problems. Across
subjects, eight different study examples appeared for each principle, so that all test
problems occurred equally often in each test condition.

principles were used. In Experiment 2b, changes were made to make
the principles less confusable. The permutations and waiting-time
principles and problems were included exactly as in Experiment
2a, but the combinations and at-least-once principles were changed.
Conditional probability was substituted for combinations, since permutations and conditional probability are very different. The

at-least-once principle was rewritten to involve the number of choices (rather than the probability of a particular choice), making it less confusable with the waiting-time principle.

The effect of superficial similarity depended not only on whether the study and test problems had similar story lines but also on the confusability of the principles. The usual advantage of the superficially similar story line between study and test examples occurred in Experiment 2a when the principles were confusable (.22, with proportions correct of .48 and .26, for the similar and different story lines, respectively). However, this advantage disappeared in Experiment 2b when all principles were distinctive (.44 vs .46). Even if one restricts the comparison to the permutations and waiting-time problems, which were exactly the same between the two experiments, a reliable advantage of similar story lines occurs only when the principles are confusable, with differences of .22 in Experiment 2a and .03 in Experiment 2b. This finding suggests that the measure of whether an earlier example will be thought of needs to take into account the similarity (in this case, the structural similarity) to other examples that the novice has learned, not just the similarity to the appropriate study example.

Finally, I hope it is clear that I do not view noticing as some special retrieval process. As the framework states, remindings occur when the retrieval process leads to an earlier example or episode. Certainly, the idea that the relative similarity of the cue and target information is important (as well as the earlier finding of interference effects in Ross, 1984, Experiment 3) is consistent with many current memory theories. The goal of this research on noticing has not been to generate new principles of memory retrieval but rather to understand how memory principles apply to these specific cases of remindings. (See also Anderson & Thompson, Gentner, and Holyoak & Thagard, all in this volume, for related ideas on noticing and memory.)

After noticing: remembering and use of remindings. Noticing an earlier example is not sufficient to affect performance. To affect performance that earlier example must be remembered and used.

Remembering and reconstruction. The original framework included a distinction between noticing the earlier example and remembering enough of that example and its solution to make use of it. Such a distinction is necessary particularly when the earlier example is complicated and not well learned. (The SAM [Search of Associative Memory] model of Raaijmakers & Shiffrin, 1981, makes a similar distinction – though the noticing may not be conscious – between sampling and recovery even in relatively simple recall situations. The suggestion that the process is reconstructive was based initially on a few protocols. Ross and Sofka (1986, Experiment 3) examined this process more thoroughly, though this study was still exploratory. After learning four probability principles and seeing one or two study examples of each principle, subjects were given test problems and asked to recall as much as they could of a study example that each test problem reminded them of. For current purposes, these are two results of interest. First, in conditions where at least one of the study examples had a story line similar to that of the test problem, remindings occurred on most problems and were usually stated as soon as the subject finished reading the test problem. Second, the recall of the earlier example was very drawn-out in time and made use of a variety of inferences and memory-probing strategies. That is, these earlier examples were not recalled all at once but seemed to be recalled in fragments. In addition, subjects would use various types of probes to stimulate recall, including earlier recalled fragments, parts of the test problem (to be discussed later), and information about other examples (e.g., in deciding whether the numbers recalled went with this example) and the formulas. Thus, although the details of this process are still to be worked out, it does appear to involve considerable retrieval beyond the initial noticing, and at least some of the retrieval is reconstructive in nature.

Use: Analogy. Assuming that novices are reminded of and remember the earlier problem, we then need to determine what knowledge is retrieved from this earlier problem and how it is applied. A claim of the original framework was that the earlier problem and solution are remembered and are applied by analogy to the current test problem, but again this suggestion was based on a few informal protocols and some post hoc analyses (see Ross, 1984). Because much instruction of new cognitive skills explicitly provides the principle, formula, or method, it is possible that remindings serve to cue this abstract information, not to set up an analogy with the earlier example. By this cuing account, once the abstract information is cued, the earlier example is no longer used. The basic idea of this account is that the abstract information can be applied to the current problem without regard to the earlier example.

Ross (1987) contrasted these two ways in which remindings could aid performance: by cuing the appropriate principles or by analogy from the earlier example. The first experiment of that paper tested these two possibilities by examining whether the similarity in the details of the study and test-example has an effect beyond the cuing of the appropriate abstract information. The story lines, objects, and object correspondences between the study and test problems were varied, using all four conditions in Table 16.4 (see Table 16.5 for an illustration). At test, when subjects were given a problem to solve, they were also given the appropriate formula. Their task was to fill in the variables correctly for this formula from the numbers given in the test problem. The logic of the experiment is as follows (see the original paper for further elaboration). If remindings are serving to cue appropriate abstract information, one would expect little difference among the four conditions, since the appropriate formula is provided. In contrast, if subjects are making an analogy from the earlier example, the similarity of the object correspondences should be important. That is, to instantiate the variables in the formula, subjects would use the details of the earlier problem. Since novices are so greatly influenced by superficial similarity, it is likely that the setting up of correspondences will be influenced by this superficial similarity. The examples in Table 16.5 that were described in detail earlier should help to make these predictions clear. If subjects are trying to assign superficially similar objects to the same variable roles that these objects had in the study example, they will assign the number of cars to be the number of items chosen from (variable n in Table 16.2) for both the same/same and the same/reversed tests. This assignment will lead to correctly instantiated formulas in the same/same condition but to incorrectly instantiated formulas in the same/reversed condition (because the object correspondences have been reversed). The two conditions with unrelated correspondence should be intermediate.

Thus, the analogy account predicts that, compared to the same/unrelated condition, the same/same condition should show higher performance (because the use of this superficial object correspondence similarity will lead to a correctly instantiated formula) and the same/reversed condition should show lower performance (because the use of superficial similarity will lead to an incorrectly instantiated formula). If the instantiation of this formula is determined solely by the object correspondence similarity, unrelated/unrelated performance should be equal to same/unrelated performance (i.e., similar story lines between study and test problems should not have an effect when the formula is provided).

The results of this experiment provide strong support for the analogy account over the cuing account. Proportions correct for the same/same, same/reversed, same/unrelated, and unrelated/unrelated were .74, .37, .54, and .56, respectively. Thus, similar object correspondences improved performance, and reversed object correspondences hurt performance, relative to the unrelated object correspondences controls. This result shows not only that subjects are using the details of the earlier problems, but also that the analogy process makes use of superficial similarities (such as the similarity of objects) for determining correspondences between the two problems.

An alternative version of the cuing hypothesis might claim that the formula is not the appropriate abstract information. This version would then assume that cuing is necessary even when the formula is provided. Hence, it would predict a difference among conditions as a function of the similarity between study and test problems, with same/same leading to highest performance and unrelated/unrelated to lowest. Thus, even this variant of the cuing hypothesis does not predict the observed results.

Reconstruction and analogy. A final result of interest from Ross and Sofka (1986) suggests that the reconstruction and analogy processes are interleaved. To understand this idea, it is necessary to point out two differences between the Ross and Sofka experiment and other studies of reconstruction (e.g., Bartlett, 1932; Kolodner, 1983; Williams & Hollan, 1981) and recall earlier examples (Mayer, 1982; Silver, 1981). First, in most other research, the people trying to remember the information have domain-related schemata that they are using to aid their recall. Novices, however, have little high-level knowledge appropriate to the domain that they can use to drive the reconstruction. Second, in other studies the subjects are simply told to recall the earlier event or example. At most, they might be provided with a cue that is a small part of what they are being asked to remember. When a reminding occurs, however, the cue is not simply the instruction to recall or a small fragment of the earlier example. Rather, another problem has reminded the learner of the earlier example.

With these two differences noted, the interleaving of the reconstruction and analogy processes may be explained. In Ross and Sofka (1986, Experiment 3), we asked subjects to recall as much as they could of any earlier example that the current problem reminded them of. As outlined above, these novices do not have the high-level knowledge that more expert subjects use to remember earlier examples (e.g., Mayer, 1982), but they do have available the current problem. What we observe is that novices use the current problem to help guide their reconstruction. In the recall of earlier examples and solutions, subjects used the current problem not only as an initial reminder but as an aid throughout the recall. This use included trying to think of objects in the earlier example that might correspond to ones in the present problem, trying to solve the present problem partially to stimulate recall of details in the earlier example, and using the numbers in the present problem to probe or make decisions about the numbers in the earlier example (e.g., "Ford sales executives, they chose the top 4 salesmen out of the 8 sounds more similar to the 6 and 9 on this one").

Thus it appears that sometimes these novices are piecing together the earlier example, using the current problem as both a probe and an instance for comparison. That is, the novices do not know the abstract structural aspects of the problem, but they do have an instantiation of the problem structure (the current problem) and are using this to help in guiding and testing their recall. It is this dual use of the current problem as both a probe and an instance for comparison that leads to the interleaving of reconstruction and analogy.

Relation of noticing to performance: types of remindings. One can think of noticing as the input to the reconstruction and analogy processes. Thus, if these inputs were to differ in some fundamental way, they might lead to differences in the output of the other processes and, hence, to differences in performance. It seems likely that remindings may be of a number of types (e.g., Schank, 1982) and that they may lead to differences in performance. An alternative view is that, given an appropriate reminding, what aspect of the earlier example was noticed is not important. This view gains some plausibility when one realizes that the reminding alone is insufficient to affect performance. Given that a great deal of reconstruction and analogy is required, it is possible that any difference in cues to the earlier problem will be small (since the cues are generated by the subject in all cases). A first step in this work (Ross & Sofka, 1986) has been to identify types of remindings based on the content of the reminding and to examine whether they result in orderly differences in performance. Finding these differences would then allow one to investigate questions about what might lead to these different remindings and how they might be used.

Ross and Sofka (1986) propose a number of reminding types, but here we will be concerned only with the broad categories of superficial and structural remindings. The basic idea is that if the reminding indicates only a general or story-line noticing of similarity (e.g., "This is like the one with the light bulbs") it is assigned to the superficial category. If, however, the reminding includes information about correspondences or difficulties in the previous problem (e.g., "4 desks, 12 airlines, like 12 cars in 4 spaces," in which all the numbers are from the test problem but the subject is clearly setting up a correspondence), we assume that the learner has noticed something more structural about the problem and we assign it to the structural category. Although superficial remindings are more common (about twice as common in those experiments), structural remindings lead to higher performance (.76 compared to .51 for superficial). Thus the category of reminding is a useful predictor of performance.

Effects on later performance. Early experiences may have a strong influence on later performance (Welford, 1958, p. 296). A possibility that makes remindings particularly important is that using one problem to help solve another might force a certain amount of generalization (see Anderson, 1986; Gick & Holyoak, 1983, for related proposals). If so, remindings may influence what is learned by determining which particular earlier example is used in making the analogy.

To approach the issue in a slightly different way, an important part of expertise appears to be the development of very specific schemata (e.g., Sweller & Cooper, 1985). Being able to recognize problem types is an important goal of any instructional program (Brown, Bransford, Ferrara, & Campione, 1983). A number of researchers have proposed that an essential part of developing these problem types or schemata is through comparison of instances of a particular problem type (e.g., Dellarosa, 1985; Holyoak, 1985). These proposals still require a means of deciding what problems to compare and how they are compared. The remindings and use of earlier examples may help in specifying both means. Remindings, when they are appropriate, serve the function of setting up the comparison. The use of the earlier example by analogy may be the means of comparison that forces a generalization. An advantage of this idea is that one does not need a separate generalization mechanism to operate over solved problems.

Although this idea has been proposed by several investigators, the evidence for the effects on later performance is meager. Holyoak (1985) cites a study done with Cantrombone in which two stories with the same underlying structure led to greater analogous solution of a target problem only if the subjects had to compare the stories. Dellarosa (1985) shows that answering questions that force a comparison of problems leads to better performance than answering questions that do not force a comparison. Pirolli and Anderson (1985) provide protocol and simulation evidence for the effects of the use of examples on later performance.

Ross (1988) examines the effect that remindings have on later tests and shows that making use of an earlier example to solve a problem

leads to better performance on the next test. To avoid the problems
of post hoc analyses, this set of recent experiments manipulates remindings by explicitly cuing (or not cuing) with the story line of the
appropriate earlier problem. All word problems had superficially unrelated story lines. At the first test, subjects either were cued with
which study example the test problem was similar to (e.g., "This is
like the golfer problem") or were not. After the first test, subjects
were shown the correct answers and given explanations of why these
answers were correct. The results of interest are what happens on the
second test of each principle, in which the story lines are unrelated
to any seen previously and no cuing is provided. Do these cued remindings on the first test have an effect on performance on the second
test? The answer is yes, with second test proportions correct of .48
when a cue was given on the first test and .30 when no cue was given.
Thus, when story lines (and, as far as possible, other superficial similarities) between study and test problems are unrelated, being explicitly reminded of the first test leads to better performance on the
second test.

This experiment shows an effect of using an example on later tests
but does not indicate what aspects of later use are affected. So far,
two possibilities have been investigated. First, this use of an earlier
example may better allow subjects to learn to access some appropriate
information with which to solve the problem. This information could
include knowledge about what type of problem the current problem
is (e.g., Chi, Feltovich, & Glaser, 1981; Hinsley, Hayes, & Simon, 1977)
and/or other associated information for solving the problem (such as
the formula). Second, this use of the earlier example may help subjects
to learn how to make better use of any appropriate information once
it is accessed. These two possibilities were examined by varying what
information the learner was provided with at test and scoring particular aspects of performance. That is, the proportion-correct scoring
presumably reflects both the access and the use of relevant information. We may make a preliminary separation in the following way
(see Ross, 1987, 1988, for further details of the logic). The first possibility, of increased access of relevant information, was tested by
scoring the performance of subjects on later problem solutions in
terms of whether the answer appeared to be making use of the appropriate formula. To do this, the data from the experiment that has
already been presented were rescored, with the scoring now reflecting
whether subjects had made use of the appropriate formula, regardless
of whether they had used it correctly. (Clearly, these data are related
to the proportion-correct data, because an inappropriate formula al-

ways leads to an incorrect answer as well. However, because there are many instances of incorrectly used formulas, this scoring of whether the formula is appropriate is not the same as the correctness scoring.) Cuing of first tests led to a .21 advantage (.69 vs. .48) on this measure of access in the second test. The second possibility, of better use of retrieved relevant information, was tested by providing subjects with the appropriate formula for the second test problems and scoring their ability to instantiate the formula correctly (i.e., put the numbers with the appropriate variables). Cuing of first tests also led to an advantage here (.75 vs. .56). Thus, from these two experiments it appears that this use of an earlier example does increase the ability both to access relevant information and to make use of such provided information.

Assuming that being reminded and using an earlier example to solve a current problem affect what one learns, there are a number of possibilities for how this process might work that are just beginning to be explored (e.g., Kolodner, Simpson, & Sycara-Cyranski, 1985). For example, Anderson (1986) proposes that the analogy is compiled, leading to a production that usually includes those features used in making the analogy. He suggests that what features are compiled into the generalization is a strategic decision. One could also imagine processes that carry over all similar features, even ones known to be irrelevant. At the other extreme, perhaps only one or two relevant features used in making the analogy are carried over. Much work remains before we will understand the effects of using examples on later performance and the means by which these effects occur.

In ending this section, I think it is important to realize that this learning mechanism is not restricted to problem solving. For instance, Susan Perkins, Patricia Tenpenny, and I have conducted category learning experiments that rely upon the idea that generalizatons are formed from using an earlier item to solve (or, in this case, categorize) a current item.

Summary. Although some aspects of the framework still require substantial elaboration, the studies reviewed here further specify how remindings are noticed and used. The noticing is affected by some (though perhaps not all) superficial similarities but also by relative structural similarities, such as the confusability of the principles. Much of my recent work has focused on the remembering and use of earlier examples. The picture that emerges from this work is of a reconstructive process that is interleaved with the analogical use, both of which are affected by specific superficial and structural similarities.

Although novices are using the earlier example to help solve the current problem, they are also using the current problem to remember enough of the earlier example to make use of it. Even when given an appropriate formula, their understanding may be poor enough that they rely upon any similarities they can find with the earlier example to determine how to instantiate the formula. Finally, it appears that this use of the earlier example also allows novices to see some commonalities of the problem type that they can make use of later.

Implications for learning

What does this work suggest about the early learning of a new domain? I would like to concentrate on three characteristics of this learning that are particularly relevant to the ideas presented earlier: context dependence, opportunism, and forcing of generalizations.

Context dependence. One major characteristic of learning is that what is learned is often less generally applicable than intended. That is, what is learned may be restricted to cases similar to the one it was learned with, rather than seen as a more general principle that was merely illustrated by the case it was taught with. The important work of Gick and Holyoak (1980, 1983) can be viewed as demonstrations of how people, when reading a story, do not abstract out the point or plan but store this information in terms of the story. When these subjects are later given a problem with a very different content, they rarely think to use the plan in the story that they just finished reading. Bransford, Franks, Vye, and Sherwood (this volume) and Brown (this volume) provide an interesting discussion on the importance of learning to transfer this "inert" knowledge. (See also Gick, 1986; Gick & Holyoak, 1987, for reviews.)

It may seem that this difficulty is largely due to extreme differences in content of the material in which the idea was learned and in which it was required at test. However, we see the same difficulty for within-domain learning, when the relevant knowledge is presumably more circumscribed. Anderson, Farrell, and Sauers (1984) give examples of this "isolation of knowledge" in the learning of LISP programming. In the very early learning, this isolation of knowledge is sometimes even "content-dependent." Not only may the information not be understood abstractly, but it is possible that any usable understanding of the principle and its associated formula is bound up with the earlier example that was used to illustrate it (Ross, 1987).

Though some of this highly contextualized knowledge is due to the lack of experience of these learners, an important idea in current conceptions of expertise is that a great deal of highly specific problem types and associated solutions are required (e.g., Brown et al., 1983; Sweller & Cooper, 1985). Although experts need general knowledge to be able to categorize and solve new and unusual problems, they may use more specialized knowledge to solve problems that are like ones they have often seen before (e.g., Hinsley et al., 1977).

An interesting parallel for future investigation is the recent work showing the unexpected (by most of us) specificity of processing, such as in the work of Jacoby and Brooks (1984). A common theme of that work is that what we had believed was accomplished by abstract processing mechanisms or rules appears to be affected by highly specific similarities across items that would not be expected to matter if these abstract mechanisms were being used. Speculatively, it is possible that some of the problem-solving behavior that appears to be rule-governed may actually be driven by more specific knowledge than we usually assume.

Opportunism. Another characteristic of novices' learning that emerges from this research is that early problem solving is very opportunistic (see Hayes-Roth & Hayes-Roth, 1979; Williams & Hollan, 1981, for similar characterizations of planning and of remembering long-term events). The point is that novices do not have deep understandings or well-learned procedures for solving these problems, so they latch onto whatever they can. Since novices are very sensitive to the superficial similarities and not very sensitive to the underlying structure (e.g., Chi et al., 1981), it should not be surprising that these superficial similarities are used in early learning. In fact, given that much of what novices learn is tied to examples and given the opportunistic quality of their problem solving, it seems likely that their learning will be sensitive to small, irrelevant changes in material and order. I think it is important to realize, however, that this sensitivity to superficial manipulations may not necessarily be due to an inability to distinguish between superficial and structural similarity (e.g., as suggested by Holyoak, 1985). Rather, it may be that novices cannot abstract out the structural similarities but realize that superficial and structural similarities are often correlated in these formal domains (e.g., Lewis & Anderson, 1985; Mayer, 1981; see Medin & Ortony, this volume, for a related argument about concepts in general). If so, and if they are unable to make use of the structural aspects, the use of superficial similarities may be the most successful course possible even when the novices are aware that these similarities are superficial.

Forcing of generalizations. Finally, though it is still under investigation, this early learning of a cognitive skill may be due partially to small generalizations forced by making analogies between problems. Given the isolation of knowledge, how to get this knowledge to be less isolated becomes a crucial question. One approach would be to posit some separate automatic generalization mechanism that acts upon instances to get less context-bound generalizations. Anderson (1986) argues against such a separate and automatic mechanism on both intuitive and empirical grounds.

An alternative view is that the generalization may be a by-product of the problem solving by analogy. That is, in an attempt to make an analogy between the current problem and the earlier example one has been reminded of, there will usually be many differences. In order to complete the analogy, certain generalizations are forced (i.e., some different aspects are allowed to be set into correspondence, essentially ignoring the differences). My proposal (see also, Anderson, 1986; Kolodner et al., 1985; Pirolli & Anderson, 1985; Schank, 1982, for related suggestions) is that this reminding-based generalization is one means by which people learn about the problem types. Such a process would often produce very conservative generalizations but, if the reminding is of an appropriate earlier example, generalizations that would help with solving some later problems. In addition, this proposal implies that the basis of the reminding will be only partially related to what is learned from the reminding. This partial dissociation occurs because the reminding is due to some similarities between the two problems, but the generalization that results from this reminding is a function of all the similarities and differences between the earlier example and the current problem (or, at least potentially, many that were not the basis of the reminding). Thus this process may be one means by which novices, though they are largely relying on the superficial aspects initially, can learn the structural aspects with practice.

This possibility has perhaps the greatest implications for learning because of its effect on later performance. Learning problem types may require comparisons of problems of the same type. The suggestion here is that remindings set up this comparison and that the analogical use of the earlier example to solve the current problem forces this comparison. If so, then the acquisition of schemata, the use of analogies, and remindings in learning are all closely related (see also Holyoak, 1985). My future work will be aimed at trying to understand this reminding-based generalization mechanism.

Differences from structural proposals

A number of recent proposals have addressed how analogies between episodes or problems may be noticed and made (e.g., Carbonell, 1983; Gentner, 1983; Holyoak, 1985; Schank, 1982; Winston, 1980). Despite considerable differences among these proposals, they have a few important commonalities that contrast sharply with the current proposal. I will first point out these contrasts and then briefly discuss their implications. Because most of these proposals have tended to focus on between-domain or far analogies, they have dealt with cases that are rather different from the ones faced in the within-domain analogies examined here. For example, the cases they examine often have no abstract principle explicitly given but rely on an example in which the principle is embedded. In addition, the earlier example (or in some cases, the source domain) is often well remembered and understood (i.e., its structure is well known). This latter aspect means that a crucial part of the analogical application involves transferring the structure from the earlier domain to the new domain. (Clearly, this is a simplification of these varied proposals, but it captures an important commonality.) Hence, these theories will be referred to as *structural* proposals. As pointed out here, however, novices are often provided with an abstract principle, do not remember the earlier problem structure well (Ross & Sofka, 1986; Silver, 1981), and have a poor understanding of the underlying structure (e.g., Chi et al., 1981, Silver, 1979). In addition, whereas the similarity between the source and target in these far analogies is almost exclusively abstract, within-domain examples often have much superficial similarity that can be, and is, made use of.

These differences in the cases dealt with by these structural proposals and the current proposal are not just minor differences but may significantly change the character of the noticing, use, and effect of these earlier examples. If a novice does not understand the structure of the problems and does not remember the earlier example well, proposals that focus on transferring relevant or systematic structure from the earlier example will be incomplete. As pointed out earlier, the remembering and use of the earlier examples are both affected by various superficial similarities that are not even considered by most of these other proposals. Any "structure" that is used for the earlier example is likely to be heavily affected by various nonstructural similarities. Given what a novice knows about examples in the new domain, it seems that the early learning is often driven more by the superficial similarity than by the structural similarity.

Remindings as tools for studying learning

Before we consider how remindings might be used in instruction, it should also be noted that remindings have proven a useful tool for examining some learning issues. In this section, I briefly outline these uses, in the hope that other researchers might be able to make use of remindings as well. Although the focus of my research has been on remindings and their effects, I realize that learners may rely on knowledge other than earlier examples. If so, then the learning performance is some unknown mixture of cases in which remindings and other types of knowledge are used. The point to be made in this section is that remindings (and their effects) can be used as a tool for understanding aspects of learning. I will discuss two general ways in which they might be used and then provide a few examples that illustrate these uses.

Protocol-based separation of remindings and non-remindings. The first way to use remindings as a tool for studying learning is to partition the solutions into cases where earlier examples were used and other cases (in which earlier examples were probably not used) by relying on the verbal protocols.[2] Remindings may be affected by various manipulations in different ways than the use of other knowledge. If they are, the overall data may provide a picture that is not an accurate portrayal of learning either by remindings or by any other means. If the data are separated into cases in which subjects mentioned an earlier example and cases in which they did not, an examination of the performance of each set may help us to understand the learning. Clearly, this separation is not perfect, but the assumption is that a case in which an earlier example is explicitly mentioned is more likely to rely upon an earlier example than a case in which an earlier example is not mentioned. This separation allows one to see how various manipulations affect performance in each of these cases, as well as the relative frequency of remindings across manipulations. Two illustrations may help make this use clearer.

In an experiment briefly discussed earlier in the chapter, I had subjects learn two methods for each task, each with a separate type of text (Ross, 1984, Experiment 1). I examined whether text-editor novices would be more likely to use the method "consistent" with the text they learned it on when they were reminded of the earlier text. Overall, the effect was in this predicted direction but very small (.61 for the first test, where .50 is chance). However, if one looks only at cases in which subjects explicitly mention an earlier text (.30 of these first tests), the effect is large (.84). The tests with no remindings showed no consistency effect.

A second illustration of the use of remindings as a tool is in examining individual differences, an important issue in both learning and instruction. Because remindings are presumed to be more likely when learners are having difficulty, I always examine performance patterns by a median split on overall performance. How remindings may be useful in this post hoc analysis is illustrated in Ross and Sofka (1986, Experiments 1 and 2), though similar analyses have proven interesting in other cases as well. Two results are of interest from those two studies. First, subjects who have lower performance tend to have more remindings, especially superficial remindings (see the section "Relation of noticing to performance," above). Second, one can look at the pattern of performance across the conditions for good and poor subjects. In both these experiments a similar pattern occurred. Because these subjects are divided post hoc on their overall performance, performance in all cases is likely to be greater for the good subjects, but the differences between good and poor subjects may change as a function of the condition. In these experiments, the condition in which a single example was studied and the test problem had a similar story line showed a much greater difference between good and poor subjects than did the other conditions. When the data were divided into reminding and no-reminding cases, almost all of the difference from other conditions was due to the cases in which no remindings occurred. That is, good subjects had higher performance than bad subjects on tests in which they mentioned an earlier example, but the size of the difference was similar to that of the other conditions (about .30). When no remindings occurred, however, the difference in this condition was .58. Though the exact interpretation suggested in that paper (that one difference between good and poor subjects is their ability to extract schematic information from a single example) is open to argument, it provides a hypothesis that would not have been evident except for the protocol-based division into remindings and no remindings.

Performance-based use of remindings. A second use of remindings as a tool for studying learning does not rely on protocols. This method may be useful in cases in which talking aloud is difficult, in which converging evidence is sought for protocol-based interpretations, and in which testing in groups is either necessary or preferred. The basic idea is that the difference in performance between appropriate and unrelated conditions (i.e., conditions in which the study and test example have similar or unrelated superficial contents, respectively) provides a performance-based index of the reliance on an earlier episode. To the extent that performance differs as a function of this superficial similarity, subjects must be relying upon some aspects of the earlier episodes. If, on the other hand, the subjects are using appropriate rules (or, for example, are experts), there should be no difference as a function of this superficial similarity (i.e., between the appropriate and unrelated conditions). So this difference reflects some (unscaled) measure of the reliance upon the earlier episodes or information learned from these episodes. To see how this idea might be used, suppose that this superficial similarity manipulation is crossed with some other manipulation. If the effect of superficial similarity (appropriate minus unrelated) decreases from one condition to a second condition of this other manipulation, one can conclude that there is less reliance on the earlier episodes in this second condition. Note that this does not tell you whether that difference is due to less noticing and equal use, equal noticing but less use, or less noticing and less use, just that the earlier episodes are having less of an effect on performance. Two cases may illustrate the usefulness of this performance-based method.

In one case, I varied whether the story lines in the study examples were shared with two other principles or were unique (Ross, 1984, Experiment 3). The reasoning was that in the shared condition the advantage of using a similar story line at test should be attenuated because the details of the earlier example would be harder to remember (but note that it is possible to tell by performance only whether there is less effect, not why). The .24 difference found in the unique condition fell to .05 in the shared condition, which suggests that the earlier examples were less relied upon in the latter condition.

A second example comes from some unpublished work with Michael Sofka that examined the representation of editing commands during early learning. In one experiment we found that the effect of superficially similar text on the probability of accomplishing an editing task was small. However, when we separated tasks that had shared commands from ones with unique commands, we found little effect of the superficially similar text when the task had commands shared with other tasks but large effects when the task had commands unique to it. After verifying this post hoc finding experimentally, we used this difference to help examine what was learned about these editing commands from their instructional examples.

Remindings in instruction

Introduction

The first part of this chapter dealt with remindings in the learning of new cognitive skills. I claimed that remindings are important both in accomplishing the current task and in learning the new domain. Given this characterization of remindings in learning, what are the implications for instruction? I present some speculations about how these results might prove to be useful. As we find out more about the learning of new cognitive skills, the opportunities for instructional benefits should increase. Currently, however, the relevant data are dismally sparse compared to the importance of the instructional issues. Before focusing on how remindings and their effects may be used to improve instruction, there is a more general controversy to deal with.

Are analogies helpful in learning? It is important to distinguish between-domain and within-domain uses of analogy. There is considerable debate about the good and the harm of teaching one domain by analogy to another (e.g., see Rumelhart & Norman, 1981; Halasz & Moran, 1982, for arguments pro and con). Many of the arguments against between-domain analogies, such as that inappropriate aspects of the source may be transferred as well, do not apply to within-domain analogies. Even so, there is a question about the usefulness of within-domain analogies. Anderson, Boyle, Farrell, and Reiser (1984) argue that though analogies to earlier examples do occur often, they should not be encouraged. They suggest that often what people learn when making an analogy is how to make the analogy, not how the problems are related in a general way. In this chapter and elsewhere (Ross, 1984), I have suggested that analogies to earlier problems may help lead to more general knowledge of problem types. Sweller (e.g., Sweller, Mawer, & Howe, 1982) has taken the view that inducing rules requires a history-cued learning (that is, learning in which earlier examples are used). Pirolli and Anderson (1985) suggest that a useful procedure might be to have analogies made not to earlier examples but to structural models that will lead to appropriate use being made. In addition, Anderson (1986) proposed a knowledge compilation mechanism that works by compiling the analogy that was made into a production. It appears that within-domain analogies may be useful but that there is still much to be learned about how best to use these analogies in instruction.

Remindings as aids in instruction

In this section, I examine the idea that remindings can be used to aid learning. I will emphasize how novices' sensitivity to superficial similarities can be used to improve instruction, though other means of remindings (e.g., by cues) could also be used. Currently, there is a great deal of variation in how superficial similarities are used in instruction. As two examples, one very good text-editing manual (Kernighan, 1979) uses the same text to illustrate every editing operation. Most math textbooks, however, have correlations between superficial similarities and problem types (e.g., Lewis & Anderson, 1985; Mayer, 1981).

Two ideas influenced the implications to be discussed. The first idea is that learning problem types and associated solutions is an important part of learning in a new domain (e.g., Brown et al., 1983; Chi et al., 1981). As has been often mentioned (e.g., Larkin, 1981), textbooks are good about teaching solution methods but often provide few clues on when to use the different possible methods. Textbooks often segregate problem types by chapter so that the focus of a particular lesson is on solving problems of a particular type, not on what problem aspects make this method the appropriate one to use. The second idea is that novices are going to be affected by superficial similarities. Given these two "truths," how can instruction be improved? I have chosen a few possibilities that I hope will provide a flavor for the set.

First, remindings can be used to break down the many parts of learning into more manageable units (Ross & Moran, 1983, provide an elaboration of this view to the learning of computer methods). For example, learners faced with a new domain may be overwhelmed by the great number of problem types and the difficult solutions for each. The common solution is to segregate by problem type, but rarely is anything done to teach learners how to recognize these types. In addition, this procedure has the disadvantage of massing practice, a usually inefficient procedure. One possibility would be to mix up the problem types but use remindings (by superficial similarity) to insure that learners are using appropriate methods. This would allow concentration first on the methods, but in a less segregated environment. As the learners become more able and confident, they could be weaned away from reliance on superficial similarities until they are able to categorize the problems by structural aspects only. (This technique is related to the fading training technique of Terrace, 1963.)

Second, remindings might be used to address particular difficulties. For example, a difficult aspect of learning problem types is determining the relevant distinctions between types and deciding how to categorize problems as a function of these distinctions. This difficulty is often compounded by segregated instruction that focuses the learners' attention on the individual types and not on their commonalities and differences. Suppose there are two problem types that are similar but have an important distinction (e.g., permutations and combinations). It might be useful to have initial worked-out examples in each involve similar contents, so that the learner is more likely to notice the similarities and the distinctions. A slight variation of this is to use these similar contents to force learners into a mistake. In solving later problems, this may increase the likelihood that they will be reminded by these problems and hence remember the crucial distinction (Riesbeck, 1981; Ross & Sofka, 1986). Bransford et al. (this volume) address the learning of distinctions and propose a method for its instruction.

After presenting these two possibilities, I should mention that I am not convinced that superficial similarity is are useful as an instructional tool. The advantages are that it can be combined with other instructional methods and that it requires little investment of time, because examples are used in almost all instruction. However, it is possible that using superficial similarities will take subjects' attention away from more important aspects. My real point is that remindings are occurring during instruction and that various instructional programs promote them more or less, but in a generally haphazard way. I cannot believe that this is the best state. If remindings are unhelpful, instructional materials should minimize them. If remindings are helpful, instructional materials should take advantage of them. We need to consider the specifics of the instructional sequence as well as the general form of the instruction.

Whatever the usefulness of reminding by superficial similarities as an instructional tool, it does seem that the ideas and distinctions from this and other research (e.g., Gentner & Landers, 1985; Holyoak, 1985) can be used to help teach problem-solving aids. Remindings might be used to point out to learners how irrelevant similarities affect their behavior. Although I do not believe one can avoid noticing by superficial similarity, careful instruction may provide the novice with tools that could lead to more appropriate remindings and less use of inappropriate remindings. The basic idea is that instruction on how to separate superficial and structural aspects of problems can have a number of potential benefits. I briefly mention three possibilities as illustrations. (a) Novices could learn to compare any example they were reminded of to the current problem to insure that the superficial similarities do not lead them to use an inappropriate earlier example. (b) Novices could make better use of appropriate remindings if they knew how to compare problems so as to lead to useful generalizations. They could be given instruction on how to set up correspondences and identify superficial aspects that can be generalized over. (c) When a test problem has left them at an impasse, novices could be taught how to look for structural aspects that might increase appropriate and useful remindings. It seems likely that learners will always make use of earlier examples, so techniques for helping them to use appropriate examples in a useful way might significantly improve learning.

Conclusion

In this chapter, I have examined the remindings of earlier examples that occur during the learning of a new cognitive skill and how they might be used. The first part of the chapter, "Remindings in learning," dealt with trying to understand how these remindings are noticed and used and what their effects are on later performance, by providing details on noticing, reconstruction, and analogy, as well as the effects on later tests. Three reasons were offered for why the study of remindings is important. First, because these remindings appear to be a common means novices use in solving problems, any account of the learning of a new cognitive skill will need to incorporate them. Second, the remindings affect performance not only on the current problem but on later problems as well. Third, this research allows an examination of some interesting processes. Although the type of knowledge being studied, an earlier example, is very restricted, the processes required include memory retrieval, reconstruction, analogy, and generalization. Each of these processes is often studied separately, but this research is trying to understand better how these processes affect each other. As examples, the interaction of reconstruction and analogical processes has been mentioned, as well as preliminary data on how what is noticed might affect how it is used (i.e., types of remindings).

The second part, "Remindings in instruction," contained some brief speculations as to how remindings might be used as instructional tools. Although the effects of remindings within an instructional program are not yet known, I hope that future work will address this issue. In addition, instruction about the distinction of superficial and structural similarity and how it might be exploited in problem solving may prove useful for helping students to learn a new domain.

In ending, I would like to mention an integrative theme that has emerged from the many interesting studies of problem solving and learning which are well represented in this volume. That integration stems from a combination of ideas on problem solving and learning. As the work on problem solving moved away from isolated puzzles and became more dependent upon the problem solver's knowledge and as the work on learning began to deal with cognitive skills, the two areas of research had a number of important issues in common. This combination has helped to further ideas on analogies and their effects, as well as on how similarities might affect problem solving and learning.

NOTES

The research reported in this paper was supported by National Science Foundation Grant IST–8308670. Preparation of the manuscript was aided by this grant and an appointment as a Beckman Fellow to the University of Illinois Center for Advanced Study. I thank Doug Medin and Cheri Sullivan for their comments on an earlier version. I also thank Dedre Gentner and Doug Medin for their discussions of this research and Michael Sofka for his contributions.

1 Although one could argue about whether any particular correspondence is natural or not, all that is important is that the probability of setting up the appropriate correspondence with the study example be less than in the same/same condition and that the probability of setting up the inappropriate correspondence be less than in the same/reversed condition.
2 In some experiments, subjects are asked to "talk aloud" during their problem solving (adapted from Ericsson & Simon, 1984, pp. 376–377).

REFERENCES

Anderson, J. R. (1986). Knowledge compilation: The general learning mechanism. In R. S. Michalski, J. G. Carbonell, & T. M. Mitchell (Eds.), *Machine learning: An artificial intelligence approach* (Vol. 2, pp. 289–310). Los Altos, CA: Kaufmann.
Anderson, J. R., Boyle, C. F., Farrell, R., & Reiser, B. (1984). Cognitive principles in the design of computer tutors. *Proceedings of the Sixth Annual Conference of the Cognitive Science Society*. Boulder, CO.
Anderson, J.R., Farrell, R., & Sauers, R. (1984). Learning to program in LISP. *Cognitive Science, 8*, 87–129.
Bartlett, F. C. (1932). *Remembering: A study in experimental and social psychology*. Cambridge: Cambridge University Press.

Brown, A. L., Bransford, J. D., Ferrara, R. A., & Campione, J. C. (1983). Learning, remembering, and understanding. In J. H. Flavell & E. M. Markman, *Handbook of Child Psychology* (Vol. 3, pp. 77–166). New York: Wiley.

Carbonell, J. G. (1983). Learning by analogy: Formulating and generalizing plans from past experience. In R. S. Michalski, J. G. Carbonell, & T. M. Mitchell (Eds.) *Machine learning: An artificial intelligence approach* (Vol. I, 137–161). Palo Alto, CA: Tioga.

Chi, M. T. H., Feltovich, P. J., & Glaser, R. (1981). Categorization and representation of physics problems by experts and novices. *Cognitive Science, 5,* 121–152.

Dellarosa, D. (1985). Abstraction of problem-type schemata through problem comparison (Rep. No. 146). Boulder: Univeristy of Colorado, Institute of Cognitive Science.

Ericsson, K. A., & Simon, H. A. (1984). *Protocol analysis: Verbal reports as data.* Cambridge, MA: MIT Press.

Gentner, D. (1980). *The structure of analogical models in science* (BBN Rep. No. 4451). Cambridge, MA: Bolt, Beranek & Newman.

Gentner, D. (1983). Structure-mapping: A theoretical framework for analogy. *Cognitive Science, 7,* 155–170.

Gentner, D., & Landers, R. (1985, November). Analogical reminding: A good match is hard to find. *Proceedings of the International Conference on Systems, Man, and Cybernetics,* Tucson, AZ.

Gick, M. L. (1986). Problem-solving strategies. *Educational Psychologist, 21,* 99–120.

Gick, M. L., & Holyoak, K. J. (1980). Analogical problem solving. *Cognitive Psychology, 12,* 306–355.

Gick, M. L., & Holyoak, K. J. (1983). Schema induction and analogical transfer. *Cognitive Psychology, 15,* 1–38.

Gick, M. L., & Holyoak, K. J. (1987). The cognitive basis of knowledge transfer. In S. M. Cormier & J. D. Hagman (Eds.), *Transfer of learning: Contemporary research and applications.* Orlando, FL: Academic Press.

Halasz, F., & Moran, T. P. (1982). Analogy considered harmful. *Proceedings of the Human Factors in Computer Systems Conference.* Gaithersburg, MD.

Hayes-Roth, B., & Hayes-Roth, F. (1979). Cognitive processes in planning. *Cognitive Science, 3,* 275–310.

Hinsley, D. A., Hayes, J. R., & Simon, H. A. (1977). From words to equations: Meaning and representation in algebra word problems. In M. A. Just & P. A. Carpenter (Eds.), *Cognitive processes in comprehension* (pp. 89–106). Hillsdale, NJ: Erlbaum.

Holyoak, K. J. (1985). The pragmatics of analogical transfer. In G. H. Bower (Ed.), *The psychology of learning and motivation: Advances in research and theory* (Vol. 19, pp. 59–87). New York: Academic Press.

Jacoby, L. J. & Brooks, L. R. (1984). Non-analytic cognition: Memory, perception, and concept learning. In G. H. Bower (Ed.), *The psychology of learning and motivation: Advances in research and theory* (Vol. 18, pp. 1–47). New York: Academic Press.

Kernighan, B. W. (1979). A tutorial introduction to the UNIX text editor. In *Unix Programmers Manual* (7th ed.), Bell Laboratories.

Kolodner, J. L. (1983). Reconstructive memory: A computer model. *Cognitive Science, 7,* 281–328.

Kolodner, J. L., Simpson, R. L., & Sycara-Cyranski, K. (1985). A process model of case-based reasoning in problem-solving. *Proceedings of the Ninth International Joint Conference on Artificial Intelligence*. Los Angeles.

Langley, P., & Simon, H. A. (1981). The central role of learning in cognition. In J. R. Anderson (Ed.), *Cognitive skills and their acquisition* (pp. 361–380). Hillsdale, NJ: Erlbaum.

Larkin, J. H. (1981). Enriching formal knowledge: A model for learning to solve textbook physics problems. In J. R. Anderson (Ed.), *Cognitive skills and their acquisition* (pp.311–334). Hillsdale, NJ: Erlbaum.

Lewis, M. W., & Anderson, J. R. (1985). Discrimination of operator schemata in problem solving: Learning from examples. *Cognitive Psychology, 17*, 26–65.

Mayer, R. E. (1981). Frequency norms and structural analysis of algebra word problems into families, categories, and templates. *Instructional Science, 10*, 135–175.

Mayer, R. E. (1982). Memory for algebra story problems. *Journal of Educational Psychology, 74*, 199–216.

Novick, L. R. (1986). *Analogical transfer in expert and novice problem solvers.* Unpublished doctoral dissertation, Stanford University.

Pirolli, P. L., & Anderson, J. R. (1985). The role of learning from examples in the acquisition of recursive programming skill. *Canadian Journal of Psychology, 39*, 240–272.

Polya, G. (1945). *How to solve it.* Princeton, NJ: Princeton University Press.

Raaijmakers, J. G. W. & Shiffrin, R. M. (1981). Search of associative memory. *Psychological Review, 88*, 93–134.

Reed, S. K., Dempster, A., & Ettinger, M. (1985). Usefulness of analogous solutions for solving algebra word problems. *Journal of Experimental Psychology: Learning Memory, and Cognition, 11*, 106–125.

Riesbeck, C. K. (1981). Failure-driven reminding for incremental learning. *Proceedings of the Seventh International Joint Conference on Artificial Intelligence*, Vancouver, B. C.

Ross, B. H. (1984). Remindings and their effects in learning a cognitive skill. *Cognitive Psychology, 16*, 371–416.

Ross, B. H. (1987). This is like that: The use of earlier problems and the separation of similarity effects. *Journal of Experimental Psychology: Learning, Memory, and Cognition, 13*, 629–639.

Ross, B. H. (1988). *Learning from the use of earlier examples during problem solving.* Manuscript submitted for publication.

Ross, B. H., & Moran, T. P. (1983). Remindings in learning a text editor. *Proceedings of CHI'83 Human Factors in Computing Systems* (pp. 222–225). Boston.

Ross, B. H., & Sofka, M. D. (1986). *Remindings: Noticing, remembering, and using specific knowledge of earlier problems.* Unpublished manuscript, University of Illinois, Department of Psychology, Urbana-Champaign.

Rumelhart, D. E., & Norman, D. A. (1981). Analogical processes in learning. In J. R. Anderson (Ed.), *Cognitive skills and their acquisition* (pp. 335–359). Hillsdale, NJ: Erlbaum.

Schank, R. C. (1982). *Dynamic memory.* Cambridge: Cambridge University Press.

Silver, E. A. (1979). Student perceptions of relatedness among mathematical verbal problems. *Journal of Mathematical Education, 10*, 195–210.

Silver, E. A. (1981). Recall of mathematical information: Solving related problems. *Journal for Research in Mathematics Education, 12,* 54–64.

Sweller, J., & Cooper, G. A. (1985). The use of worked examples as a substitute for problem solving in learning algebra. *Cognition and Instruction, 2,* 59–89.

Sweller, J., Mawer, R. F., & Howe, W. (1982). Consequences of history-cued and means–end strategies in problem solving. *American Journal of Psychology, 95,* 455–483.

Terrace, H. S. (1963). Discrimination learning with and without errors. *Journal of Experimental Analysis of Behavior, 6,* 1–27.

Welford, A. T. (1958). *Ageing and human skill.* Westport, CT: Greenwood, Press.

Wickelgren, W. A. (1974). *How to solve problems: Elements of a theory of problems and problem solving.* San Francisco: Freeman.

Williams, M., & Hollan, J. D. (1981). The process of retrieval from very long-term memory. *Cognitive Science, 5,* 87–119.

Winston, P. H. (1980). Learning and reasoning by analogy. *Communications of the Association for Computing Machinery, 23,* 689–703.

17

New approaches to instruction: because wisdom can't be told

JOHN D. BRANSFORD, JEFFERY J. FRANKS,
NANCY J. VYE, and ROBERT D. SHERWOOD

The subtitle of this chapter is borrowed from an article published in 1940 by Charles L. Gragg. He begins with the following quotation from Balzac:

> So he had grown rich at last, and thought to transmit to his only son all the cut-and-dried experience which he himself had purchased at the price of his lost illusions; a noble last illusion of age.

Except for the part about growing rich, we find that Balzac's ideas fit our experiences quite well. In our roles as parents, friends, supervisors, and professional educators we frequently attempt to prepare people for the future by imparting the wisdom gleaned from our own experiences. Sometimes our efforts are rewarded, but we are often less successful than we would like to be and we need to understand why.

Our goal in this chapter is to examine the task of preparing people for the future by exploring the notion that wisdom can't be told. Our arguments are divided into four parts.

First, we consider in more detail the notion that wisdom cannot be told. The argument is *not* that people are unable to learn from being shown or told. Clearly, we can remind people of important sets of information and tell them new information, and they can often tell it back to us. However, this provides no guarantee that people will develop the kinds of sensitivities necessary to use relevant information in new situations. Several sets of experiments will be used to illustrate how instructional procedures that result in learning in the sense of being able to recall relevant information provide no guarantee that people will spontaneously use it later on.

Second, we discuss some successful attempts to facilitate the spontaneous use of relevant information. These involve the use of problem-oriented learning environments, rather than the mere presentation of factual information. These data emphasize the importance of enhancing the similarity between the problem-solving environments used during training and the problem-solving processes that will be necessary at the time of transfer. We also present data that suggest that these are similarities in *problem-solving* requirements. Problem-solving similarities seem less important when the task is intentional recall rather than problem solving.

Third, we note that assessments of similarities change as a function of the development of expertise and that novices need to become sensitive to features and dimensions that otherwise might escape their attention. Many approaches to instruction fail to develop these sensitivities. As a result, novices frequently fail to appreciate how new situations are similar to ones encountered before.

Finally, we discuss how an emphasis on the importance of noticing relevant features of problem situations can be translated into recommendations for instruction. We argue that new advances in technology make it possible to teach in new and more effective ways.

The problem of inert knowledge

As noted earlier, the idea that "wisdom can't be told" does not imply that people are unable to learn something by being told or by being shown examples. As an illustration, consider college students who are taught about problem solving from the perspective of the IDEAL model. This model emphasizes the importance of *I*dentifying and *D*efining problems, *E*xploring strategies for solution, *A*cting on the basis of strategies, and *L*ooking at the effects (Bransford & Stein, 1984). The model is based on the wisdom of pioneers such as Dewey (1933), Wertheimer (1959), Polya (1957), and Newell and Simon (1972), so it seems worth teaching. Students find that the material is easy to learn; all of them can paraphrase the model and provide examples of its usefulness. They have, therefore, learned something by being told. Nevertheless, after several years of teaching from this problem-solving model, it has become clear that there are numerous instances in which students could profit from the model yet fail to use it. For example, unless explicitly prompted to do so, students may fail to realize how attempts to formulate the topic of a paper relate to discussions of problem identification and definition. They can think *about* the model, but they tend not to "think in terms of the model" (Bransford, Nitsch & Franks, 1977) or "think with" the model (Broudy, 1977). The model has not become what we shall call a *conceptual tool* (Bransford & Stein, 1984).

Bereiter (1984) provides an additional illustration of failure to utilize important information. He notes that a teacher of educational psychology gave her students a long, difficult article and told them they had 10 minutes to learn as much as they could about it. Almost without exception, the students began with the first sentence of the article and read as far as they could until the time was up. Later, when discussing the strategies, the students acknowledged that they knew better than simply to begin reading. They had all had classes that taught them to skim for main ideas, consult section headings, and so forth. But they did not spontaneously use this knowledge when it would have helped.

The problem of knowing something but failing to use it when it is relevant is ubiquitous. Many years ago, Alfred Whitehead (1929) warned about the dangers of *inert knowledge* – knowledge that is accessed only in a restricted set of contexts even though it is applicable to a wide variety of domains. He also argued that traditional educational practice tended to produce knowledge that remained inert (see also Bereiter & Scardamalia, 1985; Brown & Campione, 1981).

An implication of Whitehead's position is that some ways of imparting information result in knowledge that is not especially accessible. As an illustration, consider the following question that was posed to college freshmen (Bransford, Sherwood, Kinzer, & Hasselbring, 1987): "Try to remember what you learned about the concept of logarithms. Can you think of any way that they might make problem solving simpler than it would be if they did not exist?"

The college students who were asked this question were able to remember something about logarithms. However, most viewed them only as exercises in math class, rather than as useful inventions that simplify problem solving. These students had not been helped to understand the kinds of problems for which logarithms are useful. It is interesting to contrast their understanding of logarithms with that of the English mathematician Henry Briggs who, in 1624, heralded them as welcome inventions.

Logarithms are numbers invented for the more easy working of questions in arithmetic and geometry. By them all troublesome multiplications are avoided and performed by addition. In a word, all questions not only in arithmetic and geometry but in astronomy also are thereby most plainly and easily answered. [cf. Jacobs, 1982, p. 211]

Imagine telling a modern-day Henry Briggs that he will win prizes depending on the number of multiplication problems he can solve in 4 hours – problems involving very large numbers. He has no access to calculators or computers but can take anything else with him. Briggs will probably take a table of logarithms. In contrast, students who have no understanding of the function of logarithms will not think of such a possibility when confronted with the above-mentioned multiplication tasks. Similarly, many students seem to learn to calculate the answers to physics problems, yet fail to apply their formal physics knowledge when encountering everyday phenomena. They need to learn more about the conditions under which their formal knowledge applies (e.g., di Sessa, 1982).

Studies of access

A number of investigators have begun to conduct controlled studies of relationships between access and the nature and organization of knowledge. For example, studies conducted by Asch (1969), Gick and Holyoak (1980), Simon and Hayes (1977), Perfetto, Bransford, and Franks (1983), Reed, Ernst, and Banerji (1974), and Weisberg, Di Camillo, and Phillips (1978) provide evidence that relevant knowledge often remains inert, even though it is potentially useful.

An experiment conducted by Asch (1969) illustrates how the issue of spontaneous access is related to questions about learning new information. Asch first had subjects study a list of paired-associates until they had mastered all of them (all materials were letter–number pairs such as C-21, F-18, L-34). Following mastery of the first list, subjects were presented with a second list of letter–number pairs to learn. Unknown to the subjects, one pair on the second list (e.g., C-21) was a pair that had been on the first list – the list the subjects had just mastered. Asch was interested in the number of trials it would take to "learn" this old pair compared to new pairs that occurred on the second list. Results indicated that the old pair (e.g., C-21) took just as many trials to learn as did entirely new pairs (e.g., X-28) *if* students failed to notice that the old pair was one they had just learned (63% of them failed to notice). Experiments conducted at Vanderbilt University suggest that this lack of noticing was not due to forgetting. When a group of students was explicitly asked to recognize any old pairs in the new list, recognition scores were almost perfect. There are important differences between explicit, informed memory tests and "uninformed" access to information that was previously acquired.

A number of researchers have also found that knowledge of general *strategies* may remain inert unless people are explicitly prompted to use them. For example, children may be taught to (*a*) organize lists of pictures and words into common categories, (*b*) rehearse the category names during learning, and (*c*) use the names as retrieval cues

Table 17.1. *Problem solving (Trial 1) and memory (Trial 2) for informed versus uninformed groups*

	Trial 1 Problem solving	Trial 2: Memory	
		OLD	NEW
Informed	73%	81%	69%
Uninformed	18%	43%	63%

at time of test. Data indicate that, when the children are explicitly encouraged to use such strategies, their memory performance improves. However, when later provided with new lists and asked to learn them, the children frequently fail to use their clustering strategies spontaneously unless they are explicitly prompted to do so. Their knowledge of relevant strategies remains inert (e.g., Brown, Bransford, Ferrara, & Campione, 1983; Brown, Campione, & Day, 1981).

Other researchers have focused on the degree to which knowledge of the solution to one set of problems enables students to solve analogous problems. Simon and Hayes (1977) note that students who learned how to solve the Tower of Hanoi problem did not spontaneously realize that it is structurally isomorphic to the "tea ceremony" problem. Similarly, Gick and Holyoak (1980) show that, unless students are explicitly prompted to do so, they do not spontaneously use information that they just learned about the solution to the fortress problem to solve an analogous problem (Duncker's X-irradiation problem, 1945).

In the Perfetto et al. studies (1983), an attempt was made to provide students with cues that were very closely related to problems to be solved later. The problems to be solved were "insight" problems such as the following:

> Uriah Fuller, a famous Israeli superpsychic, can tell you the score of any baseball game before the game starts. What is his secret?

> A man living in a small town in the United States married 20 different women in the same town. All are still living, and he has never divorced one of them. Yet, he has broken no law. Can you explain?

Most college students have difficulty answering these questions unless provided with hints or clues. Prior to solving the problems, some students were given clue information that was obviously relevant to each problem's solution. Thus these students first received statements such as "Before it starts the score of any game is 0 to 0"; "A minister marries several people each week." The students were then presented

Table 17.2. *Interference as a function of generate versus read*

Condition	Trial 1	Trial 2 OLD	NEW
Generate	Generate answers to OLDs	41%	72%
Read	Read answers to OLDs	56%	70%

with the problems and explicitly prompted to use the clue information to solve them (we call this group the *informed group*). Their problem-solving performance was excellent. Other students were first presented with the clues and then given the problems, but they were not explicitly prompted to use the clues for problem solution (the *uninformed group*). Their problem-solving performance was very poor. Data from one experiment are presented in Table 17.1. For present purposes, the relevant data are the solution rates for informed versus uninformed subjects on Trial 1.

The data in Table 17.1 also illustrate another pervasive finding in our research. Subjects in the experiment try to solve problems on their own during Trial 1. Prior to Trial 2, those in the uninformed groups are informed that information provided earlier in the experiment is relevant to problem solving. By being informed, subjects improved their performance on Trial 2; they were able to remember many of the problem solutions that were presented to them prior to Trial 1. Nevertheless, there is still evidence for a decrement in their performance on Trial 2.

This decrement is illustrated by the OLD versus NEW columns for Trial 2 in Table 17.1. Note that informed and uninformed subjects are equivalent on NEWs. NEWs are problems that (a) had answers provided in acquisition but (b) were not presented for problem solving in Trial 1. In contrast, OLDs are problems that subjects tried to solve on Trial 1. Here, the uninformed group performs more poorly than the informed group. We argue that the uninformed subjects generate inadequate solutions to the problems on the first trial and that these generated answers interfere with subsequent access to the more appropriate acquisition answers. Informed subjects access the acquisition answers during Trial 1 and thus do not show the interference.

In further research we have shown that the degree of interference depends on the nature of the processing required during Trial 1 (Perfetto, Yearwood, Franks, & Bransford, 1986). Table 17.2 illustrates that interference effects for OLDs on Trial 2 are greater for uninformed subjects who *generate* wrong answers than for a yoked-control group of subjects who read the wrong answers generated by the former subjects. The data suggest that subjects who merely read answers provided by others are more flexible in their processing. They may exceed Generate subjects both in spontaneous noticing of the relevance of the acquisition answers during Trial 1 and in being to able to let go of the inappropriate answers during Trial 2.

Attempts to facilitate spontaneous access

Data demonstrating failures to utilize relevant knowledge have led to questions about ways to facilitate access (e.g., Gick & Holyoak, 1983). One approach has been to increase the similarity between the acquisition information and subsequent test materials (e.g., Stein, Way, Benningsfield, & Hedgecough, 1986). In one study, Stein et al. attempted to increase spontaneous access to information through the use of "copy cues." This involved the placement in the problems to be solved of key words and phrases that were identical to those in the initially presented information about problem solutions. During problem solving, subjects received copy cues in some problems but not in others. Somewhat to their surprise, the presence of copy cues facilitated performance on copy-cue items but actually hurt performance on the non-copy-cue items.

In another series of experiments, Stein et al. attempted to facilitate spontaneous access by providing subjects with preexposure to the problems prior to acquisition. There was some evidence that preexposure did indeed help spontaneous access in some cases. However, there was also evidence of a counterbalancing negative effect on performance due to interference from inadequate answers generated during the prior problem solving.

Our most successful and theoretically interesting attempt to facilitate spontaneous access involves the use of problem-oriented acquisition experiences. In the studies described above, the information was generally presented as descriptions of facts to be learned. Under these conditions, students failed to access the relevant information unless explicitly prompted to do so. Theorists such as John Dewey (1933) and Norman Hanson (1970) argue that students need to understand how new information can function as a tool that makes it easier to solve subsequent problems. Similarly, modern theories that emphasize organized knowledge structures focus on the importance of acquiring "conditionalized knowledge" – knowledge that includes information about the conditions and constraints of its use (e.g., An-

Table 17.3. _Problem-oriented versus fact-oriented acquisition_

		Trial 2	
Condition	Trial 1	OLD	NEW
Fact-oriented	36%	48%	62%
Problem-oriented	56%	72%	76%

Note: Fact-oriented item: "A minister marries several people each week." Problem-oriented item: "It is common to marry several people each week – if you are a minister."

derson, 1983; Bereiter, 1984; Glaser, 1984, 1985; Simon, 1980; Sternberg & Caruso, 1985).

Our studies (Adams, Kasserman, Yearwood, Perfetto, Bransford, & Franks, 1986) were designed to explore whether problem-oriented activities that help students experience the usefulness of information can facilitate access. We contrasted declarative, fact-oriented processing with a problem-oriented processing condition. The former condition is essentially the same as the acquisition conditions in the studies discussed above. The latter condition engaged subjects in problem solving during acquisition. The conditions merely varied the nature of the items that were rated for comprehension during acquisition. Table 17.3 illustrates the different kinds of acquisition items and also some of the results that were obtained.

Problem-oriented (as compared with fact-oriented) acquisition results in much greater spontaneous use of the acquisition information to aid in problem solving on Trial 1. Furthermore, the fact-oriented group showed much greater interference on OLDs during Trial 2 than did the problem-oriented group. The difference between the NEWs on Trial 2 was in fact not significant, and in follow-up work the difference between the NEW rates was slightly in the opposite direction. This latter result is important because it suggests that the performance differences between fact and problem-oriented processing are not due to memory-strength differences or to some general similarity effects. Such factors would lead to performance differences on NEWs on Trial 2. Rather, the differences seem to be attributable to the greater spontaneous access in the problem-oriented condition.

Additional research on fact- versus problem-oriented processing has demonstrated that the benefits of problem-oriented processing are specific to information processed in this mode; the results are not due to general set effects. In this study, the same subjects received some information in a fact mode and other information in a problem-oriented mode. Spontaneous access occurred only for those problems in which the acquisition information was processed in a problem-oriented format. These results are important because in many studies demonstrating spontaneous access the reason may be that exposure to multiple problems creates momentary set or expectation effects (e.g., see Brown, this volume; Gick & Holyoak, 1983).

We also find that conditions that facilitate access seem to generalize to semantically rich and complex materials involving concepts from science (Sherwood, Kinzer, Bransford, & Franks, 1987). They are not limited to the somewhat artificial insight problems that we used in our initial research. For example, in one experiment college students were provided with 13 short passages about topics that might be encountered in middle school science classes. Examples included topics such as (a) the kinds of high-carbohydrate foods that are healthy versus less healthy, (b) the use of water as a standard for the density of liquids plus the fact that, on earth, a pint of water weighs approximately 1 pound, (c) the possibility of solar-powered airplanes, (d) ways to make a Bronze Age lamp using clay and olive oil.

Students in one condition simply read about each of 13 topics with the intent to remember the information. Those in a second condition read the same information but in the context of problems that might be encountered during a trip to a South American jungle. For example, students in this second condition were first asked to consider the kinds of foods one should bring on a trip and then asked to read the passage about different types of high-carbohydrate foods. Similarly, the passage about the density and weight of water was read in the context of attempts to estimate the weight of fresh water needed for four people for 3 days; the possibility of solar-powered airplanes was discussed in the context of finding transportation in areas where fuel was difficult to obtain, and so on. The goal of this type of presentation was to help students understand some of the kinds of problems that the science information could help them solve.

Following acquisition, all participants received one of two types of tests. For present purposes, the most important was a test of uninformed access. This test was disguised as a filler task to be completed before memory questions would be asked about the previously read topics. Students were asked to imagine that they were planning a journey to a desert area in the western part of the United States and to suggest at least 10 areas of information − more if possible − that would be important for planning and survival. They were also asked to be as explicit as possible. For example, rather than say "You would need food and supplies," they were asked to describe the kinds of food and supplies.

The results were analogous to those reported by Adams et al. (1986) in the experiment described above. Students who had simply read facts about high-carbohydrate foods, the weight of water, and so on, almost never mentioned this information when providing their answers. Instead, their answers tended to be quite general such as "Take food and take fresh water to drink." In contrast, students in the second acquisition condition made excellent use of the information they had just read. When discussing food, for example, most of them focused on the importance of its nutritional contents. When discussing water, they emphasized the importance of calculating its weight. Similarly, constraints on the availability of gasoline versus solar energy were discussed when the importance of transportation (e.g., airplane, car) was mentioned. Overall, students who received information in the context of problem solving were much more likely to use it spontaneously as a basis for creating new sets of plans.

Problem-oriented acquisition and issues of noticing

Taken as a whole, studies of access suggest that students need to understand how concepts and procedures can function as tools for solving relevant problems. Our data suggest that fact-oriented acquisition permits people to remember information when explicitly prompted to do so, but it does not facilitate their ability to use this information spontaneously to solve new problems. These findings support Gragg's original argument in "Wisdom Can't Be Told" (1940). He emphasized that the goal of education was to "prepare students for action," and he proposed to do this by presenting them with cases that illustrate complex business problems. The basic thesis of this approach to instruction seems to be that, when students confront similar problems later, they will be more likely to solve them on their own.

The emphasis on preparing students to solve "similar" problems in the future is not new (e.g., Thorndike, 1913). However, we noted in our earlier discussion of the Adams et al. study (1986) that the constraints on similarity that operate in an intentional memory paradigm are not necessarily equivalent to those that are important for spontaneous access. Furthermore, it seems clear that the same set of events may not appear to be equally similar to different individuals. In the area of physics, for example, experts categorize problems in ways that

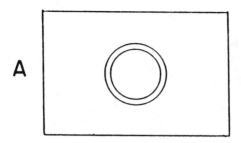

Figure 17.1. A standard stimulus (adapted from Garner, 1974).

differ considerably from novices (Chi, Feltovich, & Glaser, 1981). Similarly, imagine drawings of different structures that may or may not permit flying (e.g., shapes like birds' wings). Assumptions about similarities among these structures have changed considerably as people have developed expertise in areas such as aerodynamics (Hanson, 1970). Illustrations such as these suggest that experts and novices frequently focus on different features of events.

Many years ago, the philosopher Ernst Cassirer (1923) argued that a major problem with many theories is that they presuppose the existence and salience of particular features. In theories of concept formation, for example, the focus was on discarding dissimilar features and retaining only those that were common to members of a concept; little emphasis was placed on the issue of noticing features in the first place. Cassirer argued that, rather than presuppose their existence, it is the noticing of features that must be explained.

Following the lead of Cassirer (1923), Garner (1974), and J. Gibson and E. Gibson (E. Gibson, 1982; J. Gibson, 1977; Gibson & Gibson, 1955), we argue for the importance of focusing on the issue of noticing. Given that experts often notice features of events that escape the attention of novices, how can the learning of novices be enhanced? For example, how can novices be helped to notice relevant features of a current problem that are necessary for recognition of similar problems they may encounter later on?

Perceptual contrasts

The ability to notice relevant features of both acquisition and test events is not easy for novices dealing with complex situations. Modern theories of perceptual learning are important for clarifying how noticing can be facilitated. These theories emphasize the importance of contrasts that allow people to notice features they might otherwise

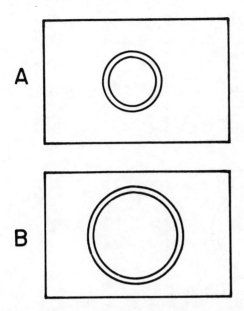

Figure 17.2. The standard in the context of Stimulus B (adapted from Garner, 1974).

miss. A demonstration from Garner's chapter on critical realism provides an excellent illustration of the role of contrasts in noticing (Garner, 1974). He asks readers to look at the stimulus in Figure 17.1 and to assume that the rectangle is simply the border around the figure. He then asks, "How would you describe the figure?" Garner notes that most people describe it as a circle or a circle with two lines. Some may describe it as two concentric circles.

Garner continues his demonstration by considering the same figure (we shall call it the standard, designated by *A* in Figure 17.2). However, this time the standard is described in the context of Stimulus B. Now features such as the size of the circle become relevant. When people see the standard in isolation, they generally fail to mention anything about size.

Garner continues his demonstration by considering the standard in a new context such as Stimuli C and B in Figure 17.3. Now features such as the location of the circles within the border become salient. Garner notes that one could continue indefinitely so that additional features become salient – features such as the thickness of the lines, the fact that the lines are solid rather than broken, the color of the ink. Garner's conclusion from his demonstration is that the single

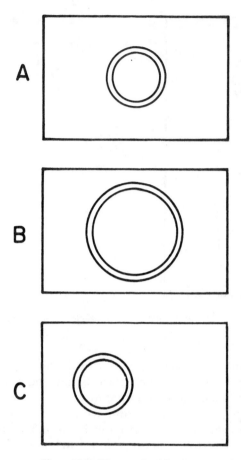

Figure 17.3. The standard in the context of Stimuli B and C (adapted from Garner, 1974).

stimulus has no meaning except in the context of alternatives. These contrasts affect the features that one notices about events. The emphasis here is quite different from theories of discrimination learning that focus primarily on learning which features are "positive" and which are "negative" (e.g., Levine, 1975). Such theories are important, but they presuppose the salience of features rather than ask how features are noticed in the first place. The ability to notice relevant and often subtle features is a consistent characteristic of expertise in a domain (e.g., Bransford, Sherwood, Vye, & Rieser, 1986; Chase & Simon, 1973; Siegler, 1986).

Verbal contrasts

Contrasts can occur with verbal as well as visual materials. For example, in pilot studies designed to be an analog of the Garner demonstration, we asked subjects to describe the relevant features of a "general and a fortress" story similar to the one used in the access research conducted by Gick and Holyoak (1980). Features mentioned included the fact that the general won the battle by dividing his forces. However, most subjects did not spontaneously mention more subtle aspects of the situation such as the location of the fortress relative to a surrounding community of farmers, yet it was this feature that made a divide-and-conquer strategy necessary.

The features mentioned by subjects were quite different when the target story was presented with two contrasting stories about a general and a fortress. In one story, the fortress was not surrounded by farmers, so it was possible to explode a set of land mines by shooting boulders with a catapult (there were no farmers in the vicinity to be harmed). In another version, the fortress was surrounded by farmers, but the general did not use a divide-and-conquer strategy and his plan failed. In the context of alternative stories, critical features of the target story were noticed by subjects. They appeared to understand the problem situation at a more precise level than did those subjects who simply read the same target story three times. Ongoing research is exploring the effects of these contrasts on subsequent problem solving.

Contrasts seem to play an important role in the success of the problem-oriented acquisition studies that were described earlier. For example, consider the first part of a problem-oriented statement such as "It is easy to walk on water." Subjects are aware that the statement seems false, but most are unaware that this is due to a basic assumption they are making, namely, that the water is in liquid form. When they next hear "if it is frozen," the idea that water can take a number of forms becomes salient. When subjects later encounter problems that hinge on similar information about alternative states of water, they are much more likely to notice the ambiguities and hence solve the problems than are those who receive only fact-oriented acquisition information such as "Water can be frozen to form ice." In general, we assume that experts in a particular domain have experienced a range of situations that provide relevant contrasts. In Garner's (1974) terminology, the experiences of the experts provide internal contexts of alternatives that enable them to notice and understand important features that novices often miss.

The importance of perceptual learning

An emphasis on the use of contrasts to facilitate noticing suggests another concern. To what extent do typical approaches to instruction and testing help people learn to notice the types of features that will be important in their everyday environments? We argue that even problem-oriented instruction often takes place in contexts that are too dissimilar from those that students will encounter later on.

This latter point can be clarified by returning to an earlier part of our discussion. There, we argued that a common form of instruction involves attempts to prepare people for the future by telling them what they might experience and how to deal with it. As a somewhat far-fetched example, imagine a parent trying to help her 20-year-old son acquire the procedural knowledge (Anderson, 1983) necessary to deal with problems in restaurants, such as when to accept versus reject a wine he orders with his meal. The parent may attempt to help the son learn by providing problems such as: "Imagine that you sip the wine and it tastes overly dry and brittle. What should you do?" Clearly, a novice can learn to respond appropriately to a verbal vignette such as this, but that does not mean that he can actually identify instances of dry and brittle wine. Similarly, clinical students are often trained to assign diagnoses based on verbal vignettes. Thus a patient might be described as "slightly defensive," "moderately depressed," and so forth, and students might learn to assign a diagnosis. However, once these students enter everyday practice and see real patients, they are often at a loss. They have not learned to recognize symptoms such as "slightly defensive" and "moderately depressed" on their own. Because of the exclusive reliance on verbal vignettes, the students have received clues that represent *the output of an expert's pattern recognition process.* In order to perceive the relevant features of wines, clients, and other situations, a great deal of perceptual learning must occur. This requires experiences with a set of contrasts so that the features of particular events become salient by virtue of their differentiation from other possible events (see also Simon, 1980).

The importance of providing perceptually based contrasts can be illustrated by considering a typical attempt to teach someone new information. A common method involves "telling," either orally or through the use of text. For example, elsewhere we discuss a text that used contrasts to attempt to teach children about different types of Indian houses (Bransford, 1984). It contained statements such as "The Indians of the Northwest Coast lived in slant-roofed houses made of cedar plank. . . . Some California Indian tribes lived in simple, earth-covered or brush shelters. . . . The Plains Indians lived mainly in tee-pees," and so on. This type of information seems quite arbitrary to the novice. It is unclear why each house has the features that it does (in the Gibsons' terminology, the affordances are unclear). For example, novices may fail to understand how features such as portability relate to the life styles of different tribes of Indians, how features such as earth-covered and slant-roofed relate to factors such as temperature and rainfall, availability of raw materials, and so forth. Arbitrary contrasts such as these occur quite frequently, but they are far from ideal.

Consider an attempt to teach about different types of houses that more carefully provides information about structure and function (note that here we are providing a contrast to the preceding scenario). In this example we focus on stationary houses (rather than teepees) that have different designs depending on different sets of needs.

The first house is designed to accommodate needs created by living in a cold, northern climate. This house is equipped with a large chimney because the house has back-to-back fireplaces in the living and family rooms. The fireplaces provide a cheap, supplemental heat source during the long and cold winter.

The second house was custom-built with tall doors. Tall doors were installed for the owner who is 6 feet, 8 inches tall, and a professional basketball player.

The third house is located in the southern Gulf Coast area of the country. Standard features of houses in the region are large-capacity gutters. These are necessary during spring and summer when the likelihood of heavy rains and flash flooding is high.

The fourth house is equipped with a large window in the living room that provides added light. This is a cheerful environment for the occupants, who enjoy spending time together.

The fifth house is designed with large families in mind. It contains a large den where family members can comfortably gather.

The sixth house has a large kitchen window. The owners of the house spend a great deal of time in the kitchen because they are gourmet cooks. The window affords added light and a pleasant view.

Given the ability to study the preceding descriptions, students can learn a considerable amount from them. For example, if given a verbal description of a house (e.g., large chimney, special gutter, or large kitchen window), they will be able to identify the type of house (e.g., designed for the cold North, the rainy South, or an avid cook).

There are also limitations of the preceding approach to instruction. In particular, assume that we teach information about house design

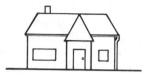

Figure 17.4. A standard house.

in the context of verbal descriptions from a text or lecture and then send our students out into the field. They will frequently encounter actual houses and pictures of houses rather than verbal descriptions, and they will often be unprepared to deal with these. Our students may often feel that our instruction "did not prepare them for the real world."

As an illustration, consider the picture of the house illustrated in Figure 17.4. How would you describe its relevant features? What was it designed for? Basically, you cannot tell. Even though you read the previous verbal descriptions, and even though you could identify different houses based on verbal descriptions of them, you have not been prepared to deal with drawings of the houses or with actual houses. You cannot tell whether the house in Figure 17.4 has the big chimney or the regular chimney, the big windows or the small windows, and so on, because since these must be defined relative to alternatives or contrast sets. Your verbally based training involved cues such as "big chimney," "smaller windows," which represent the *output* of an expert's pattern recognition processes; you have had no training in the perceptual learning necessary for pattern recognition and hence have a difficult time transferring your previously acquired knowledge. With different approaches to instruction, much of the necessary information could have been supplied in the context of formal instruction. This should reduce transfer problems later on.

Procedures for improving instruction in our demonstration involving house designs seem clear: Provide drawings of each house during instruction, and help students discover how various features become salient as a function of the context of alternatives. In addition, help students understand why each house is designed in a particular way. Figure 17.5 illustrates several different houses plus an indication of what they were designed for. People who explore these drawings begin to discover a number of features that would tend to remain unnoticed if only a single house had been observed. Readers should be able to experience these noticings for themselves by comparing the houses in Figure 17.5.

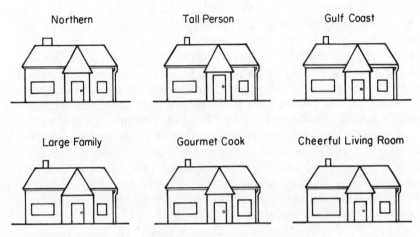

Figure 17.5. A format for discovering important features.

Implications for instruction

The idea of helping people notice relevant features and dimensions of information by providing a series of contrasts seems so straightforward that it may appear mundane. Don't most people teach this way? Our answer is, "Yes, occasionally, but generally no." Several examples are provided below.

Example 1. Consider first the part of our demonstration experiment with houses that involved the use of verbal scenarios for training. We argued that students can learn to deal with these yet fail to develop the abilities necessary to function in the everyday world. Elsewhere, we claim that problems such as these arise in a number of settings (e.g., Bransford, Sherwood, Vye, & Rieser, 1986). As already mentioned, clinical psychologists are often trained to diagnose cases based on verbal descriptions of symptoms and behaviors. They can learn to do this in the classroom context but once they enter the real world of therapy they need to develop the sensitivities necessary to recognize patterns (e.g., of "anxiety," "defensiveness," etc.) that previously were described verbally. Similarly, it is one thing to understand the importance of a client's definitions of his or her problems but quite a different matter to notice such behavior in the context of a therapy session.

We could, of course, show films in order to facilitate learning – and instructors often do. For example, in conjunction with Dan Rock at

Vanderbilt University, we have been informally exploring the benefits of viewing tapes depicting therapy sessions in order to teach people about therapy. The tapes are useful, but it is also clear that novices do not really know what to look for in them. An instructor can stop the tape and point out various events (e.g., "Notice how the client is defining her problem; notice how the therapist is responding to the client"), and this can facilitate noticing. Nevertheless, there are limits to this approach. The expert, by virtue of a wealth of experiences, has a powerful set of contrasts (e.g., other therapist styles and client styles) that set the stage for noticing important features of the interaction. The novice learner lacks such contrasts and hence lacks a clear understanding of suggestions such as "Notice the therapist's style here." In an analogous manner, imagine seeing only one house from our house demonstration (e.g., Figure 17.4) and being told "Notice the chimney" or even "Notice the large chimney." Without experience with other houses in the contrast set, one's perceptions lack the precision that is characteristic of the expert.

With new technology, it is possible to use video in ways that are more likely to help students discover features and dimensions of information that are informative. In particular, with random-access videotape and videodisc technology, parts of videos can be accessed almost instantly; hence, different segments can be compared. For example, in the therapy tape that Dan Rock is working with, there are some striking contrasts between the client's definition of her problem early in therapy and near the end of the 50-minute session. It is extremely useful to isolate these segments, let students compare them, and see how their noticings evolve. Similarly, the therapist's responses to the client change considerably throughout the course of the therapy. Segments of these provide an informative contrast set.

A particularly nice feature of a contrast-set approach to instruction is that people can experience the difference in their own perceptions and understandings – just as, on a simpler level, people can experience the noticings that occur with our demonstration involving houses. Furthermore, these types of activities set the stage for unanticipated discoveries. For example, our colleague Rich Johnson is working on a project with young children that involves videotaping them while they watch segments from the movie *Swiss Family Robinson*. He began working with 5-year-olds, and we were all fascinated to see the children's intense interest in the film as they watched it during the experiments. However, Rich then filmed some 7-year-olds watching the same tape and noticed a difference in their behavior. They, too, were intensely interested in the film segment, but they laughed aloud at certain scenes – scenes that in retrospect were funny (to adults) but relatively subtle. These differences would probably not have been noticed if Rich had worked only either with 5-year-olds or 7-year-olds. Of course, developmental researchers who have worked with children of various ages could probably have told us this information. Nevertheless, simply being told about these differences is not the same as discovering them for oneself.

Example 2. If seems useful to explore the idea of contrast-set teaching in more detail by contrasting it with a second illustration of typical approaches to teaching. For this illustration, we consider the first chapter of Gage and Berliner's *Educational Psychology* (1984). This chapter discusses characteristics of good teachers and begins by asking people to try to remember characteristics of good teachers and poor teachers they have had and to compare the two (they therefore attempt to create a contrast set). The chapter is well written and quite good as far as texts go, but there are several disadvantages with such a procedure. First, many people may have poor memories of good and poor teachers. Even more important, whatever memories they have will presumably include only those features that they noticed at earlier points in their lives. There are undoubtedly many subtleties of good versus poor teaching that were not noticed by individuals. If one relies only on memories, it is hard for new noticings to occur.

Imagine an alternative approach to teaching about teaching. Assume that we have relatively short video segments of a teacher doing a fair job of teaching something. We then see the teacher doing a worse job, a better job, and so forth. With appropriate contrasts, new insights into components of effective teaching should emerge. For example, a teacher's lag time after asking questions could emerge as a relevant feature, given some types of contrasts. Different types of nonverbal communication and their effects on impressions of the teacher could become apparent as well. This invitation to notice new features as a function of contrast sets is quite different from the typical approach, which simply lists characteristics of good versus poor teachers. It should result in a better ability to notice important characteristics of classroom events.

The use of contrast sets should result in even more powerful learning if students are helped to view them from a multiplicity of perspectives. Many traditional methods of instruction do not encourage students to take multiple perspectives on the same set of events; hence, they do not promote multiple access to a variety of relevant concepts. For example, most texts on educational psychology contain different chapters on motivation, cognitive development, the nature of testing, instruction, processes underlying learning, and so forth. Each of the chapters provides examples, but students usually receive *a different example for each concept.* This is very different from the experience of seeing how a variety of different concepts can apply to the same event or set of events.

An emphasis on the application of multiple concepts to the same set of events is a characteristic of case methods of instruction. For example, in Gragg's (1940) approach students are presented with complex cases involving businesses and are asked to use a variety of concepts in order to solve important business problems. These methods of instruction are quite different from standard forms of instruction because the case methods attempt to facilitate multiple access (e.g., Gragg, 1940; Spiro, Feltovich, Coulson, & Anderson, this volume). The goal is to have students bring a multitude of perspectives to bear on a single case. Even here, however, the instruction has been verbally based rather than verbally plus perceptually based. As noted earlier, verbally based instruction often contains clues that represent the output of experts' pattern recognition processes. When these clues are removed, novices often fail to perform effectively because they have not developed the perceptual sensitivities necessary to notice important features of complex events.

As a thought experiment (we plan to conduct actual experiments soon), imagine simulating traditional approaches to instruction by asking students to read 14 short passages describing different concepts such as research on attention, the degree to which people are often unaware of aspects of their own behavior, the general nature and purpose of educational assessment tasks, and so on. Each passage includes examples, but the examples differ for each concept that is discussed.

Contrast the traditional format of instruction with one that encourages students to apply each of the 14 concepts to a common set of exemplars involving videotapes of teaching segments. These can be used to illustrate concepts such as research on attention (children in our tapes frequently need to have guidance with respect to their attention), the degree to which people are often unaware of their own behavior (several of our teachers on video were not aware of mistakes they were making), effects of previously acquired knowledge of performance on assessment tasks (people who view our tapes invariably make inferences about children's general abilities), the concept of "scaffolding" (this involves teaching activities that continually assess the child's current level of functioning), and so forth.

A third form of instruction could encourage the kinds of multiple access emphasized in the preceding paragraph, but the instruction would be purely verbal. No visual segments would be used.

After acquisition, assume that students in all three groups – the standard acquisition group, the video-based multiple-access group, and the verbally based multiple-access group – receive (a) verbal tests and (b) video tests (the latter involve new videos of teaching segments, and students are asked to describe what they notice about these segments). For the verbal tests that ask about individual concepts, we suspect that all three forms of instruction will result in equivalent performance. For verbally described problem-solving situations that require the application of knowledge, we expect the two case-oriented, multiple-access groups to perform better than the standard instructional group. When the test involves video segments, the video-based multiple-access condition should produce the best performance. Students in this condition should be better able to notice important features of complex situations – features that involve access to a variety of concepts that were learned. Advantages of the video-based multiple-access condition should be most pronounced under conditions of uninformed access; for example, under conditions in which subjects are asked to comment on new video segments that they believe are filler tasks or are unrelated to the experiment. These are the kinds of conditions that students will often face when they leave the classroom. If they fail to notice important features of the situation, they will fail to access information that is relevant for solving problems they may face.

Conclusion

Our goal in this chapter has been to explore the idea of preparing students for the future. As Gragg (1940) notes, a typical form of instruction is simply to tell people facts and principles that one day may be important. Gragg argues against this approach because "wisdom can't be told."

We have tried to clarify the claim that wisdom can't be told by relating it to existing literature in cognitive psychology. Our argument was that telling works to some extent, but it has drawbacks as well. The drawbacks are that people can frequently tell information back to us when explicitly prompted yet they fail to use relevant information in unprompted problem-solving situations. In Whitehead's terminology (1929), their knowledge remains inert. Several laboratory demonstrations of inert knowledge were reviewed.

We also discussed studies that explored ways to overcome the inert knowledge problem. The use of problem-oriented acquisition activities had important effects on people's propensities to use spontaneously what they had learned. These results provide support for Gragg's (1940) arguments. In order to prepare students for future action, Gragg felt that they needed to experience problem situations that were similar to ones they might encounter later. We emphasized that this similarity was along a dimension of problem-solving requirements. When we used measures involving intentional memory rather than problem solving, fact-oriented versus problem-oriented acquisition had no measurable effects.

The emphasis on problem-oriented acquisition led to concerns with another issue involving similarity. Experts' perceptions of similarity often differ from those of novices. In order to facilitate the development of expertise, novices must be helped to notice the important features of various situations. However, we also argued that novices are often trained in ways that fail to facilitate subsequent noticing. For example, when we present novices with verbally described problems, the descriptions often contain verbal clues (e.g., the client is "mildly defensive") that represent the output of experts' pattern recognition processes. When these clues are absent, novices are unable to perceive problem situations in useful ways.

In the final section of this chapter we considered how new approaches to instruction might facilitate people's abilities to develop usable knowledge. New technology such as random-access videodisc technology makes it possible to use a perceptual learning approach with sets of semantically rich materials. Through exposure to relevant sets of contrasts, students can be helped to notice important features of events that they might otherwise miss. A major assumption underlying this approach is that, through a variety of experiences, experts have experienced sets of contrasts that provide internal contexts of alternatives (cf. Garner, 1974) for perceiving subsequent events. However, the contrasts experienced by experts are often haphazard due to the nonsystematic nature of their training and experience. It is hoped that, through systematic exposure to sets of relevant contrasts, the development of expertise can occur in a shorter time span than would normally be the case. Of course, the use of random-access videodiscs is merely one way to facilitate the development of expertise. We have emphasized the value of videodiscs for noticing *visual* features, but many other sources of information can be important for guiding our actions (e.g., what we hear, feel emotionally, touch, taste, etc.). Contrasts can be helpful for any modality.

An important issue for this volume involves the degree to which a general concept of similarity can provide a guide for the design of effective instructional environments. Given important constraints, we think that it can. The constraints involve the fact that there are many possible ways to define similarity. For example, it seems clear that similarities in wordings between facts at acquisition and facts at test can facilitate access, but the goal of education goes considerably beyond attempts to help people retrieve facts.

As noted above, we argue that the important similarities to pursue are similarities in *requirements for problem solving*. Like Gragg (1940), we assume that the most important goal of education is to prepare students for action – to prepare them to use relevant knowledge to solve important problems. The best way to do this is, presumably, to provide students with problem-solving experiences that are similar to situations they will encounter later on. An emphasis on similaritites in problem-solving requirements has a number of implications for the design of educational experiences.

First, fact-oriented acquisition does not involve problem solving. It falls far short of the goal of providing experiences that are similar to problem-solving situations that students may encounter later in their lives.

Second, problem-solving practice that is based exclusively on verbal problems is often quite dissimilar to the kinds of conditions that will be encountered in everyday practice. In particular, we noted that verbally communicated problems often contain words that act as cues for access. These cues represent the output of experts' pattern recognition processes. If students do not develop similar competencies – competencies that are often based on nonconscious processes (e.g., Lewicki, 1986) – their ability to notice relevant features of new situations will be impaired.

Third, an important part of everyday problem solving involves *discovery* and *problem finding* (e.g., Bransford & Stein, 1984; Sternberg, 1985). Even visually based presentations of problems will not necessarily develop the skills required to find and discover important features, issues, and questions. For example, when video is used people frequently employ a "tell and show" technique. They mention a concept verbally and then show students an example ("Next I want to show you this Gulf Coast house with the extra-large guttering"). This approach is quite different from one in which students are helped to discover features on their own. Similarly, students can be encouraged to use video as a context for creating their own problems and issues (see Bransford, Sherwood, & Hasselbring, 1986). This problem-generation approach to learning emphasizes features of problem solving that will almost undoubtedly be important later in life.

Related to the third point is a fourth one. Problem-solving situations often seem overwhelming and frustrating when they are initially encountered. People with experience can often deal with these situations because they have "been there before." They realize that, eventually, their feelings of being overwhelmed by complexity and frustration will change. However, these types of realizations presumably involve experiences with change; they are not the types of beliefs that come simply from being told that "things will get better." Perhaps the most important implication of Gragg's notion that wisdom can't be told is its emphasis on the importance of *experiencing the changes* (contrasts) in our perceptions, understandings, beliefs, and feelings as a function of new information. Perhaps wisdom arises from the opportunity to experience changes in our own beliefs and assumptions – changes that help us realize that the ideas and priorities that seem so clear today will probably be modified as a function of new experiences. These realizations seem healthy. They help us maintain some degree of humility with respect to our current beliefs, and they provide us with the conviction that we will not run out of things to discover and understand.

NOTE

Research reported in this paper was supported by Contract MDA903–84–C–0128 from the Army Research Institute. We are grateful to Beverly Conner for her outstanding editorial help.

REFERENCES

Adams, L., Kasserman, J., Yearwood, A., Perfetto, G., Bransford, J., & Franks, J. (1986). *The effects of fact versus problem-oriented acquisition.* Unpublished manuscript, Vanderbilt University, Department of Psychology, Nashville.
Anderson, J. R. (1983). *The architecture of cognition.* Cambridge, MA: Harvard University Press.
Asch, S. E. (1969). A reformulation of the problem of associations. *American Psychologist, 24,* 92–102.
Bereiter, C. (1984). How to keep thinking skills from going the way of all frills. *Educational Leadership, 42,* 75–77.
Bereiter, C., & Scardamalia, M. (1985). Cognitive coping strategies and the problem of "inert" knowledge. In S. F. Chipman, J. W. Segal, & R. Glaser (Eds.), *Thinking and learning skills: Current research and open questions* (Vol. 2, pp. 65–80). Hillsdale, NJ: Erlbaum.

Bransford, J. D. (1984). Schema activation versus schema acquisition. In R. C. Anderson, J. Osborn, & R. Tierney (Eds.), *Learning to read in American schools: Basal readers and content texts* (pp. 259–272). Hillsdale, NJ: Erlbaum.

Bransford, J. D., Nitsch, K. E., & Franks, J. J. (1977). Schooling and the facilitation of knowing. In R. C. Anderson, R. J. Spiro, & W. E. Montague (Eds.), *Schooling and the acquisition of knowledge* (pp. 31–55). Hillsdale, NJ: Erlbaum.

Bransford, J. D., Sherwood, R. S., & Hasselbring, T. (1986). *Computers, videodiscs, and the teaching of thinking* (Tech. Rep. 86.1.1). Nashville, TN: Peabody College, Vanderbilt University.

Bransford, J. D., Sherwood, R. D., Kinzer, C. K., & Hasselbring, T. S. (1987). Macro-contexts for learning: Initial findings and issues. *Applied Cognitive Psychology, 1,* 93–108.

Bransford, J. D., Sherwood, R., Vye, N. J., & Rieser, J. (1986). Teaching thinking and problem solving: Suggestions from research. *American Psychologist, 41,* 1078–1089.

Bransford, J. D., & Stein, B. S. (1984). *The IDEAL problem solver.* New York: Freeman.

Briggs, H. (1624). *Arithmetica Logarithmica.*

Broudy, H. S. (1977). Types of knowledge and purposes of education. In R. C. Anderson, R. J. Spiro, & W. E. Montague (Eds.), *Schooling and the acquisition of knowledge* (pp. 1–17). Hillsdale, NJ: Erlbaum.

Brown, A. L., Bransford, J. D., Ferrara, R. A., & Campione, J. C. (1983). Learning, remembering, and understanding. In J. H. Flavell & E. M. Markman (Eds.), *Carmichael's manual of child psychology* (Vol. 1, pp. 77–166). New York: Wiley.

Brown, A. L., & Campione, J. C. (1981). Inducing flexible thinking: A problem of access. In M. Friedman, J. P. Das, & N. O'Connor (Eds.), *Intelligence and learning* (pp. 515–530). New York: Plenum Press.

Brown, A. L., Campione, J. C., & Day, J. D. (1981). Learning to learn: On training students to learn from texts. *Educational Researcher, 10,* 14–21.

Cassirer, E. (1923). *Substance and function.* Chicago: Open Court.

Chase, W. G., & Simon, H. A. (1973). The mind's eye in chess. In W. G. Chase (Ed.), *Visual information processing* (pp. 215–281). New York: Academic Press.

Chi, M. T. H., Feltovich, P. J., & Glaser, R. (1981). Categorization and representation of physics problems by experts and novices. *Cognitive Science, 5,* 121–152.

Dewey, J. (1933). *How we think* (rev. ed.). Boston: Heath.

di Sessa, A. A. (1982). Unlearning Aristotelian physics: A study of knowledge-based learning. *Cognitive Science, 6,* 37–75.

Duncker, K. (1945). On problem solving. *Psychological Monographs, 58* (Whole No. 270).

Gage, N. L., & Berliner, D. C. (1984). *Educational psychology* (3rd ed.). Boston: Houghton Mifflin.

Garner, W. R. (1974). *The processing of information and structure.* Potomac, MD: Erlbaum.

Gibson, E. J. (1982). The concept of affordances in development: The renaissance of functionalism. In W. A. Collings (Ed.), *The concept of devel-*

opment: The Minnesota symposium on child psychology (Vol. 15, pp. 55–81). Hillsdale, NJ: Erlbaum.

Gibson, J. J. (1977). The theory of affordances. In R. E. Shaw & J. D. Bransford (Eds.), *Perceiving, acting, and knowing: Toward an ecological psychology* (pp. 67–82). Hillsdale, NJ: Erlbaum.

Gibson, J., & Gibson, E. (1955). Perceptual learning: Differentiation or enrichment. *Psychological Review, 62*, 32–51.

Gick, M. L., & Holyoak, K. J. (1980). Analogical problem solving. *Cognitive Psychology, 12*, 306–355.

Gick, M. L., & Holyoak, K. J. (1983). Schema induction and analogical transfer. *Cognitive Psychology, 15*, 1–38.

Glaser, R. (1984). Education and thinking: The role of knowledge. *American Psychologist, 39*, 93–104.

Glaser, R. (1985). All's well that begins and ends with both knowledge and process: A reply to Sternberg. *American Psychologist, 40*, 573–574.

Gragg, C. L. (1940, October 19). Wisdom can't be told. *Harvard Alumni Bulletin*.

Hanson, N. R. (1970). A picture theory of theory meaning. In R. G. Colodny (Ed.), *The nature and function of scientific theories* (pp. 233–274). Pittsburgh: University of Pittsburgh Press.

Jacobs, H. R. (1982). *Mathematics: A human endeavor* (2nd ed.). New York: Freeman.

Levine, M. (1975). *A cognitive theory of learning*. Hillsdale, NJ: Erlbaum.

Lewicki, P. (1986). *Nonconscious social information processing*. Orlando, FL: Academic Press.

Newell, A., & Simon, H. A. (1972). *Human problem solving*. Englewood Cliffs, NJ: Prentice-Hall.

Perfetto, B. A., Bransford, J. D., & Franks, J. J. (1983). Constraints on access in a problem solving context. *Memory & Cognition, 11*, 24–31.

Perfetto, G., Yearwood, A., Franks, J. J., & Bransford, J. (1986). *The effects of generation on memory access*. Unpublished manuscript, Vanderbilt University, Department of Psychology, Nashville.

Polya, G. (1957). *How to solve it*. Princeton, NJ: Princeton University Press.

Reed, S. K., Ernst, G. W., & Banerji, R. (1974). The role of analogy in transfer between similar problem states. *Cognitive Psychology, 6*, 436–450.

Sherwood, R. D., Kinzer, C. K., Bransford, J. D., & Franks, J. J. (1987). Some benefits of creating macro-contexts for science instruction: Initial findings. *Journal of Research in Science Teaching, 24*, 417–435.

✓ Siegler, R. S. (1986). *Children's thinking*. Englewood Cliffs, NJ: Prentice-Hall.

Simon, H. A. (1980). Problem solving and education. In D. T. Tuma & R. Reif (Eds.), *Problem solving and education: Issues in teaching and research* (pp. 81–96). Hillsdale, NJ: Erlbaum.

Simon, H. A., & Hayes, J. R. (1977). Psychological differences among problem isomorphs. In N. J. Castelan, D. B. Pisoni, & G. R. Potts (Eds.), *Cognitive theory* (Vol. 2). Hillsdale, NJ: Erlbaum.

Stein, B. S., Way, K. R., Benningsfield, S. E., & Hedgecough, C. D. (1986). Transfer in problem solving tasks. *Memory & Cognition, 14*, 432–441.

Sternberg, R. J. (1985). Teaching critical thinking: 1: Are we making critical mistakes? *Phi Delta Kappan, 67*, 194–198.

Sternberg, R. J., & Caruso, D. R. (1985). Practical modes of knowing. In E.

Eisner & K. J. Rehage (Eds.), *Learning and teaching: The ways of knowing.* Chicago: University of Chicago Press.

Thorndike, E. L. (1913). *Educational psychology* (Vols. 1 & 2). New York: Columbia University Press.

Weisberg, R., DiCamillo, M. & Phillips, D. (1978). Transferring old associations to new situations: A nonautomatic process. *Journal of Verbal Learning and Verbal Behavior, 17*, 219–228.

Wertheimer, M. (1959). *Productive thinking.* New York: Harper & Row.

Whitehead, A. N. (1929). *The aims of education.* New York: Macmillan.

18

Multiple analogies for complex concepts: antidotes for analogy-induced misconception in advanced knowledge acquisition

RAND J. SPIRO, PAUL J. FELTOVICH,
RICHARD L. COULSON, and
DANIEL K. ANDERSON

Few would disagree that analogy is an important tool in the acquisition of new knowledge. Indeed, work in cognitive science and educational psychology in the last dozen years provides ample evidence of the usefulness of analogy in learning and has substantially advanced our understanding of the psychological mechanisms responsible for that utility (e.g., Burstein, 1986; Carbonell, 1986; Collins & Gentner, 1987; Gentner, 1983; Gentner & Gentner, 1983; Gick & Holyoak, 1980; Rumelhart & Norman, 1981; Vosniadou & Ortony, 1983). Yet, as this chapter will demonstrate, the use of analogies in learning is far from straightforward and, surprisingly, often results in deeply held erroneous knowledge.

Our intention is to offer a more temporized and cautionary alternative to the general enthusiasm for learning by analogy, especially in its most common form: the use of a single mapping between a source and a target concept (the "topic") – what we shall refer to as a *single analogy*. (For exceptions that address more complex uses of analogy, see Burstein, 1986; Collins & Gentner, 1987). We argue that simple analogies that help novices to gain a preliminary grasp of difficult, complex concepts may later become serious *impediments* to fuller and more correct understandings. Specifically, although simple analogies rarely if ever form the basis for a full understanding of a newly encountered concept, there is nevertheless a powerful tendency for learners to continue to limit their understanding to just those aspects of the new concept covered by its mapping from the old one. Analogies seduce learners into reducing complex concepts to a simpler and more familiar analogical core.

Our position is not antagonistic to analogy; again, there is no doubt-

498

ing the value of apt analogies in introducing unfamiliar concepts. However, we are not as sanguine about the benefits of single analogies at later, more advanced stages of learning about complex concepts. Therefore, sensing an unhealthy imbalance in the attention devoted to the nature and benefits of analogical learning, we attempt to address some of the more neglected hazards. On a more positive note, we discuss *two antidotes* for what we have found to be an insidious tendency of analogies to block more advanced knowledge acquisition: (a) Pay more attention to the ways that analogies fail or mislead or are incomplete; learners and teachers are more likely to be able to avoid pitfalls if they have explicit warning of what those pitfalls are. And (b) employ integrated multiple analogies to convey more of the necessary complexity of difficult concepts; the more complex and ill-structured the new concept, the greater the need for a finely tuned synthesis of the relations between it and *several* already known concepts.

Overview

We begin with a brief introduction to the overarching orientation that guides our remarks on analogy. Then, in the first main section of the chapter we illustrate the danger of misuse of single analogies in the learning of complex concepts, using examples drawn from the biomedical domain. We demonstrate several common misconceptions held by medical students that are traceable to a cognitive (and sometimes instructional) overreliance on single analogies. Eight varieties of analogy-induced misconception are identified. We then examine the circumstances of learning and instruction that promote the uncritical acceptance and entrenchment of learning based on inadequate analogies.

The second section of the chapter presents our approach to the use of multiple analogies to capture correctly, yet manageably, the complexity of difficult concepts and illustrates the approach with the example of force production by muscle fibers. In this approach, multiple additional analogies are chosen to correct the problems introduced by any single analogy, without canceling its beneficial effects. In order to mitigate the additional cognitive load that multiple analogies introduce in learning, we describe a technique for context-dependent *selective and contingent composite imaging* of the productive features of the multiple analogies.

In the third major section we present a more detailed picture of the variety of ways that adding analogies can affect the earlier learning outcomes derived from previously encountered analogies. We develop a nine-part taxonomy of the functions of new analogies and modifications of old analogies in promoting understanding.

Thus the three primary sections of the chapter can be thought of as addressing (a) what can go wrong in the use of single analogies (and often does); (b) how a set of multiple analogies can counter the hazards of single analogies and how such a set should be selected, integrated, and psychologically managed; and (c) the various functions in promoting understanding accomplished by combining analogies.

The perspective of advanced knowledge acquisition

The work on analogy that we discuss in this chapter is part of a larger program of research concerned with *advanced knowledge acquisition.* Detailed accounts of our theory of advanced knowledge acquisition in complex and ill-structured domains and applications of the theory to topics other than analogy may be found in Coulson, Feltovich, and Spiro (1986); Feltovich, Coulson, and Spiro (1986); Feltovich, Spiro, and Coulson (in press); Spiro (in press); Spiro, Feltovich, and Coulson (1988); Spiro and Jehng (in press); Spiro and Myers (1984, last two sections); and Spiro, Vispoel, Schmitz, Samarapungavan, and Boerger (1987). Here we present just a bare sketch of some general issues. At the end of the chapter, we situate the analogy research within our encompassing theoretical orientation. The use of analogy is just one area of cognition and instruction critically affected by the relative complexity of the material to be learned. Our theoretical approach to the problems posed by complexity takes a similar generic form whether the concern is with analogies, prototype examples, schemata, or overall organizational schemes for the presentation of large bodies of material.

Advanced knowledge acquisition refers to the learning that follows initiation into the rudiments of a knowledge domain and precedes the attainment of expertise. This intermediate stage, falling between the novice and the expert, is often neglected. We argue that this neglect has serious consequences because the aims of advanced knowledge acquisition are different from those of introductory learning, and those differing aims are best attained by qualitatively opposed means – what helps at the introductory stage may hurt at the advanced stage, and vice versa. In other words, success at the introductory stage may sometimes result in forms of entrenched fundamental understanding that interfere with the eventual attainment of expertise.

The main aims of advanced knowledge acquisition are: (a) *mastery of complexity*, the acquisition of those aspects of conceptual complexity that are necessary for a correct understanding of important concepts (rather than the attainment of a superficial familiarity with simplified versions of concepts, which is often the goal at introductory stages of learning in a knowledge domain); and, relatedly, (b) *knowledge applicability*, development of the ability to apply or transfer acquired knowledge adaptively, especially to realistic situations, as those situations present aspects of novelty (rather than merely being able to reproduce content material from memory in just the way that it was learned, the criterion too often employed at all stages of learning).

The present chapter is concerned with the first aim. We report on misconceptions held by advanced learners (medical students) that involve a failure to master important complexities in concepts (because of interference from an analogy); and we present an approach to mental representation, learning, and instruction that is designed expressly to address the difficulties posed by complexity. (Although full apprehension of conceptual complexities is often a necessary but not sufficient condition of knowledge application – the second aim – that issue is not addressed here.) Of course, not all concepts are so important that their complexities must be mastered. However, at some stage in knowledge acquisition a point is reached where certain concepts are so central that they must be correctly understood. Furthermore, we argue that the complexities of a knowledge domain become much more centrally important to the extent that that knowledge must be *applied* in unconstrained, naturally occurring situations (rather than learned in the abstract or for application in artificial instructional settings). At some point during the progress of learning in a content area, it becomes important that the learner "get it right," even if the associated difficulties place burdensome demands on learners and teachers.

To insure our not being misunderstood, it is worth repeating at this point that we are not advocates of complication for its own sake. Well-structured subject matter can and should be taught in much simpler ways than we recommend for complex and ill-structured material; every kind of reductive use of analogy that we criticize has a counterpart that is a strategy for *usefully* stripping away complexities – either at the early stages of learning some topic (especially for learners who will not be going further in a subject area) or when complicating factors are not especially important. Furthermore, we realize that the *premature* introduction of complexity may confuse learners. However, we do argue that complexity should be introduced as soon as learners are ready for it, because early simple frameworks often act as impediments to grasping complexities introduced later (as we shall see in the next section). Furthermore, new approaches to learning and instruction are now being developed that will advance the time at which learners are ready to deal with complexity – that is, procedures are being created for making the learning and instruction of complex information more tractable at an earlier stage of knowledge acquisition. One example of such a procedure is the use of integrated multiple analogies, made psychologically manageable with composite images; this procedure is dealt with at length in the section, "Antidotes for analogy-driven misconception."

The reductive force of analogy and analogy-induced misconceptions

Those who study analogy offer frequent reminders that the useful applicability of an analogy is never total; only some relational aspects of a *source* domain may be transported to a target domain (the *topic*). For example, only a subset of the relationships in the domain *solar system* are representative of the domain of *atoms* (Gentner & Gentner, 1983). Although this point is obvious to those who study analogy, it unfortunately fails to characterize the state of affairs with respect to the actual employment of analogies in learning and instruction. In fact, as we shall see, there is evidence that analogies exert a powerful "reductive force": When a striking, pedagogically efficient analogy is employed that incompletely represents some target of understanding, the incomplete representation often remains as the *only* representation of the target concept. We have found that misconceptions attributable to the reductive effect of analogies occur even when teachers and texts are explicit in stressing the inadequacy of an analogy. In other words, when analogies are used to "start simple," the knowledge ultimately acquired often *stays* simple. Well-intended analogies often result in *oversimplified knowledge*.

Analogy-induced misconception: a typology of varieties, with biomedical examples

We have used directed, open-ended discussion probes to assess medical students' knowledge. (The probe procedure is discussed in Coulson et al., 1986, and in Feltovich et al., in press.) The probes have uncovered several instances of commonly held misconceptions connected to cognitive and instructional aspects of the use of analogies.

We shall simply refer to these misconceptions without presenting methodological details and specific results of the various studies that they have been culled from (i.e., the examples of analogy-induced misconception have been taken from research in which issues related to analogy happened to emerge in the context of probes with a more open-ended focus or a focus directed toward matters other than analogy). More detailed treatments of the misconceptions discussed here and the procedures in the studies that revealed them are available elsewhere (Coulson et al., 1986; Feltovich et al., 1986, in press; Spiro et al., 1987).

Eight ways that analogies can induce misconceptions are identified below. Each type is illustrated by an example of a biomedical misconception that we have observed to be common among medical students (and, occasionally, among physicians and popular medical textbooks). Since the analogy-based misconceptions involve very technical subject matter, our characterizations will stress the form or structure of the fallacious knowledge and how it develops, rather than going into the specific content of the misconception. (Again, references in which more substantive discussions are provided for each misconception have already been supplied.)

All of the examples have two features in common: (a) The source (or base) domain information in the analogy is inadequate or potentially misleading for understanding the target domain (the topic); and (b) in practice, the knowledge acquired about the topic is reduced to just that information mapped by (inadequate) analogy from the source domain. This includes both incorrect *overextensions* from the source (derived from misleading aspects) and *omissions* in the source of information important for understanding the topic.

This list of types of analogy-induced misconception is intended to call attention to such effects of analogy and, as a step toward prevention, to provide a somewhat detailed analysis of the forms in which these deleterious effects are manifest, thereby making learners and teachers more alert to their occurrence. It is not claimed that the eight types identified form an exhaustive list or that some misconceptions may not be characterizable according to more than one type. Also, the order in which the types are presented is dictated primarily by sequencing requirements related to the biomedical examples, rather than by any natural ordering of the misconception types.

1. Indirectly misleading properties. Some salient characteristic of the source domain that is not central to the pedagogical point of the analogy adversely influences understanding of a parallel characteristic

504   SPIRO, FELTOVICH, COULSON, ANDERSON

in the topic domain. Roughly put in schema-theoretic terms, there is a prominent variable "slot" in the source domain that has a different instantiation in the topic domain (Rumelhart, 1980). As will become clear after the following example, it is not the case that the slot's value is changed in the topic domain to be identical to its value in the source; rather, misconceptions develop regarding the topic that derive from properties *entailed* by the mismatched slot instantiation in the source.

Example: A common analogy used to teach opposition to blood flow (impedance) uses rigid pipe systems such as household plumbing as the source domain. This analogy promotes understanding of that aspect of impedance due to resistance, which primarily depends on the radius of the vessel. However, unlike plumbing pipes, blood vessels are flexible. Related to that flexibility is an additional source of impedance, compliant reactance. Further, a third source of impedance exists, inertial reactance, which also derives from the pulsatile (beating) nature of the heart, accelerating the mass of blood on every beat. These latter two forms of impedance are jointly referred to as reactance. Aspects of impedance that involve reactances are frequently misunderstood by medical students (Feltovich et al., 1986, in press). The misunderstandings take the form of either ignoring reactance or (mistakenly) reinterpreting reactance phenomena in terms of their limited aspects that bear resemblance to resistance (where, again, resistance is the only aspect of impedance supported by the plumbing analogy). For example, compliance (the stretchiness of vessels – related to compliant reactance) is erroneously thought to contribute to impedance through the ability of a stretchy vessel to change radius and thereby affect resistance; and blood density, which directly affects inertance (and inertial reactance), is either neglected by students or equated with blood viscosity, which is, again, a contributor to resistance. This family of misconceptions connected to the rigid-pipes analogy occurs despite the fact that students usually are exposed to a complete account of the factors contributing to impedance.

It is very important to note that the students do *not* have the misconception that blood vessels are rigid. The misconceptions that we have referred to come from those aspects of the analogy to household plumbing pipes that are *entailed* by their rigidity. So, for example, the rigidity of plumbing pipes (as well as the constant, as opposed to pulsatile, pressure head that is usually associated with plumbing) makes resistance the only factor substantially opposing flow, and misconceptions about impedance to blood flow tend to involve the erroneous conversion of nonresistance phenomena to ones that are resistancelike. Thus the effects of the misleading slot instantiation in the source (rigidity) on the development of misconceptions of the topics are *indirect*. Of course, there may be cases where the learner mistakenly adopts for the topic domain the actual value of a mismatching variable slot from the source domain. This is more likely to happen when the instantiation of the variable slot is not especially important or salient (in contrast to the obvious actual flexibility associated with blood vessels).

2. Missing properties. An important aspect or characteristic of the topic domain has no counterpart in the source domain, and that missing aspect or characteristic does not get incorporated in the understanding of the topic.

Example: Medical students frequently have trouble attaining a sophisticated understanding of pressure in the cardiovascular system. A contributing factor is, again, the analogy to household plumbing, water taps, and so on. Because these more familiar fluid systems have a constant pressure head, there is no need in these systems to think about the variable acceleration of water. When the plumbing analogy is used in the heart domain, this missing aspect leads students to omit from their thinking contributions to blood pressure deriving from the pulsatile acceleration of blood. The conception of pressure and the factors that influence it are thereby reduced to ones that would be captured by analogy to Ohm's law applied to plumbing.

3. Exportation of base-domain properties. A salient characteristic of the source domain that has no analog in the topic domain is nevertheless exported to the topic. A nonexistent slot is *created* in the topic to correspond to a slot in the source.

Example: Starling's relationship between end diastolic *volume* in the heart and cardiac *output* is seen as analogous to the relationship between the *length* to which an individual muscle fiber is stretched and the *tension* it can produce. This is partly because the graphs of both relationships (volume–output and length–tension) have similar ascending left limbs and plateaus. However, whereas the length–tension relationship for an individual (skeletal) fiber has a descending limb reflecting decreased tension at long lengths, the Starling relationship (in the *in vivo* heart) has no corresponding descending limb at large volumes. A common error made by medical students, physicians, and some medical texts is to assume that the Starling relationship has a descending right limb like that of the length–tension curve for skeletal muscle (Coulson et al., 1986).

This mistaken importation of the source domain's descending limb has serious consequences: It plays a central role in the development of a major misconception about the nature of congestive heart failure. Heart failure is erroneously attributed to "falling off the plateau of the Starling curve" as the collection of individual muscle fibers gets stretched too far (thus losing tension), resulting in reduced cardiac output, further stretching because of blood accumulation in the heart, further reduced output, and so on. In fact, there are physiological limitations preventing the cardiac muscle fibers from reaching a "descending limb" on the Starling curve (for an *in vivo* heart). In contrast to this misconception, the heart enlarges due to hypertrophic mechanisms while it weakens as a result of the breakdown of muscle activation mechanisms – the heart does not fail because it is getting enlarged (stretched too far), as the analogy to the individual skeletal muscle fiber length–tension relationship mistakenly suggests; it gets enlarged in response to its failing. (See Coulson et al., 1986, for further explication.)

As we shall see in the next subsection, "The analogical bias," length–tension : Starling's volume–output is a false analogy; the circumstances of its mistaken adoption will be discussed later. Our present point only examines its consequences *after* it has been mistakenly adopted.

4. Directly misleading properties. A nonsalient aspect of the source domain in an analogy has a different value than the parallel aspect of the topic domain. The variable slot in the topic is incorrectly assigned the instantiated value of the slot in the source.

Example: Recall the misconception that heart failure is due to collective (ventricular) overstretching of individual muscle fibers, "falling off the plateau of the Starling curve," in much the same way that such falling off could be achieved in an individual skeletal muscle fiber's length–tension curve (Coulson et al., 1986). The correct explanation involves biochemical *activation* or energizing of the components of the system. One reason that activation is neglected by medical students as a possible cause of heart failure is that cardiac muscle fibers are understood by analogy to skeletal muscle fibers. The implicit assumption is that "all striated muscles are alike." In reality, the two kinds of muscles differ greatly in their activational properties, in ways that are important with regard to heart failure. Skeletal muscle always functions at full activation, so that the activation level of the muscle is not an issue. If cardiac muscle is taken to be like skeletal muscle, and the level of activation is not an issue for skeletal muscle, then it follows that activation is not an important issue for cardiac muscle either. Unfortunately, in contrast to skeletal muscle, the degree of activation of cardiac muscle is *variable*. And degree of activation is the key to the correct account of heart failure (in a way that would not be similarly manifested in skeletal muscle failure). The analogy of cardiac to skeletal muscle brings along with it an incorrect instantiation of the variable slot, *type of activation*, and adopting that property of the source domain for the topic has serious ramifications.

5. *Focus on surface descriptive aspects with corresponding mistreatment of underlying causation.* Some analogies are very effective at characterizing surface features and relationships but gloss over underlying causal mechanisms. The result is that learners tend either to fill in a convenient but incorrect causal account of their own or just to leave the causal mechanism unexplained, as a kind of "black box." (It might be said that a comparison based primarily on surface descriptive aspects is more metaphorical than analogical. However, our point here is that an underlying relational structure is indeed transferred – that is, people have a tendency to interpret metaphors analogically.)

Example: The failing heart is often compared by medical students to a stretched-out, saggy balloon (or to overstretched Silly Putty). In fact, this analogy gives a very good picture of representational correlates in the two domains: Both heart and balloon get big, but the heart gains passive tension whereas the balloon loses it. The stretched-out balloon, when underinflated for its enlarged size, exhibits floppy walls (low tension); but in the enlarged heart, although each individual fiber exhibits the low active tension associated with heart failure, the increased mass of the enlarged heart and the decreased compliance of pathological origin allow the bearing of increased tension in the walls (via the law of Laplace). However, the analogy is pitched to mere description and leaves the causal mechanisms in both the balloon and the heart situations unaddressed. Medical students then fill the causal vacuum by employing the convenient assumption that the stretching in the heart causes the failure, as it causes the failure in the balloon. As was indicated earlier, activational problems are responsible for heart failure; enlargement (mistakenly likened to overstretch) is merely a later *consequence* of a variety of processes associated with failure. Correlation can easily be mistaken for causation in this case because causation is not represented in the analogy.

6. *Magnification to the wrong grain size.* An important aspect of the topic domain is missed because the analogy is pitched at the wrong

level of magnification or elaboration. It is not that the source domain does not address the aspect, as in number 2 but, rather, that the analogy is cast in such a way that the relevant aspect is not noticed.

Example: Certain applications of the law of Laplace to lung function are demonstrated using an analogy to soap bubbles. In particular, soap bubbles are used to demonstrate what does *not* happen in the lungs (due to an agent secreted by the lungs called surfactant): Little air sacs of the lung do not empty into larger air sacs, as happens when small and large soap bubbles are in communication. However, it is difficult to understand why this does not happen in the lungs without knowing why it does happen in soap bubbles. And it is here that grain size is a problem. You would need to magnify the structure and dynamics in the *walls* of the soap bubble considerably to appreciate what happens differently in the lungs (due to the surface-tension-lowering effects of surfactant). The magnification would focus on the nature of the wall as two concentric circle layers with fluid in between them. In other words, the important lesson is in the "fine grain" of the soap bubble wall rather than in the typical, grosser image of soap bubbles connected by a pathway.

7. *Misleading properties derived from common language meanings of technical terms.* Ordinary language concepts are often employed analogically as technical terms. Their everyday, "public" connotation is overextended to their technical use in the topic domain.

Example: In its technical usage the "compliance" (stretchiness) of vessels in the cardiovascular system is important because it contributes to the vessels' ability to exchange potential and kinetic energy. This ensures smooth movement of blood under the influence of the pulsatile beating of the heart. Students develop misconceptions that reflect the adoption of analogies for compliance that are consistent with common, ordinary language uses of *compliance* and that clash with its technical meaning. These include analogies of compliance as a "giving way" (surrender) of vessels under the onslaught of blood and even analogies that reflect the vessels' willingness to respond to orders from the nervous system – to, for example, dilate or contract (Feltovich et al., 1986).

(This misconception type, as well as number 8, might be considered to be based more in metaphor than in analogy. However, because the metaphorical descriptions lead to the adoption of specific source exemplars the features of which are mapped to the topic, the designation of these misconception types as analogical seems appropriate.)

8. Misleading properties due to connotations of nontechnical descriptive language. Inappropriate analogies are induced by the loose use of poorly chosen, connotatively loaded nontechnical descriptors.

Example: The arterial vessels and other sections of the circulation system are active contributors to blood flow. During the period of the heart's ejection (systole), blood from the heart is stored under pressure in the distended walls of the arterial vessels so that when the heart is no longer actively ejecting (diastole) the recoil of these elastic vessels continues to propel blood. Perhaps to make a contrast to the period of active ejection of blood from the heart, *diastole* is often referred to loosely in instruction as a period of "runoff" or "drainage." These terms do not convey active motive force but, rather, passive flow from a region of high to low static energy density. Students tend to think of the arterial vessels as passive receptacles and also tend not to consider adequately the active propulsion of blood during diastole, viewpoints more consistent with a notion of passive "seepage" than with the reality of blood flow during diastole.

It is interesting to note that a similar misconception occurs on the venous side of blood circulation due to the use in instruction of such language as "pooling" of blood in the veins, a term that carries the connotation of stagnation or lack of interaction with the surround. Students develop the notion that some major components can (at least temporarily) be removed from the active stream of circulation. Components of the venous circulation take on characteristics of reservoirs, "pools" that can be augmented and drained according to circumstantial needs for blood delivery but that are not continuous parts of the overall circulation of blood.

Multiple-based misconceptions. A single analogy may in fact lead to a variety of misconceptions, each involving a different influence from the list above.

Example: The analogy of a rowing crew is commonly used to represent the functioning of the contractile units (sarcomeres) of muscle fibers. This analogy captures some aspects of the topic domain of muscle function well, particularly anatomic aspects of force production by oarlike ratcheting elements within the fiber. At the same time, the analogy (*a*) *indirectly misleads* (number 1) with regard to some aspects of muscle ultrastructural function (e.g., conveying erroneously that the force-producing units act in synchrony); (*b*) *misses* (number 2) some aspects (e.g., sarcomere characteristics related to their width as opposed to their length); and (*c*) *exports* (number 3) still other misleading aspects (e.g., the idea that the force-generating units can get entangled and thus fail to produce force). Much more will be said about the strengths and weaknesses of this particular analogy in the section on multiple analogies.

Summary of analogy-induced misconception. Several ways that analogy can induce misconceptions have been presented. Although they differ in many respects, they have in common the characteristic that students' understanding of a topic domain is too exclusively determined by properties of an analogous source domain. In the various ways that we have illustrated, the mental representation of the topic domain is *reduced* to the source domain. It is in that sense that the misconceptions involve *reductive analogies*. In the next section we address the influences that contribute to the ready acceptance of analogical reductions.

The analogical bias: patterns of psychological support for the uncritical acceptance of deficient analogies

Where do maladaptively reductive analogies originate? We have observed three sources. In the first, teachers and textbook authors recognize the pedagogical value of analogies in introducing difficult concepts and employ a conventional analogy for just that introductory purpose (while providing disclaimers about the limitations of the analogy and descriptions of appropriate corrections). They then find that their students have simplified their understanding of later, more advanced treatments of the concept to just what was covered by the introductory analogy. The second source is teachers and textbook authors who themselves have misconceptions. These may be associated with mistaking conventional approaches to introducing a complex concept for complete accounts of the concept. In the third scenario, learners independently adopt analogies that, despite being both unconventional and incorrect, are nevertheless seductive in some way.

However, regardless of their origin, reductive analogies all share certain features. All of the scenarios involve a *bias* to overrely on analogies: in the first case by students/learners in their implicit strategies for assimilating externally provided instructional information, in the second case by teachers, and in the third case by students/learners as regards their self-generated cognitive strategies. A further feature of the reductive analogies that we have observed is that they seem to lull the learner into an unquestioning acceptance that leads to a durable entrenchment of the misconception. Why, then, are maladaptively reductive analogies so readily adopted and so durably held? We will offer a partial account of the factors contributing to this bias, including its motivational origins and the methods implicitly employed for its self-justification. We will take an example of the third kind, an inappropriate analogy that is frequently adopted spontaneously. Understanding the sources of such especially maladaptive analogies will also provide clues to why reductive analogies seem to be held so uncritically; that is why they are so *seductive* of the belief that a full and accurate understanding has been achieved.

Support for false analogy in the Starling length–tension example. The *length–tension* relationship of a single skeletal muscle fiber (studied in the laboratory, isolated from other muscles it normally interacts with *in vivo*) is essentially *irrelevant* to Starling's relationship between ventricular *volume* and cardiac *output* for the *whole* heart in vivo. (See the earlier discussion of number 3 in the typology of ways analogies induce misconceptions.) Thus, when people adopt the analogy they are doing it largely on their own. Despite its irrelevance, students give no sign that they consider the analogy at all controversial. What contributes to this unquestioning acceptance? More specifically, why would students want the analogy to be a useful one, and what causes them not to be suspicious of it? The following is a partial set of contributing forces.

1. *Bolstering due to similar-appearing objects*: Volume is like length; force that produces ventricular (cardiac) output is like tension.

2. *Bolstering due to similar-appearing relations*: The graph of the relationship between cardiac volume and output (Starling) has a similar shape to that of the relationship between skeletal muscle length and tension; they both have ascending slopes to a plateau.

3. *Reciprocating effects of separate bolstering elements*: The extent to which the similar-appearing objects in the source and the topic bolster the analogy (number 1) is increased by the fact that those similar objects also have a similar pattern of relationship in the source and the topic (number 2). In a circular fashion, each is used to increase the credibility of the other.

4. *Bolstering due to assumptions of ontological similarity*: Why does it sound so initially plausible that the collective function of muscle fibers in the whole heart would be analogous to that of individual, isolated muscle fibers? Here we have what can fairly be described as a fundamental ontological assumption about the natural world, namely, that the world is structured in such a way that it is legitimately reducible by analogy: *Wholes are like parts*. The relational functioning of

collections of fibers will be analogous to that of individual fibers (even though the objects involved, hearts and heart muscle cells, are markedly dissimilar): They will have the same-shaped curve mapping their size aspects (i.e., length/volume) to their force aspects (i.e., tension/output), and the latter relationship will have the same theoretical explanation invoking the same mechanism (in particular, the sliding-filament theory of muscle contraction; see Coulson et al., 1986).

Note further that this ontological bias can be reached through presuppositions deriving from two different ways of theorizing about the world: organicism and mechanism (Pepper, 1942). Organicist accounts are noted for their attention to the symmetry of relationships found in microcosms and macrocosms (here, wholes are like parts). Mechanistic accounts would reach the same conclusion via such presuppositions as additivity and atomism: The collective Starling function "sums over" individual fiber length–tension functions (additivity); and individual fibers function the same when placed in context (in vivo) as when they are studied in isolation (atomism; i.e., the primary units of analysis are the individual components of a system and not the whole system itself – a fundamental bias of mechanistic approaches).

5. Indirect bolstering by convenience of explanation: In students' learning about heart failure, the well-known sliding-filament account of the length–tension relationship has a plausible-sounding (but incorrect) extension to volume–output relationships in the heart. In other words, you don't need to learn a new underlying mechanism. Furthermore, you get to use a well-learned concept; the situation is akin to that of the person trying to improve his or her vocabulary who learns a new word and then orchestrates opportunities to use it. The conveniently overextended sliding-filament theory then invokes a theme of over-stretching for heart failure that (misleadingly) corresponds to a prominent and well-known clinical sign of heart failure, enlargement.

In fact, as we have discussed, heart failure has more to do with biochemical *activational* or energizing operations than with mechanical and anatomical (stretching) causes, a point that has implications for number 6.

6. Indirect bolstering by elimination of potential analogy blockers: We have seen that activational/energizing operations are neglected in favor of mechanical overstretching operations (sliding-filament theory), in the account of heart failure commonly proffered by medical students and by some physicians and popular textbooks. This elimination of activation cleans up a bit of potential untidiness in adopting the length–tension : volume–output (Starling) analogy. The absence of an activational component reinforces the idea that only mechanical factors are involved, and are involved in the same way, in the production of the two curves. That is, if heart failure is a mechanical phenomenon, and it is caused by "falling off the Starling curve," then mechanical rather than activational factors account for Starling. This consideration of Starling as being entirely mechanical makes it easy to ignore fundamental differences between the length–tension relationship and the Starling relationship that are due to the role of activation. Without an understanding of the differential roles of activation in the two curves, the length–tension : volume–output analogy gains strength.

But how does activation become neglected in the first place? One contributing factor is presented in number 7.

7. *Bolstering due to shared name:* Degree of activation of muscle is not an issue if cardiac muscle is taken to be like skeletal, since skeletal muscle fibers always function at *full activation* (tetanic activation). So, if cardiac is like skeletal, variable activation is not an issue. Unfortunately, in this respect cardiac muscle fibers are *not* analogous to skeletal – the former are in fact *variably activated* (twitch activation).

So the analogy between length–tension and volume–output is supported by the overreliance on the analogy of skeletal and cardiac muscle, which in turn is supported by the implicit (and reductive) bias that is described in the heading of this subsection and may be roughly instantiated in the present case as the belief that "all muscles are alike."

This neglect of activation in the cardiac volume–output relationship of course contributes to the mistaken acceptance of the length–tension : volume–output (Starling) analogy; without activation as an alternative account of volume–output and heart failure, volume–output is left with no competition for the mechanical overstretching account derived from the length–tension relationship.

8. *Bolstering due to overall convergence of support*: When many factors converge to support an analogy, as in the present length–tension : volume–output (Starling) example, the analogy is bolstered to a greater degree than if it had fewer supporting factors. "If so many things point to it, it must be right."

Summary

We have argued in this section that (a) single analogies induce misconceptions involving the reduction of the topic domain to the source, and (b) there are certain mutually reinforcing biases that increase the likelihood that such reductive analogies will be uncritically adopted.

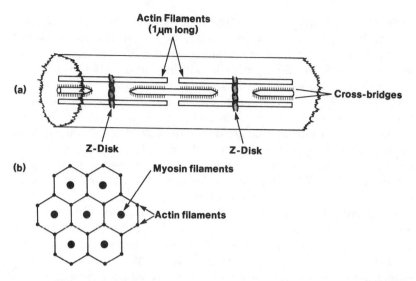

Figure 18.1. Schematic representation of the sarcomere. The sarcomere is the functional contractile unit of the muscle cell (fiber). The sarcomere is usually thought of as the unit contained between two of the z divisions in Figure 18.1(*a*). Actually a great many actin filaments are attached to each z-disc and a great many myosin filaments are interspersed among them. A schematic cross-section through a muscle fiber is presented in Figure 18.1(*b*). It shows a hexagonal array in which each myosin filament is surrounded by actin filaments and each actin filament is surrounded by myosin filaments.

If one adopts reductive analogies, they cause trouble; and one is likely to adopt them.

Antidotes for analogy-driven misconception: multiple analogies and composite images

What should be done to counter the tendencies toward oversimplification that come with the use of analogy and lead to misconceptions? The reductive force of analogies appears to be so great that it is not enough merely to tell people what the limitations of an analogy are. When teachers or texts provide such caveats for an instructional analogy, the result over time tends to be the same: The analogical core is what is retained. The remedy that we propose is to combat the power of a limited analogy with *another powerful analogy* that counteracts the limitations of the earlier one. In general, the antidote to *any* kind of reductive analogy might be the use of appropriately integrated *multiple analogies*, designed to vitiate the effects of three generic types of shortcomings in the use of single analogies (for a more detailed treatment

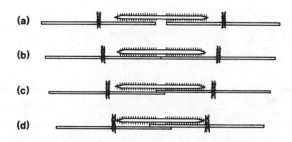

Figure 18.2. Schematic representation of a sarcomere during shortening. The illustrations (*a–d*) represent the sarcomere at various stages of a shortening contraction, between the rest length (*a*) and the maximum shortened length (*d*). The sarcomeres in a muscle cell (fiber) fill the cell from end to end. When they all shorten at once, the whole cell shortens.

of such shortcomings, see the earlier section on analogy-induced misconceptions): (a) information that is *missing* from the source, (b) information in the source that is *misleading* about the topic, and (c) information that is *inappropriately focused* in the source. In this section we discuss an approach for *selecting, integrating, and managing* multiple analogies to promote full understanding of complex concepts in advanced stages of knowledge acquisition.

The discussion of our multiple analogy approach uses as an example the concept of muscle function introduced earlier. When the topic of force generation in a muscle is taught using the analogy to rowing teams, we see that the resulting knowledge contains the seeds for various misconceptions. Some could be attributed to what the analogy *misses* (e.g., reduction in width with elongation of a muscle fiber) and some to aspects of the analogy that *mislead* (e.g., the synchronicity of movement across rowers).

Our approach to using multiple analogies is simply to introduce new analogies targeted at emending the missing, misleading, or misfocused information contained in earlier analogies. Then, as we will see in the next subsection, the various analogies are integrated in a *composite image* that has selective instantiations of the correct and useful information found in each analogy but suppresses the inappropriate information. In other words, our procedure permits the retention of each analogy's strengths while discarding its weaknesses.

A multiple analogy set for muscle fiber function

We begin with a brief treatment of some of the more essential features of muscle fiber function, with reference to the muscle fiber portrayed in Figure 18.1.

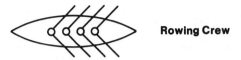

Figure 18.3. Force production to create movement (contraction): the rowing crew analogy.

Table 18.1. *The rowing crew analogy: strengths and weaknesses (see Figure 18.3)*

Captures	Misses or misleads
1. Anatomy of force producers: the little arms	1. Conveys synchronicity: idea that all producers act in unison
2. Nature of the movement of the force producers: back and forth, hitting a resistance	2. Conveys notion that oars can get tangled (e.g., if boat too short) (locus of length–tension bug)
3. Many individual force producers	3. Misses actual nature of gross movement (see Fig. 18.4 and Table 18.2)
	4. Misses things related to *width* (see Fig. 18.6 and Table 18.4)

The contraction of a muscle ultimately is accomplished by microstructures within the muscle called cross-bridges. Cross-bridges are tiny "arms" that reach from one part of the muscle (myocin) out to an adjoining muscle structure (actin). The cross-bridges deliver the pulling force that accomplishes the contraction of a muscle. During a shortening contraction (nonisometric) each cross-bridge head releases from its site on the actin and moves to the next slot, possibly just vacated by its neighbor, while another cross-bridge pulling elsewhere prevents backsliding. The actin structures are thus pulled in toward the center of the myocin filament (see Figure 18.2). Each release and rebinding is called a *cross-bridge cycle*. After a cross-bridge releases and rebinds, the cycle repeats until muscle deactivation occurs. That is, cross-bridge cycling continues over and over unless activating material (e.g., calcium) and/or usable energy (ATP) needed to energize the releases and rebindings become limited. The duration of the contraction is dependent on the degree of availability of these materials. The strength depends upon the number of cross-bridges pulling on actin filaments at any instant during the contraction. The

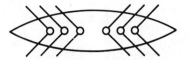

**2 Rowing Crews Facing
Each Other in the Same Boat**

Figure 18.4. The nature of overall gross movement of parts in relation to each other (pulling toward the middle): the analogy of two crews facing each other in a longboat.

Table 18.2. *The analogy of two crews facing each other in a longboat: strengths and weaknesses (see Figure 18.4)*

Captures	Misses
1. Notion that action tends to pull something toward middle (the water)	1. Attachment to some *structure* that gets pulled toward middle (problem is that oars slip through water)

somewhat simplified description presented here does not do justice to the real complexity of the process. The mechanisms by which the repeated cross-bridge cycles are accomplished involve intricate electrostatic, chemical, and physical processes and exchanges.

The processes of muscle function are clearly quite complex. As we have already seen, much of this complexity is not captured by the rowing team analogy (although the analogy is very helpful for conveying some of the anatomical aspects). Some strengths and weaknesses of the rowing team analogy (Figure 18.3) are listed in the left-hand and right-hand columns, respectively, of Table 18.1. Analogies relevant to other aspects of muscle fiber function are found in Figures 18.4–18.7 and Tables 18.2–18.5, each with the same two-column structure of strengths and weaknesses.

The missing, misleading, and inappropriately focused information found in the right-hand column of each of the analogy tables guides the selection of additional analogies used to promote fuller understanding; new analogies are chosen that convey the correct knowledge not conveyed by the old analogies. For example, one of the misconceptions engendered by the rowing team analogy concerns the nature of the gross movement of the main structures in relationship to each other. To produce contraction, the "oars" must in fact pull something toward the center. Figure 18.4 (Table 18.2) modifies the analogy in Figure 18.3 to correct this incorrect aspect.

However, the analogy in Figure 18.4 (Table 18.2) still has the prob-

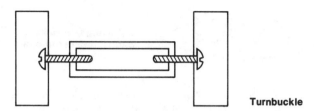

Turnbuckle

Figure 18.5. The nature of overall gross movement: the turnbuckle analogy.

Table 18.3. *The turnbuckle analogy: strengths and weaknesses (see Figure 18.5)*

Captures	Misses
1. Notion that action pulls something toward middle, with no change in length of puller	1. Cross-bridges
2. Notion that there are limits to shortening	2. Individual force producers
	3. Weak on limits to lengthening (see Figure 18.6 and Table 18.4)

lem that it misses the crucial notion of attachment of the cross-bridges to some structure (the actin; see Figure 18.1) that gets pulled toward the middle. Oars, in contrast, slip through water. This shortcoming suggests the analogy of the turnbuckle in Figure 18.5 (Table 18.3). This analogy captures the correct idea of something being pulled toward the middle, without any change in the length of the structure doing the pulling (the myosin) or the structure being pulled (the actin). It also conveys the notion that there is a limit to the shortening process, which has also been missed by the earlier analogies. However, the turnbuckle analogy has nothing corresponding to the cross-bridge anatomy depicted so well by the rowing team analogy; hence, the new analogy is not a complete substitute for the old one. It is for such reasons that multiple analogies must often be maintained, rather than new ones simply supplanting old ones.

Another failing of the turnbuckle analogy is that it provides no useful guidance on the limits to *lengthening* of the fiber (an aspect that is important, for example, in understanding heart failure). Here the analogy of the Chinese finger cuffs shown in Figure 18.6 (Table 18.4) provides a (partial) corrective: The double-wound spiral structure of the muscle covering (the collagen and elastin) produces a length limit

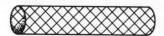

Chinese Finger Cuffs

Figure 18.6. Structure and function of the casing (elastin) surrounding the force producers (i.e., sarcomeres are contained within the casing): the Chinese finger cuffs analogy.

Table 18.4 *The Chinese finger cuffs analogy: strengths and weaknesses* (*see Figure 18.6*)

Captures	Misses
1. Anatomy of the covering: the double-wound spiral	1. Anything about force producers, etc.
2. Thinning with stretch (the dimension missed in Fig. 18.3; important in right side of length–tension function)	2. Anything about the stuff inside the casing (Where's the beef?)
3. Limits to length: (*a*) wall beyond which one cannot go; (*b*) At wall, will break before it lengthens	

(a kind of wall). Here again, some of the elements that the new analogy is weak in conveying are covered by earlier analogies (e.g., the anatomical information about individual force producers covered well by the rowing team analogy and the limits to shortness covered by the turnbuckle).

We have now progressed considerably from the initial rowing team analogy, but essential information has still not been conveyed. Most prominently, there is still nothing about the recruitment of force producers (rowers and oars) to act in any given contraction cycle; not all force producers need act on any cycle, and there is a process of selection from those available. (Note also how this analogy might serve to correct a notion that all rowers must be rowing at any one time, which is conveyed by the rowing team analogy.) This variable recruitment aspect of the topic is conveyed by the galley ship analogy in Figure 18.7 (Table 18.5).

More could be added about how muscle cells work. For example, the metabolic and energetic "life processes" of the muscle's force producers have not been addressed. (The processes are important in understanding muscle activation, which, in turn, is important in understanding cardiac failure.) Furthermore, analogies for them are not

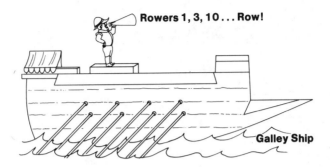

Figure 18.7. Recruitment of force producers: the galley ship analogy.

Table 18.5. *The galley ship analogy: strengths and weaknesses (see Figure 18.7)*

Captures	Misses
1. Control that selects and recruits which force producers are to work (on any stroke)	1. Communication mechanisms
2. Recruitment aspects of activation	2. Anything about internal metabolic, energetic life processes of the force producers (the galley ship rowers)

easily created. (Note, however, that we have been talking about the force producers as *people* rowing. This may actually be a fairly good analogy for the processes under discussion here.)

At this point of the analysis a plateau of sorts has been reached. Many essential aspects of the topic have been covered. And if one considers that much of what medical students understand (and mis-understand) about muscle function is guided by the rowing team analogy, the advance in understanding easily enabled by the additional analogies is very substantial indeed. A complex topic that typically is oversimplified can now be more readily grasped.

Integrating multiple analogies

The most important step in the integration of multiple analogies has already been covered by the selection procedure discussed in the previous subsection. The multiple analogies in a set are *interlocking*, because each new analogy is chosen to correct the negative aspects (the right-hand columns in Tables 18.1–18.5) of the preceding analogies. The remaining discussion of integration is merely an unpacking of the integrative machinery implicit in the procedure for selecting analogies.

Once a set of analogies has been selected, such that the unproductive missing, misleading, or poorly focused information for each analogy has been modified or canceled out by some aspect of a succeeding analogy, then the multiple analogy set must be integrated. There are two main ways of adding new analogies to earlier analogies. These will have an impact on how the additions function to produce new understanding. (A more detailed taxonomy of the functions of new analogies and modification of old ones is presented in the next subsection. Although there are relationships between the *functions of new analogies* discussed there and the *patterns of combination* described here, they are distinct topics. We restrict ourselves here to the smallest number of types of combination necessary for introducing the composite imaging procedure in the next subsection.) In one of the two combination patterns, *modified analogies*, new analogies merely emend an earlier one (e.g., correcting the rowing crew analogy to have two sets of rowers pulling toward the middle; Figure 18.3 and 18.4). In the second pattern, *new analogies*, a totally new analogy is added (e.g., introducing the turnbuckle analogy following the rowing crew analogy).

The class of modified analogies contains two subtypes: *simple* and *complex*. With the addition of a simple modified analogy there is no need to retain the old analogy; the new analogy emends incorrect information from the old one but loses none of its essential information. This type of modified analogy is the easiest to deal with. First, the modified analogy is merely *substituted* for the earlier one (e.g., replace the drawing in Figure 18.3 with that in Figure 18.4). Second, the critical new aspect of the substituted modified analogy is accentuated. For instance, the image of two sets of rowers *facing each other* and *rowing toward the middle* is marked for special notice. This may be accomplished, for example, by suggesting to students that they envision one of the sets of rowers as colored red and the opposed set as blue; or by placing eyeglasses on the rowing team members to accentuate the directions they are facing. The point, again, is to accentuate the features of the modified analogy that constitute the main change from the prior analogy.

In a complex modified analogy, the analogy used for correction of the earlier analogy contains seeds of misconceptions that are best mitigated by *maintaining* an aspect of the earlier analogy. Here the prior analogy cannot simply be "updated." Analogies of this type do not occur in our muscle fiber example. However, integration would be handled by the same *selective instantiation* feature of our composite imaging technique that is illustrated with new analogies, discussed next.

Making multiple analogy representations cognitively tractable: composite images with context-dependent selective instantiation

How should one keep track of several analogies and the complicated pattern in which they are combined (i.e., the patterns by which the left-hand columns of Tables 18.1–18.5 are retained and the right-hand columns overridden as successive analogies are introduced)? The cognitive demands are considerable. To make the psychological management of this complexity more tractable, we introduce the technique of "composite imaging with selective contingent instantiation" (CISCI). Although conventional means of teaching concepts will not receive attention, it must be emphasized at the outset that *the composite images are perceptual adjunct aids that supplement rather than replace verbal instruction* (see also Bransford et al., this volume).

In the CISCI procedure, a complete set of images, each corresponding to one of the multiple analogies (other than those superseded by a simple modified analogy), is available in a latent state. That is, all of the images that are to be combined are represented as potentials in a state of readiness for instantiation. (We intend for these representations to refer both to latent mental images and to displayable external images, e.g., computer graphic displays. Thus our discussion refers *both* to mental representation and to its parallel in instructional support systems.) Which of the latent images (analogies) of the total composite image are actually instantiated at any one time is *aspect-dependent*. That is, a component of the (latent) total composite image will be a part of an actual instantiated composite image as a function of the aspects of muscle fiber function under consideration. For example, in contexts where it is important to focus on the way muscle fiber is affected by longer lengths and length limitations, the Chinese finger cuffs image would become salient; when thinking is directed at muscle functioning under short lengths and toward the limits to shortening, the turnbuckle image would be "programmed" for high salience. Component images that are not activated are suppressed; either they may not be visible (in "the mind's eye" or in an external support system) or, preferably, they may be instantiated very faintly, as a kind of background to the aspect-dependent focal images.

Finally, at the same time that either the turnbuckle or the Chinese finger cuffs image (continuing the last example) is relatively salient within the instantiated CISCI, images corresponding to the other analogies that are not being actively suppressed (i.e., that retain their usefulness for the conceptual aspect under consideration) will simultaneously be superimposed within the total image. So, if the Chinese finger cuffs are active, that image would be overlaid by the double rowing team image; an image of two sets of rowers pulling toward the center would be superimposed on the cylinder of the finger cuffs, enabling the positive properties of both analogies to make a simultaneous contribution.

In sum, the characteristic of aspect-dependent *selective and contingent instantiation* of component images (along with the initial motivation and basis for selecting each of the analogies, i.e., overcoming some inappropriate information in an earlier analogy – the right-hand columns in Tables 18.3–18.7) makes it possible for understanding of the concept to be supported only by the correct and productive features of each analogy, with the incorrect and unproductive features canceled out. The CISCI can be thought of as a montage of simultaneous ways that muscle fiber function can be *"seen as"* (Wittgenstein, 1953) something else. Parts of the montage are emphasized in visualization as a function of the productive left-hand-column information that needs to be stressed and the unproductive right-hand-column information that needs to be suppressed, given the conceptual aspects under consideration at any one time.

The CISCI method we have described is thus one of *nonabstractive integration.* By using a *composite* of several analogies, understanding is not abstractively reduced either to a superordinate system or to any one of the analogies acting as privileged with respect to the others. In contrast, in *abstractive integration* the individual elements are *replaced* by a subsumptive abstraction that *stands for* the elements and/or their combinations. By presenting the composite analogies as simultaneously overlapping images, the composite leads to a *perceptual* integration. Thus, as in the perception of complex objects like human faces, a whole is psychologically graspable without loss of information about parts – although one's image of the face of a close friend is typically perceived as a simultaneous physiognomy, the components of the face are recoverable (i.e., perceptual focus can shift to individual facial features, such as the size of the nose or the distance between the eyes). The physiognomy is perceptually integrated while the component parts continue to make their contributions individually (in contrast to the supplanting of individual elements in an abstractive integration).

The kinds of perceptual composites or "integral visual displays" for representing nonreducible multidimensional information that we are proposing have been receiving increasing support in recent years (Chernoff, 1973; Spiro & Myers, 1984; Spiro et al., 1987; Wainer & Thissen, 1981). The more complexly structured the domain, the more it becomes impossible in principle to chunk large groups of information conceptually; so, instead of a conceptual chunking of information to lessen the cognitive load, we employ a perceptual chunking.

Although formal experimental tests of the CISCI procedure have not yet been completed, there is evidence from its informal employment that the procedure is (a) effective in fostering in novices a sophisticated understanding of the complexities of force production by muscle fiber (think about the effects on you the reader of having stepped through the figures and having received just partial guidance as to how to compose an image of the set) and (b) easily managed psychologically.

Regarding psychological manageability, it should not be surprising that such a small number of analogy images and aspectual contingencies can be grasped and memorized fairly readily. Furthermore, the component images are fairly familiar ones (rowing crews, Chinese finger cuffs, etc.). Also, the *incremental* introduction of the analogies (see also Burstein, 1986) leads to only gradual increases in the complexity of the target concept; by the time the final analogy is introduced, the concept will already be comprehended fairly well. Then, when the CISCI is introduced, support for learning it will come from the conceptual understanding of the concept already established (through the incremental procedure). That is, incremental introduction of multiple analogies that are individually pedagogically effective helps the understanding of the complex concept, and understanding of the complex concept then helps to encode durably the CISCI that corresponds to the concept – the composite image is not arbitrary. The concept supports the initial acquisition of the CISCI, and then the CISCI supports the concept. (It should be quite clear from what we have said that CISCI is very dissimilar to the "method of loci," which involves memorizing lists of unrelated items by placing them against the backdrop of familiar sequentially ordered scenes; Yates, 1966.)

A taxonomy of functions of additional analogies in promoting conceptual understanding

There are many reasons why new analogies might reasonably be introduced to augment earlier analogies in promoting understanding.

Earlier, for purposes of illustrating the mechanics of the composite imaging technique, we presented a very simple classification of the kinds of analogy additions that can be made. Here we offer a more detailed accounting of the ways that additional analogies can contribute to understanding. A preliminary and nonexhaustive classification of such functions of multiple analogy is given below (mostly carrying over examples from muscle fiber function).

1. *Supplementation (with new analogy)*. Aspects of a topic domain that are *missed* by earlier analogies are covered by a supplementary analogy (also see Burstein, 1986). *Example*: adding the turnbuckle analogy to cover the information missing from the rowing crew analogy about attachment to some structure that gets pulled (Figure 18.5; Table 18.3).

2. *Correction (with new analogy)*. Aspects of a source domain that *mislead* about the topic domain are corrected (without altering the correct information in the earlier analogy). *Example*: replacing the turnbuckle with Chinese finger cuffs in the context of understanding muscle fiber function at *long* lengths (Figure 18.6; Table 18.4).

3. *Alteration (of an earlier analogy)*. Sometimes an incorrect element in an earlier analogy can be dealt with by modifying or "patching" it, rather than by fundamentally changing it or replacing it altogether. *Example*: modifying the rowing crew analogy to have the crew split in half and row toward the center (Figure 18.4; Table 18.2).

4. *Enhancement (of an earlier analogy)*. Enhancement is a refinement of an earlier analogy that *deepens* the understanding of the topic domain – that overcomes some earlier superficiality, without either altering the existing components of the earlier analogy (number 3) or changing its magnification (number 5). *Example*: having the cockswain call out the numbers of the rowers (recruitment of cross-bridges) to convey the notion of asynchronous movement and degrees of recruitment (Figure 18.7; Table 18.5). Note that the enhancement impresses an appropriate new layer of mechanism on the phenomenon. As a side effect, the enhancement also repairs a misleading *implication* of an earlier analogy (Table 18.1, first item in the right-hand column), without repairing the earlier analogy itself. Thus it differs from number 3. In terms of the rules for constructing composite images, this is a *simple* modified analogy, whereas alteration is a *complex* modified analogy.

5. Magnification (or elaboration). An aspect of the topic domain that is not correctly captured because of the grain size of the analysis (and corresponding image) evoked by the source analogy is addressed by scale alterations (i.e., changes in grain size). *Example*: Although the introduction of the cockswain (Figure 18.7; Table 18.5) captures the notions of recruitment of force producers and asynchronous movement, it is simply opaque regarding the biochemical life processes involved in variably energizing the force producers. Perhaps the best way to remedy this problem is by the many-times magnification of an individual rower in the rowing crew (i.e., "people" and their intake, breakdown, and utilization of energy, as an analogy for the metabolic aspects of the force producers).

Note that there are two possibilities following magnification: introduction of a *new* analogy for the magnified section of the old analogy and retention of the *old* analogy on a different scale. An example of magnification involving the retention of an earlier analogy but with change of scale was encountered earlier in the law of Laplace example, where magnification of the soap bubble wall was a key step.

Of course, when a more synoptic view is required, grain size may be decreased in a "reverse magnification." Also, a function related to magnification would be served by rotating the image of the source domain so that previously obscured elements are brought into view (e.g., as would happen if the first image involved the front of a thing and one needed to augment understanding by later looking at the back of the thing).

6. Perspective shift. Complex domains can often be thought of in fundamentally different ways. In such cases, a new analogy may convey a different perspective than that conveyed by earlier ones. *Example*: The rowing crew represents well the perspective of *movement production*. The finger cuffs represent well the perspective of *limits to movement*.

A related use of new analogies for contributing to understanding involves the introduction of an analogy that addresses underlying causal mechanisms after an earlier analogy that was more concerned with the surface form of a situation. *Example*: When heart failure is taken as analogous to an overstretched balloon that has lost its tensile strength, some aspects of superficial similarity are captured: Two things have become enlarged and have lost their ability to produce force. However, as we saw when this kind of reductive analogy was discussed earlier, despite the fact that the underlying causes are greatly different, students mistakenly assume they are the same. Introduction of an analogy that more correctly characterizes the cause of heart failure (e.g., a dying car battery) would make it less likely that students would mistake gross input–output correlation for causation in the development of the misconception about heart failure.

7. *Competition.* More than one analogy competes as an overall account of the same domain. One analogy eventually supersedes its competitor, which is discarded. Only one analogy occupies a specific analogical niche. *Example*: A common analogy employed by medical students in understanding congestive heart failure is that of an overstretched, "bagged-out" balloon incapable of generating force (Coulson et al., 1986; also see the earlier discussion of the false analogy between the length–tension relationship for individual muscle fibers and Starling's relationship between cardiac volume and output). Since heart failure is really due more to impotence within energetic activational factors of cardiac muscle than to anything related to mechanical overstretching, a more appropriate overall analogy would involve something like the dying battery (or perhaps a fouled spark plug or broken distributor wire) introduced under *perspective shift* (number 6).

8. *Sequential collocation.* Successive stages in a process are each represented by an analogy. In other words, a single analogy is used for each identifiable "segment" of a phenomenon, and the analogies are simply collocated (without any integration being necessary).

The last two categories are the main ones addressed by Collins and Gentner (1987) in one of the few discussions of multiple analogies in the literature (see also Burstein, 1986). A brief discussion of their work on evaporation models will help to clarify our own approach. Again, Collins and Gentner deal with multiple analogies in two different ways. In the first, they divide the water cycle into successive stages (e.g., what happens in bodies of water; what happens in the sky; and so on). This is number 8, *sequential collocation.* A multiple analogy set would then be the group of analogies for each stage. Their second use of multiple analogies involves choosing the best analogy for each stage. That is, they discuss alternative analogies for each stage (e.g., alternative analogies for what happens in bodies of water), with the ultimate goal of selecting the most appropriate analogy for that stage. This is number 7, *competition.*

The fundamental difference from our approach should be clear: Our multiple analogies are all applied to the *same* stage of a process, and all of the analogies in the set are *partially correct* – they are all "best" at conveying something about the topic domain. More generally, we claim that for most domains of any complexity the "pieces" (e.g., stages, sectors, aspects, etc.) into which the domain is divided will each need to be covered by more than one analogy. And this is what our *aspect dependencies* do. However one compartmentalizes a complex domain, the pieces cannot usually be effectively treated with a single analogy. (A related issue that we have not addressed here concerns the extent to which pieces of a complex domain can be adequately treated separately from each other at all.)

Conclusion

There are two main conclusions to be derived from the work that we have presented. First, there are serious hazards involved in the use of analogies. In particular, the employment of a single analogy for a complex concept may impede the acquisition of more advanced understandings of that concept and engender misconceptions. Second, access to a fuller and more immediate comprehension of conceptual complexities may be achieved by the systematic employment of integrated sets of multiple analogies.

With regard to the first conclusion, a theme of our recent research has been the recurring empirical observation of a pervasive tendency in cognition and instruction toward oversimplification of complex concepts (Coulson et al., 1986; Feltovich et al., 1986, in press; Spiro et al., 1988; Spiro et al., 1987). This tendency, which we have referred to as the *reductive bias*, has been identified in both biomedical and historical domains and has been shown to take a great variety of forms. In this chapter we have confined our inquiry to just one cognitive arena, analogical learning, where we have provided several illustrations of the reductive force of analogies and the ramifications of that reductive force in the development of fallacious knowledge. Eight different ways that analogy can induce misconception were identified, and each was illustrated by an important misconception commonly held by medical students who have already had courses in the relevant content area.

This demonstration clearly indicates that analogies must be used with great caution. Even when they are used judiciously to initiate learners into a difficult subject area with appropriate caveats about their limitations, reduction of the topic domain to the source domain appears to be a too common occurrence. It is hoped that our typology of ways that analogy can induce misconception can serve to alert learners and teachers to these potential hazards. However, the reductive force of analogies appears to be so great that even very detailed warnings are probably not sufficient by themselves. More positive measures may be needed, which brings us to the second main conclusion of this chapter.

Analogies have traditionally been seen as a powerful *positive* force in learning new material. We have shown a countervailing tendency: In more advanced forms of knowledge acquisition, the power of analogies is often *negatively* exercised. We have argued that the best way to counter this powerful negative force is with equally powerful positive forces: In order to combat the elements that induce misconceptions in an otherwise useful single analogy, import new analogies that powerfully convey the correct knowledge.

In order to lay the groundwork for such an approach, we have offered a detailed conceptualization of the diverse functions of multiple analogies in learning, a procedure for selecting and integrating multiple analogy sets so that they convey complexity without inducing misconceptions, and a composite imaging technique to lessen the cognitive load of working with a multiple analogy set. Taken together, these elements constitute a comprehensive program for the employment of multiple analogies in support of advanced forms of complex knowledge acquisition.

A final note: simplicity and complexity in advanced knowledge acquisition

This chapter has dealt explicitly with the reductive force of single analogies in the development of misconceptions and with the role of multiple analogies in promoting correct understandings of complex concepts. However, it has a more general purport as well. It can also be treated as a kind of apologue about learning in complex domains. The detailed treatment of hazards of analogy use and remedies for them has close parallels in the use of *any* mode of cognitive support for complex new learnings. In the findings of our other studies, the maladaptive reductive force of single analogies is paralleled by misconception-inducing reductive forces of a single schema, single mode of organization, single line of argument, single precedent example, single prefigurative "world view," and so on. The antidote for these maladaptive forces of simplification is in each case the *systematic assembly of multiple knowledge sources* – integrated multiple analogies, compiled fragments from diverse schemata, re-presentations of the same information under different organizational schemes, multilinear lines of argument, and multiple precedent examples. So it could be said that this chapter, besides being about analogy per se, is also in an important sense about the seductive force of all singular approaches to complex learning, the prevalent role of oversimplification in the development of entrenched fallacies of conceptual understanding, and the general importance of assembling multiple knowledge sources to support the mastery of complex concepts at advanced stages of knowledge acquisition.

NOTE

This research was supported in part by grants from the Basic Research Division of the U.S. Army Research Institute (Contract MDA903–86–K–0443) to the first author, from the Josiah Macy Foundation (B8520001) to the second author, and from the U.S. Office of Educational Research and Improvement to the Center for the Study of Reading (Contract 400–81–0030). The authors wish to thank Andrew Ortony, Stella Vosniadou, Judith Orasanu, John Schmitz, Angela Boerger, and Marlene Schommer for their helpful comments.

REFERENCES

Burstein, M. H. (1986). Concept formation by incremental analogical reasoning and debugging. In R. S. Michalski, J. G. Carbonell, & T. M. Mitchell (Eds.), *Machine learning: An artificial intelligence approach* (Vol. 2, pp. 351–370). Los Altos, CA: Kaufmann.

Carbonell, J. G. (1986). Derivational analogy: A theory of reconstructive problem solving and expertise acquisition. In R. S. Michalski, J. B. Carbonell, & T. M. Mitchell (Eds.), *Machine learning: An artificial intelligence approach* (Vol. 2, pp. 371–392). Los Altos, CA: Kaufmann.

Chernoff, I. (1973). The use of faces to represent points in k-dimensional space graphically. *Journal of the American Statistical Association, 68*, 361–368.

✓ Collins, A., & Gentner, D. (1987). How people construct mental models. In D. Holland & N. Quinn (Eds.). *Cultural models in language and thought* (pp. 243–265). Cambridge: Cambridge University Press.

Coulson, R. L., Feltovich, P. J., & Spiro, R. J. (1986). *Foundations of a misunderstanding of the ultrastructural basis of myocardial failure: A reciprocating network of oversimplification* (Tech. Rep. No. 1). Springfield: Southern Illinois University Medical School.

Feltovich, P. J., Coulson, R. L., & Spiro, R. J. (1986). *The nature and acquisition of faulty student models of selected medical concepts: Cardiovascular impedance.* Paper presented at the annual meeting of the American Educational Research Association, Montreal.

Feltovich, P. J., Spiro, R. J., & Coulson, R. L. (in press). The nature of conceptual understanding in biomedicine: The deep structure of complex ideas and the development of misconceptions. In D. Evans & V. Patel (Eds.), *The cognitive sciences in medicine.* Cambridge, MA: MIT Press (Bradford Books).

Gentner, D. (1983). Structure-mapping: A theoretical framework for analogy. *Cognitive Science, 7,* 155–170.

Gentner, D., & Gentner, D. R. (1983). Flowing waters or teeming crowds: Mental models of electricity. In D. Gentner & A. L. Stevens (Eds.), *Mental models* (pp. 99–129). Hillsdale, NJ: Erlbaum.

Gick, M. L., & Holyoak, K. J. (1980). Analogical problem solving. *Cognitive Psychology, 12,* 306–355.

Pepper, S. (1942). *World hypotheses.* Berkeley: University of California Press.

Rumelhart, D. E. (1980). Schema: The building block of cognition. In R. J. Spiro, B. C. Bruce, & W. F. Brewer (Eds.), *Theoretical issues in reading comprehension* (pp. 33–58). Hillsdale, NJ: Erlbaum.

Rumelhart, D. E., & Norman, D. A. (1981). Analogical processes in learning. In J. R. Anderson (Ed.), *Cognitive skills and their acquisition.* Hillsdale, NJ: Erlbaum.

Spiro, R. J. (in press). Building flexible knowledge structures from and for reading. In R. J. Spiro (Ed.), *Reading research into the 90s.* Hillsdale, NJ: Erlbaum.

Spiro, R. J., Feltovich, P. J., & Coulson, R. L. (1988). *Seductive reductions: The hazards of oversimplification of complex concepts* (Tech. Rep. No. 4). Springfield: Southern Illinois University Medical School.

Spiro, R. J., & Jehng, J. C. (in press). Random access instruction: Theory and technology for the nonlinear and multidimensional traversal of complex subject matter. In D. Nix & R. J. Spiro (Eds.), *The "Handy Project": New directions in multimedia instruction.* Hillsdale, NJ: Erlbaum.

Spiro, R. J., & Myers, A. (1984). Individual differences and underlying cognitive processes in reading. In P. D. Pearson (Ed.), *Handbook of research in reading* (pp. 471–501). New York: Longman.

Spiro, R. J., Vispoel, W., Schmitz, J., Samarapungavan, A., & Boerger, A. (1987). Knowledge acquisition for application: Cognitive flexibility and transfer in complex content domains. In B. C. Britton (Ed.), *Executive control processes* (pp. 177–199). Hillsdale, NJ: Erlbaum.

Vosniadou, S., & Ortony, A. (1983). The influence of analogy in children's acquisition of new information from text: An exploratory study. In P. A. Niles & L. A. Harris (Eds.), *Searches for meaning in reading: Language processing and instruction* (pp. 71–79). Clemson, SC: National Reading Conference.

Wainer, H., & Thissen, D. (1981). Graphical data analysis. *Annual Review of Psychology, 32,* 191–242.

Wittgenstein, L. (1953). *Philosophical investigations.* New York: Macmillan.

Yates, F. A. (1966). *The art of memory.* Chicago: University of Chicago Press.

19

The activation and acquisition of knowledge

WILLIAM F. BREWER

Introduction

This chapter discusses the issues of similarity and analogy in development, learning, and instruction as represented in the chapters by John Bransford, Jeffery Franks, Nancy Vye, and Robert Sherwood; Ann Brown; Brian Ross; Rand Spiro, Paul Feltovich, Richard Coulson, and Daniel Anderson; and Stella Vosniadou. The following anecdote illustrates many of the themes that appear in the discussion of these chapters.

I was in a seminar recently where we were trying to set up an overhead projector for the first time. There was no screen in the room, and the one patch of wall of reasonable size was crossed with pipes. So I said to one of the other faculty members, "Let's try aiming the projector at the blackboard." This individual said, "No, that's crazy." I immediately gave in and began helping to aim the projector toward the wall. Then I said, "Wait, let's try the blackboard – I think it will work." We did try the blackboard, and it did work reasonably well.

What was going on here? First, why did the other person immediately reject my original suggestion, and why did I give in? I think it is clear that the other person had a causal model for light which included the assumption that black surfaces absorb all the light that falls on them. As applied to the example at hand, this meant that it would be stupid to try to project the overhead on the blackboard, since no light would reflect off it and we would not be able to see the transparencies. Although this model was not made overt in our exchange, I am sure I also partially held this model, and that was why I gave in so quickly. This part of the episode looks like a good example of using old knowledge to solve a new problem.

However, as we were moving the overhead projector I went through the following line of reasoning: Moon rocks are almost as black as the

532

blackboard. The light from the moon is reflected. The moon looks bright white. From this I was willing to try using the blackboard as a screen. The going gets a little complex here, but it looks as if I was trying to find some fact that would support my original suggestion. My retrieval of this particular fact was not quite as exotic as it seems since at that time I was deeply immersed in knowledge about astronomy for a project on knowledge acquisition. When I retrieved the moon example I knew that I had some counterevidence for the light-absorption model and was willing to reason by analogy from the moon example to the projector problem. Notice the fluid nature of the interplay between the particular examples and the underlying models. I first found a *fact* that was counterevidence for a *general model* and then used the *fact* to form a *new general model*, which I transferred to the problem at hand.

After we saw the first transparency projected on the blackboard we both modified our models for light to include the belief that even black objects can reflect back some of the light that hits them. Thus, in addition to solving the problem and remembering the facts in the incident itself, we each acquired a small amount of new, more general knowledge in the form of a slightly modified psychological model of the reflection of light.

The example shares a number of characteristics with the problems treated in the chapters in Part III: (a) the knowledge is complex; (b) the incident is taken from everyday life; (c) some of the knowledge was in the form of a causal model; (d) there were multiple, and in this case inconsistent, models; (e) the example required a crucial memory retrieval; (f) the individual making the structural analogy had considerable knowledge of the relevant domain; (g) there was between-domain analogical transfer; (h) old knowledge was used to support new knowledge; (i) there was recourse to both specific and general knowledge; (j) a particular problem was solved; and (k) some more general knowledge acquisition took place during the episode. The rest of this chapter will examine these and related issues as they occur in the five chapters that make up Part III.

Development, learning, and instruction. The research and ideas in the chapters on development, learning, and instruction have considerable continuity with the work reported in the other parts of the book; nevertheless, there is clearly a different flavor to these chapters. It is hard to characterize the difference, but one major aspect is the decision by this set of researchers to study real-world tasks.

Real-world tasks. Each of the researchers in this section has taken some complex real-world instructional problems and brought them into the laboratory. Ross has studied the learning of text editors and probability theory by undergraduates. Spiro and his collaborators have studied the problems that occur in the learning of physiology by students in medical school. Brown has studied the acquisition of aspects of natural selection by elementary school children. Vosniadou has studied the acquisition of observational astronomy in elementary school children. Bransford and his colleagues have studied the learning of science material by children and the acquisition of skill in therapy by clinical psychology students.

Real-world tasks and theory. It seems to me that the confrontation of established beliefs and theory with the characteristics of real-world problems gives rise to some of the distinguishing characteristics of these chapters. The crisp, clear models of the earlier parts of the book often become much more complex. Extreme parsimony is *not* one of the sins of the researchers in Part III – they tend to use a variety of theoretical constructs to deal with the phenomena they have chosen to study. They postulate a wide range of different forms of knowledge. These chapters show a pervasive concern with the impact of already acquired knowledge on the psychological processes under study. There is a general concern with the issue of how different procedures for presenting knowledge affect the knowledge acquisition process.

The remainder of this chapter will be divided into four sections. The first deals with the issues of similarity and knowledge. The second deals with the representation of knowledge. The third deals with the issues of development. The fourth treats the issues of instruction.

Similarity

Physical similarity. The issue of physical or surface similarity plays an important role in the discussions in the earlier chapters. The importance of physical similarity in these theories can be seen in the assumptions behind Medin and Ortony's statement that "The criteria for category membership . . . are not necessarily always apparent on the surface as physical properties of instances of the category" (Chapter 6). For the chapters in Part III the issue of physical or surface similarity plays a considerably reduced role. It is implicit in the choice of task and materials that the major kind of knowledge these researchers are interested in studying (and in having their students learn) is abstract, structural knowledge. Physical similarity loses its privileged position and becomes just one important type of information that can play a role in the acquisition of structural knowledge.

Physical similarity and knowledge. An example of the reevaluation of physical similarity can be seen in the chapters by Brown and by Vosniadou. Both researchers discuss the hypothesis that children are "perceptually bound," the hypothesis that physical appearance is of primary importance in carrying out various psychological tasks. They both also provide evidence that young children can carry out tasks based on underlying structural information, thus suggesting that children do not have a "deficit" in processing abstract structural knowledge. Brown and Vosniadou argue that young children give the appearance of being perceptually bound because they often lack underlying abstract knowledge about a domain and so are forced to use surface (physical) similarity to respond.

Bransford et al. and Vosniadou point out that one implication of the knowledge-based approach is that the similarity of two objects is not a fixed construct but will change with changes in the learner's underlying knowledge base.

Brown extends the knowledge-based approach even further. She suggests that it may be the underlying structural information that is primary for the child. She proposes that children may come equipped with constraints that lead them to give an abstract structural interpretation to surface physical events. For example, the child may be biologically constrained to interpret the motion of physical objects within a framework of physical causality.

One of the main themes in the earlier parts of the book is the reduction of the role of physical similarity in theories of concept formation. Brown's chapter in Part III provides a dramatic example of this knowledge-based approach taken to its full extent. As a long-time member of the "knowledge Mafia" it is hard for me to disagree with this strong knowledge-based approach to these problems.

The concept of similarity. The core concept of similarity still plays a major role in the chapters in Part III, but the focus of theoretical attention seems to shift. Here, the researchers tend to emphasize the structural properties of the materials or representations that are being studied. Ross is concerned about the way in which surface and underlying similarity can be independently varied to facilitate or hinder knowledge acquisition. Bransford et al. stress the importance of having the acquisition conditions of a form of knowledge be similar to the way in which the knowledge is to be used. Brown reports several studies in which she presents pairs of tasks that are related by structural similarity. She attempts to eliminate all surface and structural similarity across pairs of tasks, so all that is left for the child to acquire across pairs of tasks is the very abstract construct that within each pair of tasks there will be some form of underlying structural similarity. Thus, although each of these researchers uses similarity, the strong differences between these lines of research result from the differences in what is being related by similarity and in how the relation is applied.

Tasks. One of the issues that appears in the earlier parts of this book is the problem posed for theories of categorization by Rips's finding that subjects give a different pattern of responses in similarity tasks than they do in category tasks. This issue appears to be of only indirect importance for the chapters in Part III, since essentially all of the experiments reported in these chapters consist of presenting the subject with some form of information and later giving a test that requires the use of the earlier information. The difference in tasks used by the researchers in Part III compared to those used by the researchers in Parts I and II seems to be a reflection of differences in their goals and strategies. The researchers represented in Part III are interested in problem solving and the acquisition of knowledge, and they have chosen to study the issue directly by using tasks that involve complex forms of knowledge.

Knowledge

Forms of knowledge. One striking aspect of these chapters taken together is that they suggest the need to introduce a wide variety of types of knowledge in theory development. Ross's chapter reports data that reinforce the need for a distinction between surface information and underlying structural information. He finds that surface similarity leads to more remindings than does structural similarity but that the remindings based on structural knowledge are more successful in enabling the student to solve a new problem. Brown argues for a distinction among forms of knowledge in terms of the breadth and depth of the knowledge. She proposes to distinguish among pieces of arbitrary knowledge (canaries are yellow), locally meaningful knowledge (birds that eat seeds have thick beaks), principled knowledge (evolution leads to birds' having appropriate beaks for their food), and broad theory-based knowledge (birds are animate). She points out that as one moves up this scale the amount of transfer possible increases dramatically.

Spiro et al. argue that there is a basic distinction between knowledge of well-structured domains (math, physics) and knowledge of ill-structured domains (literary criticism, political theory) and that the mechanisms for knowledge acquisition may differ for these two forms of knowledge. Bransford et al. suggest that one has to distinguish between linguistic knowledge and perceptual knowledge of a topic (i.e., the difference between having been told that a certain type of disease leads to a shadow in a certain location on an X-ray radiograph and being able to identify correctly a particular picture). Bransford et al. also argue for a distinction between static declarative knowledge and more active procedural knowledge. Finally, Brown proposes that certain forms of knowledge may show constraints imposed by biology whereas others may not.

What are we to make of all this? First, as a practical matter this apparent diversity is probably due to the tendency of these investigators to look to the real world for problems to study. Investigators who adopt this research strategy seem to be drawn quickly into postulating different forms of knowledge. It is possible that this apparent diversity is merely the reflection of our current primitive understanding of these issues and that with deeper understanding much of the apparent diversity will vanish. However, I believe that nature is trying to tell us something and that, in the long run, a proper understanding of the human mind will require that we recognize a large number of very different forms of knowledge and associated psychological processes.

Instances versus abstract knowledge

Although most of the researchers in Part III explicitly propose that there are different forms of knowledge, it is not clear that they agree about the nature of the different forms of knowledge. In particular, there are some interesting differences on the issue of *knowledge of instances* versus *abstract knowledge*. Ross shows that in certain types of problem-solving tasks the learners are reminded of previous episodes and that these remindings apparently facilitate problem solving. His research involves a paradigm in which he observes undergraduate subjects' very first attempts to understand a relatively new form of knowledge. He suggests that knowledge of instances may play a large role in the very early stages of knowledge acquisition and then speculates that knowledge of instances may also play a major role in the apparently rule-governed activity of the more experienced individual.

Though Brown and Vosniadou do not make explicit statements on this issue, it seems fairly clear that they work within a framework in which knowledge is considered abstract (e.g., rules, schemata, models). Brown was quite properly pleased when one of her 3-year-old subjects spontaneously articulated the abstract analogical rule that had been embodied in the pairs of experimental tasks. Spiro et al. may be switch-hitters on this issue. There are suggestions in their chapter that they might adopt the position that the representation of well-structured domains tends to be in terms of abstract structures whereas the representation of ill-structured domains tends to be more specific. In particular, Spiro et al. propose an instructional technique that involves the use of multiple analogies in a process of "nonabstractive integration." It seems fairly clear that Spiro et al. want to give their medical students knowledge in the form of a set of specific instances (images?). However, an interesting question for Spiro et al. is: What is the form of representation of the knowledge of muscle physiology in the case of the true expert? Does the research scientist who studies muscle physiology continue to use the "nonabstractively integrated" instances, or does the information become an integrated abstract structure?

Clearly, at this stage in our understanding about the forms of knowledge representation it is not possible to resolve these issues. One of these positions may eventually be shown to be closer to the truth, or the differences of opinion may be resolved through some higher-order integration. For example, one might hypothesize that knowledge in the early stages of acquisition and/or for ill-structured domains tends to be represented in terms of instances, whereas other forms of knowledge tend to be represented in terms of abstract structures.

Knowledge acquisition. Although all of these researchers appear to want to understand how knowledge is acquired and provide much information on conditions that facilitate the solving of a particular problem, there are very few explicit attempts to propose a model of how knowledge is acquired (i.e., long-term changes in the knowledge base). Ross suggests that the use of analogies forces certain generalizations and that these make up the knowledge that is stored in long-term memory (a position that seems to be a bit at odds with his suggestion that knowledge may remain represented in terms of specific instances). Overall, one characteristic aspect of these chapters with respect to the issue of how knowledge is acquired is that they provide little overt theory on this difficult problem.

Development

Deficit in underlying structure. The chapters by Vosniadou and by Brown address developmental issues. Both researchers provide a theoretical argument against the hypothesis that children show a deficit in the ability to use underlying structural information in solving new problems based on old solutions. The basic line of attack is to argue that previous work showing such deficits may have resulted from the subject's lack of the required domain-specific structural knowledge.

Brown's chapter provides an elegant series of experiments which show that if a child knows the relevant structural information and if the experimenter points out the possible usefulness of the old information in solving the new problem then the child is clearly able to use abstract structural information. Vosniadou points out that when children are trying to use an instructional analogy (e.g., white blood cells are like soldiers) their "errors" frequently show a transfer of relatively abstract information, not surface perceptual information (e.g., they state that the white blood cells think that the germs are bad, not that the white blood cells carry guns). Thus, both of these chapters provide substantial evidence against the hypothesis of a developmental deficit in using structural information.

What develops. Although Brown uses knowledge-based arguments to attack the structural deficit hypothesis, she is not willing to attribute *all* differences shown by young children to a lack of domain knowledge. She suggests that even when care is taken to insure that the young child has the needed structural knowledge there is still evidence that young children do not perform as well as older children on a variety of transfer tasks. She tentatively suggests that what may be developing in the child is the general ability to use metacognitive strategies (the older children are able to look for underlying structure without being told). It is not clear if Brown considers this developmental change to be a developmental shift in the child's underlying ability or just another form of change due to increased (meta)knowledge. Overall, the fundamental approach in both of these chapters is that the apparent changes with age in analogy use, problem solving, and transfer are due not to the development of ability in the child but to the acquisition of knowledge.

Instruction

Detailed models of the learner. A close reading of these chapters shows that most of the researchers share a common underlying belief about research on instruction. They assume that the task of the cognitive psychologist is to work out detailed models of what the learner is actually going to do in a given learning situation. Then, they assume that this information will make it possible to improve instruction. For example, Bransford et al. provide some data showing that allowing learners to generate their own incorrect solutions to problems reduces their ability to find the correct solutions (score one for B. F. Skinner!). To the degree that one takes this as a general principle, one might attempt to design inputs to the learner that lead the learner away from incorrect solutions. Ross's chapter provides data suggesting that the surface features of problems can be used to remind the learner of either appropriate or inappropriate earlier information. Spiro et al. show what type of transfer is produced by a particular instructional analogy and suggest techniques for dealing with information that is either missing or incorrect in the analogical transfer.

It seems to me that one of the appealing aspects of these chapters is that these researchers make serious attempts to obtain detailed information about what the learner is likely to do in a particular instructional situation. It is hard to see how this can do other than improve our general understanding of knowledge acquisition and, eventually, of the practical problems of instruction.

Degree of learner expertise. One factor that probably accounts for some of the differences in the specific theories proposed in these chapters is the enormous range of expertise being investigated – from 3-year-old children to medical students. Brown points out that the theorists who have hypothesized that children are "perceptually biased" are often studying the children's performance in a domain in which they have little underlying structural knowledge. Ross's results suggesting an important role for surface remindings also occur with subjects who are extreme novices in the relevant domain. Brown's studies showing that children can transfer structural information use structural relations that even young children have thoroughly mastered. Spiro et al. find that in trying to give a very deep understanding of a domain such as muscle action a single reductive analogy can lead to incorrect or incomplete knowledge. However, note that if one were trying to teach an elementary school child the rudiments of muscle action the single reductive analogy might well be the most one would hope to achieve.

It is in the context of the advanced level of expertise expected of medical students that the possible importance of multiple analogies looms large. Clearly, much additional research across the entire spectrum of expertise is needed before it will be possible to see to what degree these various proposals are general or specific to a given range of expertise.

Advantages of underlying structural knowledge. Several chapters in Part III make the point that learning is greatly facilitated when the learner can make use of underlying structural knowledge. Bransford et al. argue that providing the learner with underlying structural information (e.g., about the purpose of certain features of houses) improves the learner's ability to acquire information about particular houses. Ross shows that if learners are reminded of underlying structural information they will display improved performance in solving problems. Brown provides a number of experiments demonstrating that techniques that lead the child to focus on the underlying structure of a domain result in greatly improved problem solving.

Inert knowledge. Bransford et al. make a strong argument for the position that much instruction leads to a collection of facts that students are not able to use when faced with new problems. This issue is part of the larger problem of the relationship of instruction to the goals of the instructor that will be covered next.

Forms of knowledge presentation and knowledge acquisition. A consistent theme running through these chapters is the impact that certain kinds of knowledge presentation have on knowledge acquisition. Brown shows that giving the learner multiple exemplars of the same structural construct and pointing out the underlying relations will allow even very young children to acquire biological constructs such as animal mimicry. Bransford et al. suggest that for the acquisition of something such as the Gick and Holyoak (1980, 1983) fortress story the acquisition conditions should contain "contrasting" stories that enable the student to work out the important aspects of the initial story. Bransford et al. also propose the technique of providing the learner with multiple perspectives on the same event. Brown suggests an instructional strategy of presenting the student with a series of exemplars of very different underlying structures.

If one looks at these different proposals in terms of the type of knowledge that the instructor is attempting to teach, there is more consistency here than appears at first. Ross suggests that the procedure of presenting problems of the same type in a common chapter with a common surface topic may be a poor procedure, because it will encourage the learner to use surface information to retrieve the underlying structure. However, if the *student's* goal is to obtain a high grade and the instructor gives homogeneous tests at the end of each chapter, this may, in fact, be a successful form of presentation for attaining this limited goal. Ross suggests as an alternative that one might apply each procedure to a common example. This approach would hold surface information constant and would thus limit the student's ability to select solutions on the basis of surface information. This type of acquisition procedure appears to be directed at facilitating the acquisition of underlying structural knowledge that will enable the students to solve problems expressed in new surface forms. Brown's use of a series of different exemplars of the same underlying structure seems to be a different procedure directed at facilitating the acquisition of a particular underlying structure. Brown notes that there can be a negative side to the schema-acquisition approach. The children taught with this form of presentation were so successful at acquiring the underlying structure that they overapplied the schema when faced with an exemplar embodying a different structure. Bransford et al. propose that the acquisition of an underlying structure will be facilitated by the use of exemplars that contrast on the crucial aspects of the underlying structure.

Both Brown and Bransford et al. make suggestions that are directed at very abstract forms of knowledge. Bransford et al. suggest that the same exemplar be presented from multiple perspectives. Here, the goal seems to be to facilitate the learner's acquisition of the idea that the same exemplar can be used in a variety of different structures. This type of knowledge presentation thus appears to be appropriate when one does not know how the exemplar is likely to be experienced in the future. Finally, Brown's procedure of giving children a variety of very different pairs of underlying structures can be seen as an attempt to improve the learner's ability to look for some form of underlying structure (as distinct from teaching a particular underlying structure). Thus, if one considers the form of knowledge that the instructor is attempting to teach, there is much more lawfulness in these very different proposals. It is, however, clear that much more research is needed before we will know whether the particular acquisition procedures proposed in these chapters are the most appropriate ones for these different forms of knowledge.

Table 19.1. *Relative ease of access to old knowledge*

	Access to old knowledge	
	Instructed	Uninstructed (spontaneous)
Within-domain	Easy	Moderately easy
Between-domain	Moderately easy	Hard

Access to old knowledge. Another important issue that comes up in these chapters is the ease of access to old knowledge for different types of tasks. Brown points out the problem that arises from two inconsistent general beliefs in this area: (a) old knowledge plays a crucial role in solving new problems, and (b) the transfer of old knowledge to new situations is very poor. It seems to me that part of this paradox can be resolved by looking at the issue in terms of within-domain transfer versus cross-domain transfer and instructed transfer versus uninstructed transfer (see Table 19.1).

Both Ross and Vosniadou point out that transfer within a knowledge domain tends to be easier than transfer across a domain. Collins and Burstein, in their chapter, suggest that one should distinguish between transfer in cases where a teacher is providing explicit instruction on the relevant structural relations and in cases where the students must access the required structural information on their own.

Brown's research demonstrates that with the use of instructed within-domain tasks even very young children show rapid access and transfer of old information. Brown's experiments on training flexibility suggest that instructed cross-domain tasks show moderate ease of access and transfer. Much instruction research focuses on the general task of teaching individuals to solve, on their own, new examples from a particular domain. Some of Ross's experiments on problem solving suggest that uninstructed within-domain tasks show moderate difficulty of access and transfer of old knowledge. Finally, there is general agreement that uninstructed cross-domain tasks are hard. (The first individual in a culture to see a very productive cross-domain analogy often finds a place in the history books.) However, this example gives a false picture of the difficulty of this type of task. It seems likely that in the course of learning a new domain ordinary students do, in fact, make cross-domain analogies. The chapters by Spiro et al. and by Vosniadou both give some partial data in keeping with this suggestion.

Conclusion

The work in this section is a reflection of the change in the type of research and theory that is produced by a concern with complex forms of representation in real-world tasks. Much of the research in the earlier section of this volume derives from the concept-learning tradition. This work tended to focus on the problem of how instances of a concept are classified. The researchers in this area typically carried out experiments using simple stimuli so that the subjects in these experiments had little opportunity to bring the full force of their background knowledge to bear on the tasks. The forms of representation used by theorists in this tradition often focused on the physical aspects of the stimuli, and the learning mechanisms that were suggested frequently made strong use of the construct of physical similarity.

The work reported in Part III diverges from the earlier work on concept formation on each of the characteristics discussed above. For the researchers in this section, the nature of the question has shifted; they have focused on the issues of problem solving and the acquisition of knowledge. These researchers have tended to adopt a research strategy of bringing complex real-world problems into the laboratory for study. These theorists tend to deemphasize the role of physical similarity in knowledge acquisition. They have chosen to investigate individuals over a wide range of expertise. The theories developed by these researchers tend to assume that there are a number of very different forms of knowledge. Some of the researchers emphasize knowledge of specific instances; others emphasize general forms of knowledge such as rules and schemata.

The differences between children and adults in their ability to solve problems are interpreted as due to differences in the amount of knowledge that has been acquired, not as differences in basic underlying abilities. These researchers attempt to provide detailed models of the learning process so that instruction can be derived from a basic understanding of the learning process. Most of them emphasize the importance of having the learner master the underlying structure of the domain being acquired. They provide a great variety of different procedures for the presentation of knowledge. These procedures can be organized in terms of the different goals of the instructors in each case. It appears that some of the difficulties in understanding how transfer occurs can be resolved by distinguishing between within-domain and between-domain transfer and between instructed and uninstructed transfer. Overall, these five chapters give the impression of a young, exciting, and vigorous area of research.

REFERENCES

Gick, M. L., & Holyoak, K. J. (1980). Analogical problem solving. *Cognitive Psychology, 12,* 306–355.
Gick, M. L., & Holyoak, K. J. (1983). Schema induction and analogical transfer. *Cognitive Psychology, 15,* 1–38.

Afterword: A framework for a theory of comparison and mapping

ALLAN COLLINS and MARK BURSTEIN

In our studies of human reasoning (Burstein, 1986; Collins, 1978; Collins & Loftus, 1975; Collins & Michalski, 1989) we have found that the processes of comparison and mapping are central to all forms of human inference. For example, comparison underlies categorization (Smith & Medin, 1981) in that the very act of categorizing involves a comparison between an instance and a concept. Categorization is of use to humans because it allows us to make inferences (mappings) about what properties the categorized instances will have (e.g., they may fly away, they can be turned on, etc.). As the chapters in this volume amply illustrate, analogies and metaphors are also heavily dependent on these processes of comparison and mapping.

The literature on similarity, analogy, and metaphor ranges over many different kinds of comparison and mapping processes. Our goal is to clarify the issues being addressed and the critical distinctions that need to be made. We will attempt to consider the entire territory over which the discussion of comparison and mapping arises, but no doubt we will miss some of the critical distinctions and issues.

Some of the disagreements arise because researchers are talking about different kinds of comparisons or the different contexts in which comparison and mapping processes are used. Indeed, one common confusion is due to the use of the term *mapping* to describe either a functional *correspondence* between conceptual entities, the process that establishes such correspondences (which we will refer to as *comparison*), or the process of transferring properties of one conceptual system to another, "similar" one. In this discussion, we will reserve the word *mapping* for the last of these, the transfer process.

We have divided the chapter into three main sections. The first distinguishes the different kinds of entities that are related by analogy and similarity, and some of their more salient properties. The second section discusses the different contexts or tasks that give rise to comparisons and mappings. The third catalogs the set of issues we have

546

identified in the literature and identifies some of the different solutions proposed or possible for each issue. In a concluding section we briefly discuss the implications of this framework for future research.

Types of correspondences

The hypothesis we offer is that there are three fundamentally different kinds of entities that are compared and mapped: systems, concepts, and properties. All the other kinds of comparisons and mappings discussed in the literature are variations on these three. The distinction among these three classes is based on the amount of internal structure of the objects compared and therefore the complexity of the correspondences that need to be established.

System correspondences. The mapping from the solar system to the atom that Gentner (1983) discusses is the classic example of a system mapping. In a system mapping it is critical to determine two types of correspondences (Gentner, this volume):

1. which components (i.e., concepts) in the source domain correspond to which components in the target domain
2. which properties of each component (including relations between components) in the source domain correspond to which properties in the target domain.

In Gentner's analysis of the solar system/atom analogy, one has to decide what components correspond (sun → nucleus, planets → electrons) and what properties correspond or can be mapped to enable correspondences (planets orbit the sun → electrons orbit the nucleus).

Concept correspondences. To answer the question "Was Nixon a crook?" (Collins, 1978) or to decide how likely Linda is to be a feminist bank teller (Tversky & Kahneman, 1980; E. Smith & Osherson, this volume) requires only a comparison of the properties of two concepts. There is no decomposition into components, as there is with a system correspondence. So, in the case of Linda in Smith and Osherson's account, you consider the properties of salary, education, and politics, comparing Linda and feminist bank tellers with respect to these properties.

Property correspondences. The simplest kind of correspondence is when a particular property of two concepts is compared, as when one judges whether an object 3 inches in diameter is more similar to a quarter or a pizza (Rips, this volume). (This is actually an example of a double comparison, discussed later under three-element comparisons, between a 3-inch object and a quarter and between a 3-inch object and a pizza. System and concept correspondences can also involve double comparisons.) Property correspondences differ from concept correspondences in that the concepts are compared with respect to a particular property rather than with respect to many properties.

The critical distinction among these three kinds of correspondences is that system correspondences involve component (or object) correspondences as well as property correspondences, that concept correspondences involve multiple property correspondences, and that property correspondences relate individual properties of two concepts. The distinction between system and concept correspondences is not entirely straightforward. For example, one elementary text we studied (Collins, Gentner, & Rubin, 1981) explained the composition of the earth by analogy to a peach. There is the crust, which is analogous to the skin, the mantle analogous to the fruit, and the core analogous to the pit. This may appear to be a concept correspondence, because it involves a comparison of the properties of the two concepts. But in fact it is a system correspondence, because it requires first decomposing the earth and peach into their components (i.e., the three layers) and then comparing the properties of each pair of components (e.g., the skin and crust are both very thin) and their relations to each other. Thus the distinction between a system correspondence and a concept correspondence rests upon whether there is a two-part process that establishes correspondences between an organized set of components and their properties or a single-stage process that just relates properties of two concepts.

To give a second example of a system mapping that may be difficult to recognize, one might hypothesize (Collins & Michalski, 1989) that a bird's pitch depends on the length of the bird's neck, which is why ducks quack and geese honk and, more generally, why small birds sing and big birds squawk (Malt & E. Smith, 1984). This hypothesis might be generated by analogy to the fact that human pitch (e.g., children's vs. adult's voices) depends on the length of the windpipe. To make the inference about birds by analogy to humans requires mapping windpipe length onto neck length, and human pitch onto bird pitch. Because the analogy involves both a correspondence between their components (e.g., windpipes and necks) and a correspondence between some of their components' properties (relative length), it is a system mapping. In this case the property mapped (e.g., "pitch is inversely related to length") is a relational property in Gentner's (this volume) terms or a mutual dependency in Collins and Michalski's (1989) terms.

There are a number of other kinds of comparisons and mappings discussed in the literature that we think are special cases of these three kinds of correspondence. We will briefly describe each:

Procedure correspondences. Van Lehn and Brown (1980) discuss correspondences between the addition and subtraction procedures we learn in school and different addition and subtraction procedures with Dienes blocks (wooden blocks in three denominations: units are small squares, tens are 10 unit blocks long, and hundreds are 10 by 10 unit blocks). Similarly, Anderson and Thompson (this volume) describe correspondences between the procedure for factorial and that for summorial. Correspondences between procedures are essentially system correspondences, where both the objects manipulated by component operations of the procedure (e.g., for Dienes blocks, units map onto the numbers in the right-hand column, etc.) and the components operations themselves are subsequently mapped or compared like properties.

Problem correspondences. Ross (this volume), Holyoak and Thagard (this volume), and Carbonell (1986), among others, discuss correspondences between a problem you are trying to solve and an earlier problem you have solved. This kind of correspondence is frequently suggested in science texts where students solve new problems by referring back to the sample problems worked in the text. Gick and Holyoak (1980, 1983) and Holyoak & Thagard (this volume) discuss the analogy between a fortress problem, where an army must split into small units to capture a fortress, and Duncker's (1945) ray problem, where a ray source must be split in order to kill a tumor without destroying healthy tissue around it. Problem correspondences require correspondences between components (e.g., ray → army units, tumor → fortress), and so they are system correspondences.

Story correspondences. Gentner and Landers (1985) and Ross (this volume) have studied correspondences between stories. These, again, are simply system correspondences, where it is necessary both to relate the characters or objects in one story to those in the other and to compare the relations or events linking these entities in each story.

Table 20.1. *Contexts in which correspondences are formed*

Type of task

1. *Comparative judgments*
    a. Similarity judgments
    b. Typicality judgments
    c. Categorization judgments
    d. Identity judgments
    e. Overlap judgments
    f. Difference judgments
2. *Mapping*
    a. Property mappings
    b. Component mappings
3. *Conceptual combinations*

Number of entities compared

1. *Two-element comparisons*
2. *Three-element comparisons*
3. *Four-element comparisons*

Undoubtedly, other kinds of mappings are made, but we think they will all be variations of the three kinds we have identified.

Contexts in which correspondences are formed

Various tasks or real-world demands require different kinds of reasoning when relating entities. Our taxonomy of contexts in which comparisons and correspondences occur consists of two dimensions: *type of task* and *number of entitites compared*. The overall structure of the taxonomy of contexts is shown in Table 20.1. These two dimensions, type of task and number of elements, define a space of possible contexts in which correspondences are considered or established. There may be some cells empty in the space, but most combinations are possible.

Type of task

Type of task breaks down into three basic categories: comparative judgments, mappings, and conceptual combinations. We will briefly describe six different kinds of comparative judgments, and then two kinds of mappings. Last, we will briefly discuss conceptual combination.

Comparative judgments. The comparative judgment types are derived primarily from the chapters by Rips and by Linda Smith. This may not be a complete list of comparison judgments, but it covers the types discussed in this volume.

1. Similarity judgment. Judging how similar two entities are is a common task in psychological experiments (Tversky, 1977; Rips, this volume; E. Smith & Osherson, this volume; Barsalou, this volume). Smith and Osherson (this volume) and Collins and Michalski (1989) argue that similarity judgments affect the certainty of many inferences people make. Similarity judgments obviously can apply to pairs of systems, concepts, or properties.

2. Typicality judgments: Typicality has been studied in psychology since Rosch (1975) and plays much the same kind of role in plausible reasoning as similarity (Collins & Michalski, 1989). Rips (this volume) has shown convincingly that typicality and similarity judgments are not always made in the same way, so they must be distinguished in any theory. Like similarity, typicality applies to pairs of systems, concepts, or properties.

3. Categorization judgments: Rips (this volume) discusses the similarity theory of categorization, which he rejects. In any case, categorization requires a comparison between properties of two entities, the thing to be categorized and the category. Categorization applies only to systems and concepts, not to single properties of concepts, except when they are treated as concepts in their own right.

4. Identity judgments: L. Smith (this volume) raises the issue of making identity judgments between entities – that is, comparing whether all their properties are the same. Of course, no two entities are ever exactly the same (e.g., her examples of identical elements are not quite the same darkness or shape), so it is necessary to learn what degree of variability of a property can be called the same. Identity judgments therefore depend on context.

5. Overlap judgments: None of the chapters in this volume mentions overlap judgments (e.g., whether therapists are psychiatrists), but logically, if one includes categorization and identity judgments, overlap and difference judgments must also be included. Evaluating a "some" statement (e.g., "Some women are doctors") requires making an overlap judgment (Meyer, 1970).

6. Difference judgments: The question of whether two entities are different (e.g., "Are whales fish?") also involves a comparison of properties. Like categorization, identity, and overlap judgments, difference judgments are contextually defined. For example, whales and fish are different, but both are animals and can be treated as the same in some contexts, such as in grouping things as plants and animals.

Mappings. The other type of task that is referred to frequently in the literature is one of mapping properties, components, or both, from the source domain to the target domain.

Property mapping: Most of the work on analogy (e.g., Anderson & Thompson, this volume; Gentner, this volume; Holyoak & Thagard, this volume) concerns itself with bringing properties (including primarily relational properties) of objects in the source domain over into the target domain. A similarity or typicality judgment between the source and target is made before mapping a property over and affects the certainty with which the property is believed to hold for the target domain. For example, before deciding that the pitch of birds depends on their neck length, based on an analogy to the human vocal tract, a person would compare humans and birds with respect to their similarity, particularly on those properties related to sound production (in this case, properties of the relevant components, such as vocal cords and necks) (Collins & Michalski, 1989). A person's certainty about whether the property holds for birds depends on this similarity judgment.

Component mapping: Sometimes in the mapping of two systems, whole components are introduced by the mapping. In the earth/peach analogy, the text introduced two new components of the earth to students (the mantle and the core) in the course of explaining the analogy. This same thing can occur when people generate an analogy in their own minds (Collins & Gentner, 1980).

Conceptual combinations. E. Smith and Osherson (this volume) raise the possibility that conceptual combination (feminist + bank teller → feminist bank teller) is another task that a theory of mapping should address. We see conceptual combination, as they have modeled it, as primarily addressing the issue of how property mappings are combined when there is prior information about the properties involved in the target system. This becomes particularly important when learning or making predictions from multiple analogies and in interpreting descriptive metaphors.

Number of entities compared

Number of entities compared is the other dimension we have identified with respect to the contexts in which analogies occur. This can

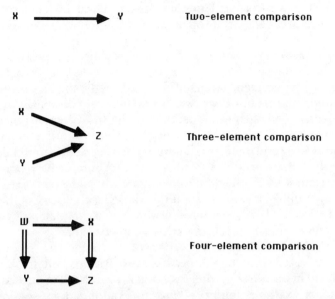

Figure 20.1. The structure of different comparisons of concepts.

range from two, as in the earth/peach analogy, to four, as in analogies like wolf : dog :: tiger : cat, and the geometric analogies considered by Evans (1968). Slightly different constraints operate in two-, three-, and four-element comparisons, shown in Figure 20.1.

Two-element comparisons. Many of the mappings discussed in the literature – for example, Gentner's (this volume) water flow–heat flow mapping, and Holyoak and Thagard's (this volume) fortress problem–ray problem – are basically two-element comparisons. In a two-element comparison there is a single source item (system, concept, or property) to be compared with a single target item, possibly resulting in a mapping of properties or components from one to the other.

Three-element comparisons. A good example of a three-element comparison is the task used by Rips (this volume) where subjects had to decide whether a 3-inch object was more likely to be a pizza or a quarter. In many tasks that appear to be two-element comparisons, there may be a comparison element implicit that subjects generate on their own. For example, if you tell a child that a whale is a mammal, he or she may compare whether whales are more like mammals or fish, which is a three-element comparison. Three-element comparisons, therefore, compare properties of X to those of Y versus Z.

Four-element comparisons. Standard analogy tests pose questions using the syntactic form $W : X :: Y : Z$. We view such problems as falling into two categories, based on whether the analogy's interpretation depends on one or two (within and between) comparisons. True four-element comparisons depend on both sets of comparisons, as in the analogy wolf : dog :: tiger : cat. The within-group comparisons (e.g., wolf : dog and tiger : cat) determine the properties or dimensions along which the pairs differ (wildness or not), and the between-group comparisons identify the dimensions along which the pairs are similar (feline or canine class membership). Evans (1968) discusses the need for both kinds of comparisons (relating the components of both W and X and W and Y) in solving some geometric analogies.

Some analogies stated in the same syntactic fashion are more properly interpreted as analogies between two systems, where W and X are related in one system, whereas Y and Z are related in an analogous system. For example, Johnson-Laird (this volume) discusses the analogy water : sluice :: gas : jet. Here, there is a between-system correspondence involving water → gas and sluice → jet, but the comparison of water and sluice or gas and jet is not useful. Instead, there are relational systems relating each pair (e.g., a sluice directs water and a jet directs gas). True four-element comparisons involve comparing each concept to two others, but in Johnson-Laird's example, a single similarity judgment is required between the functional relations in the two systems.

Issues for a theory of comparison and mapping

There are a number of issues running through the chapters in this volume and the literature more generally. In part they reflect the set of subprocesses outlined by Gentner (this volume), but they have wider scope. Our attempt here is simply to delineate the set of issues as best we can and to discuss possible resolutions to them. We start with the most microscopic issues and work up to the more macroscopic issues.

How are individual properties compared?

Potentially, there are two kinds of properties that a theory must take into account. Discrete properties (e.g., male or female) and continuous properties (e.g., size). Tversky and Gati (1982) have shown how it is possible to treat all continuous properties as if they were discrete. Another possibility is to treat all discrete properties as continuous (a person is on a continuum of male/female, and most people fall near one or the other ends of the continuum).

Rips (this volume) addresses the question of how continuous properties are compared for different kinds of three-element comparisons: similarity, typicality, and categorization judgments, which he finds are judged differently. His results suggest that categorization judgments are based on the relative height of the distribution – for example, a 3-inch object is more likely to be a pizza than a quarter, because the distribution of pizzas is higher at that point. His results for similarity judgments suggest that both height of the distribution and distance from the mean (or mode) come into play. Typicality judgments appear to fall in between categorization and similarity, as if some subjects treat them like categorization judgments and others like similarity judgments (or perhaps they are combination judgments).

There are many possible functions for computing any of these judgments: For example, similarity might be based on the relative distance between modes of the distribution compared; typicality judgments might be similarity judgments between a concept and its superconcept, as E. Smith and Osherson (this volume) assume. Rumelhart's (this volume) theory probably makes a prediction as to which of these functions will best fit the data, but he is not explicit on this point. Most of the other theories take no stand on this issue.

How are judgments from different properties combined?

Tversky (1977) proposes a combining function for similarity judgments, which E. Smith and Osherson (this volume) have adopted for their theory of decision making. The essence of the Tversky combination rule is that matching properties increase similarity and mismatching properties decrease similarity between concepts. Mismatching properties consist of two sets: property values of one concept that the other does not share, and property values of the other that the first does not share. Mismatching properties include properties where one concept has a known value and the other has no known value. Each of these three sets (one matching and two mismatching properties) is weighted appropriately depending on the direction of the judgment. Thus people think North Korea is more like China than China is like North Korea, because there are many properties they know about China that do not apply to North Korea but few properties they know about North Korea that do not apply to China (Tversky, 1977).

The Tversky rule is defined only over similarity judgments and discrete properties. If one adopts the view that all properties are continuous, then a modification of the Tversky rule is necessary. Whether it applies to other kinds of judgments (e.g., categorization judgments) is an open question. And, of course, there are an infinite number of other combination rules, some of which might still be viable given Tversky's (1977) data.

How do people access similar entities?

The question of access is fairly central to the chapters by Ross; Gentner; Bransford, Franks, Vye, and Sherwood; Barsalou; Brown; Vosniadou; and Holyoak and Thagard. It is called "noticing" by Ross. All of these papers address the access issue for the case where the source must be found in memory. As Johnson-Laird (this volume) points out, the source is often given, as when a text explains that the earth is like a peach or the atom like a solar system. In Ross's paradigm, when working problems a person may go back through a book to find a similar problem. This access may or may not be governed by the same properties as the access from memory.

Gentner (this volume) proposes that attributes (or superficial properties) govern access more than relational properties. This seems to accord fairly well with both her data and those of Gick and Holyoak (1983). Rumelhart (this volume) takes the position that access is governed by a match on all microfeatures, but in different contexts it may be attributes that match, or higher-order relational features. These positions are compatible if one posits that superficial attributes are the most available and therefore will usually dominate higher-order relations in most matches.

There is some evidence (e.g., Chi, Feltovich, & Glaser, 1981) that part of becoming an expert is learning to pay attention to higher-order relations rather than superficial attributes. This also accords with Ross's (this volume) observation that superficial properties will mislead people if the principles underlying the problem (i.e., higher-order relations) are confusable. Brown (this volume) gives evidence that functional fixedness and cognitive embeddedness of problem-solving contexts are sources of diminished accessibility to potential analogs in children as well.

How is knowledge about the source reconstructed?

Ross (this volume) points out that people often have to reconstruct their knowledge about the source domain after they have accessed an analogy. This reconstruction process is guided by the knowledge being sought about the target domain. For example, if people are told that heat flow is like water flow (Gentner, this volume), since they do not have a particularly good understanding of water flow (Gentner & Gentner, 1983) they must in part figure out what they know about water flow: that it flows from one container to another as long as there is a difference in the height of the water in the two containers, that the surface area of the water in the container does not matter, that the flow rate is proportional to the diameter of the connection between the containers. Which properties of the source domain people think of depends on what aspects of the target they are trying to understand, as Ross (this volume) has found in his studies.

What governs which properties are transferred?

This is the central argument animating most of the discussion in the analogy literature. We will briefly delineate the different positions.

Ortony (1979) advocates the position that *salience imbalance* governs transfer: That is, those properties are transferred that are important in the source domain but not important in the target domain. For example, "Sam is a hippopotamus" transfers fatness, since fatness is a typical property of hippos but not of people.

Gentner (1983) proposes a syntactic theory that states that, in analogies, relational properties are transferred but attributes (i.e., non-relational properties) are left behind. Furthermore, according to her systematicity principle, relational properties that are a part of a system of relations (e.g., the large mass of the sun attracts the planets into orbiting around it) are more likely to be mapped across.

Holyoak and Thagard (this volume), Johnson-Laird (this volume), Carbonell (1986), and Burstein (1986), although there are differences in their views, take a position on mapping that appears somewhat different from that of Gentner. Their position is that a system (or schema) of properties is mapped over, as Gentner proposes, but with two differences: (a) Attributes will be mapped if they are part of the system, and (b) the major problem is to decide which system to map over. For example, if the analogy was made between the solar system and a person tanning under a sun lamp, the properties mapped would have to do with the heat being transmitted, the person rotating to cover all sides, and the yellow color of the lamp.

It turns out that the latter criticism may be partially handled by the structure-mapping engine (Falkenhainer, Forbus & Gentner, 1986; Gentner, this volume) that was built recently to embody the Gentner theory. This system compares representations of two domains to decide which relations fit into a connected system that can be mapped into the target domain. Because it is effectively comparing all possible sets of relations in the source with those in the target, it is to some degree automatically choosing a "best system" to map. However, some pragmatic, contextual selection mechanisms will almost certainly be required as well. This is particularly true during learning, when people usually do not know enough about the target domain to pick out corresponding systems simply by matching (Burstein, 1986).

An important test of any of these computer models (Burstein, 1986; Carbonell, 1986; Gentner, this volume; Holyoak & Thagard, this volume) is whether they can select two different correspondence mappings from a source domain (e.g., the solar system) depending on what aspects of the source domain are relevant to the target domain (e.g., the atom vs. a person tanning). None of the models has, as yet, addressed this central problem directly.

Whether goals and subgoals guide the selection of the system to be mapped often arises in the debate between the different positions. But that is probably because some of the researchers are working with analogies in problem solving, whereas Gentner is dealing mainly with explanatory analogies. Certainly both sides would agree that goals are critical properties to map in problem-solving analogies and play the same central role that causal relations play in explanatory analogies.

Anderson and Thompson (this volume) rely on a set of three principles (i.e., "no function in content," "sufficiency of functional specification," and "maximum functional elaboration") to determine what is mapped. Although it is not clear to us exactly how these principles operate, they indicate the use of function as the main criterion for selecting what to map and so would fall into the problem solving camp.

In our view the position of Gentner, on the one hand, and that of Holyoak and Thagard, Johnson-Laird, Carbonell, and Burstein, on the other hand, are not that far apart, given the centrality of systems of properties or schemata that are mapped over. The Ortony theory is orthogonal to that issue and could operate in conjunction with some kind of system mapping. Whether the Anderson and Thompson position is genuinely distinct or reduces to the use of system properties as well remains to be seen.

How are multiple mappings merged together?

This issue is raised by Burstein (1985, 1986, 1988), Spiro, Feltovich, Coulson, and Anderson (this volume), and Collins and Gentner (1983). In Burstein's work, students were learning to program and were forced to combine the results of mappings of several systems. Assignment was related to both putting things in boxes and the interpretation of arithmetic equalities. The result was a mental model that could be used to understand computer statements like $A = B + I$. Collins and Gentner (1983, 1987) describe how subjects combined different analogies (e.g., billiard-ball analogy, rocketship analogy, crowded-room analogy) in understanding evaporation processes. It is clear that people frequently construct their understandings of systems by multiple mappings, and so theories will have to specify how conflicts are resolved about what properties to map from each analogy and whether, in fact, some form of conceptual combination is required to merge related properties mapped from several different sources. In Burstein's model, conflicts between mappings are usually resolved by reasoning from specific examples in the target domain that cause one or another analogical mapping to fail. However, the hypotheses that are eventually selected must still be integrated with what had been mapped previously or was otherwise known about the target domain (Burstein, 1988).

Burstein (1985) and Collins and Gentner (1983) also raise the issue of *vertical integration* of mental models. Analogies do not always map onto the same level of description of a target system. In such cases, one cannot directly merge analogs. Instead, the mapped structures must be maintained distinctly, and rules of correspondence must be formed between the different views or levels of abstraction described by the different analogical models.

How are mappings refined?

After a mapping is made, some properties carried over into the target domain will not apply. How are the correct properties identified and replaced? Burstein (1986) and Anderson and Thompson (this volume) address this question in the context of mapping computer program statements. In Burstein's model, analogically mapped predictions are compared to the actual results in target domain examples. If the predictions are wrong, alternative structures are considered for mapping, from either the same or a different source domain. Anderson and Thompson discuss several examples of failures due to overgeneralization from an analogy and suggest that they may be handled by searching for contextual features that were *not* mapped and adding them as preconditions.

Another kind of refinement occurs when successful analogies are extended to encompass new sets of corresponding systems or related causal principles. In addition to mapping new relational properties, this kind of analogical extension can lead to the introduction of new object or concept correspondences. For example, in the kinds of demonstration physics experiments that are often used to explain the diffraction and interference behavior of sound and light by using water wave tanks, a number of experimental objects are introduced to cause different wave behaviors. Each object that is introduced in these experiments must be related to an analogous object that causes a similar kind of interference with light or sound. In this sense, each new experiment described causes the refinement of the analogy between water waves and light or sound waves, because new objects and new causal implications are placed in parallel.

What is generalized from a mapping?

This is the question of how, when, and if generalizations are made based on a mapping between two domains. For example, one hypothesis might be that the corresponding components in the two systems are replaced by their common supersets, and the generalization is stored as a set of (possibly generalized) relations on these common supersets. Gentner (this volume), Anderson and Thompson (this volume), and Winston (1982) have addressed this issue to some degree, although no specific claims have been made.

It is not at all clear that analogies always lead to new generalizations. Most analogies are useful only because they map one or two specific pieces of information from one domain to another. In such cases, the generation of a new general principle may not be warranted.

At the other extreme, attempting to generalize from an analogy that relates radically different classes of objects by a new principle calls for a strong form of conceptual reclassification, as when sound and light are reclassified as waves. Very strong evidence of the analogy's pervasiveness may be needed for this kind of reclassification to occur. Alternatively, "bridging analogies" can be used to show why the analogy is justified. Clement (1981, 1986) gives examples of series of bridging analogies designed to convince people of the generality of physical laws. One set of these analogies shows how the behavior of a spring is related to the longitudinal and torsional flex of a wire by considering intermediate cases where the wire is partially bent. Clement (1986) also discusses Newton's analogy between the moon and an apple falling from a tree, with a sequence of bridging analogs where a cannonball is fired at greater and greater speeds until it is in orbit around the earth.

How does the process of mapping develop?

This is the central issue raised by Linda Smith (this volume), and it is also discussed in the chapters by Brown, Vosniadou, and Gentner. In Smith's chapter, she proposes that development proceeds from overall resemblance matches to identity matches and finally to dimensional matches. Her proposal perhaps is best summed up by saying that children learn to make finer discriminations in their comparison processing with age.

Smith's thesis raises the question of how children can make overall resemblance comparisons without being able to make individual property comparisons. This is not really a paradox, from the vantage point of the kind of microfeature theory proposed by Rumelhart (this volume). Overall resemblance comparison in Rumelhart's theory can be carried out by comparing two concepts with respect to all their microfeatures. This requires no identification of microfeatures with particular properties (like color) of entities in the world. Based on the kind of perceptual learning described by Bransford and his colleagues (this volume), dimensions or subgroups of the microfeatures will emerge as contrastive sets of microfeatures that inhibit each other. Making an identity match would seem to require learning how much variability is possible on any dimension, so that one can assess whether the difference between two entities falls below the normal range of variability on that dimension. In any case, the chapters by Smith, Rumelhart, and Bransford et al. together promote a consistent picture of how similarity matching develops.

Are analogies helpful for learning?

This issue was initially raised by Halasz and Moran (1982) and is a central focus in the chapter by Spiro and his colleagues. Halasz and Moran's position is that if you give people explanatory analogies, such as the analogy that computer addresses are like boxes (Burstein, 1986) or that heat flow is like liquid flow (Gentner, this volume), you lead them to make more wrong mappings than helpful ones. So they argue that it is better to give people descriptions of the mechanisms involved rather than analogies.

There are at least three arguments against the Halasz and Moran (1982) position. First, when people learn about novel systems, they are going to impute mechanisms to them. In order to understand any mechanistic description, they have to draw from their stock of basic mechanisms, such as Collins and Gentner (1983) have described. So, whether you give students an analogy or not, they are going to make an analogy to some mechanism they already understand. The continuum from remembering to reminding to analogy that Rumelhart (this volume) describes is operating here. Subjects will pull in the mechanism they know about that matches most closely. By giving students an explicit analogy, you then accomplish two things: (a) You make sure they impute the best matching mechanisms, and (b) you know what wrong inferences they are likely to draw, so that you can try to counter them as you explain the mechanism.

A second argument against the Halasz and Moran (1982) position is that the power of analogies for teaching derives from the fact that they provide a well-integrated structure that can be assimilated all at once. This structure may have been acquired over a long period of time, as Vosniadou (this volume) shows for the solar system. So, when people are told the atom is like a solar system, they have a well-integrated structure acquired over many years that they can map as a whole in order to understand the atom. Thus they do not have to recapitulate the same long learning process for the atom. Analogies are particularly powerful where there is a competing structure already in place that the teacher is trying to dislodge.

A third argument can be made from the observation that several partially competing analogies are often presented to students simultaneously. Although none of the analogies will be entirely correct, instruction that highlights the useful portions of each analogy may tend to reduce or cancel the harmful effects of other, competing analogies with respect to specific aspects of the target (Spiro et al., this volume; Burstein, 1985).

The Halasz and Moran (1982) position, however, has to be correct if the analogy introduces too many wrong mappings and no competing models are introduced (Spiro et al., this volume). Therefore, we would argue that the issue is not whether analogies are helpful or harmful but what determines when they are helpful versus when they are harmful for learning.

Conclusion

Most researchers are working in a little corner of this framework, which is fine. One use of the framework is to help them see what the rest of the territory looks like in order to help them extend their theory to cover the whole territory. Trying to extend their theory in this way puts additional constraints on theory construction, which will help researchers refine their theories. Furthermore, as theories are extended to cover the whole domain, they will bump up against other theories in more ways, which will lead to fruitful controversies and issues to be settled empirically. Psychology and artificial intelligence have a tendency to construct task-based theories and need to enforce on their theorists the desirability of constructing more global theories.

NOTE

The writing of this paper was supported by the Army Research Institute under Contract MDA 903–85–C–0411.

REFERENCES

Burstein, M. H. (1985). *Learning by reasoning from multiple analogies.* Unpublished doctoral dissertation, Yale University, New Haven, CT.

Burstein, M. H. (1986). Concept formation by incremental analogical reasoning and debugging. In R. S. Michalski, J. G. Carbonell, & T. M. Mitchell (Eds.), *Machine learning: An artificial intelligence approach* (Vol. 2, pp. 351–370). Los Altos, CA: Kaufmann.

Burstein, M. H. (1988). Incremental learning from multiple analogies. In *ANALOGICA: The first workshop on analogical reasoning* (pp. 37–62). Boston: Pitman.

Carbonell, J. G. (1986). Derivational analogy: A theory of reconstructive problem solving and expertise acquisition. In R. S. Michalski, J. B. Carbonell, & T. M. Mitchell (Eds.), *Machine learning: An artificial intelligence approach* (Vol. 2, pp. 371–392). Los Altos, CA: Kaufmann.

Chi, M. T. H., Feltovich, P. J., & Glaser, R. (1981). Categorization and representation of physics problems by experts and novices. *Cognitive Science,* 5(2), 121–152.

Clement, J. (1981). Analogy generation in scientific problem solving. *Proceedings of the Third Annual Conference of the Cognitive Science Society* (pp. 137–140), Berkeley, CA.

Clement, J. (1986). Methods for evaluating the validity of hypothesized analogies. *Proceedings of the Eighth Annual Conference of the Cognitive Science Society* (pp. 223–234). Amherst, MA.

Collins, A. (1978). Fragments of a theory of human plausible reasoning. In D. L. Waltz (Ed.), *Theoretical issues in natural language processing* (pp. 194–201). Urbana-Champaign, University of Illinois, Coordinated Science Laboratory.

Collins, A., & Gentner, D. (1980). A framework for a cognitive theory of writing. In L. W. Gregg & E. Steinberg (Eds.), *Cognitive processes in writing: An interdisciplinary approach* (pp. 51–72). Hillsdale, NJ: Erlbaum.

Collins, A., & Gentner, D. (1983). Multiple models of evaporation processes. *Proceedings of the Fifth Annual Conference of the Cognitive Science Society*, Rochester, NY.

✓Collins, A., & Gentner, D. (1987). How people construct mental models. In D. Holland & N. Quinn (Eds.), *Cultural models in language and thought* (pp. 243–265). Cambridge: Cambridge University Press.

Collins, A., Gentner, D., & Rubin, A. (1981). *Teaching study strategies* (Tech. Rep. No. 4794). Cambridge, MA: Bolt Beranek & Newman.

Collins, A. M., & Loftus, E. F. (1975). A spreading-activation theory of semantic processing. *Psychological Review, 82,* 407–428.

Collins, A., & Michalski, R. (1989). The logic of plausible reasoning: A core theory. *Cognitive Science, 13,* 1–49.

Duncker, K. (1945). On problem solving. *Psychological Monographs, 58* (Whole No. 270).

Evans, T. G. (1968). A program for the solution of geometric analogy intelligence test questions. In M. Minsky (Ed.), *Semantic information processing* (pp. 271–353). Cambridge, MA: MIT Press.

Falkenhainer, B., Forbus, K., & Gentner, D. (1986). The structure-mapping engine. In *Proceedings of the American Association for Artificial Intelligence* (pp. 272–277). Los Altos, CA: Kaufmann.

Gentner, D. (1983). Structure-mapping: A theoretical framework for analogy. *Cognitive Science, 7*(2), 155–170.

✓ Gentner, D., & Gentner, D. R. (1983). Flowing waters or teeming crowds: Mental models of electricity. In D. Gentner & A. L. Stevens (Eds.), *Mental models* (pp. 99–129). Hillsdale, NJ: Erlbaum.

Gentner, D., & Landers, R. (1985, November). Analogical reminding: A good match is hard to find. *Proceedings of the International Conference on Systems, Man, and Cybernetics*, Tucson, AZ.

Gick, M. L., & Holyoak, K. J. (1980). Analogical problem solving. *Cognitive Psychology, 12,* 306–355.

Gick, M. L., & Holyoak, K. J. (1983). Schema induction and analogical transfer. *Cognitive Psychology, 15,* 1–38.

Halasz, F., & Moran, T. P. (1982). Analogy considered harmful. *Proceedings of the Human Factors in Computer Systems Conference*, Gaithersburg, MD.

Malt, B. C., & Smith, E. E. (1984). Correlated properties in natural categories. *Journal of Verbal Learning and Verbal Behavior, 23,* 250–269.

Meyer, D. E. (1970). On the representation and retrieval of stored semantic information. *Cognitive Psychology, 1,* 242–300.

Ortony, A. (1979). Beyond literal similarity. *Psychological Review, 86,* 161–180.

Rosch, E. H. (1975). Cognitive representations of semantic categories. *Journal of Experimental Psychology: General, 104,* 192–233.

✓ Smith, E. E., & Medin, D. L. (1981). *Categories and concepts.* Cambridge, MA: Harvard University Press.

Tversky, A. (1977). Features of similarity. *Psychological Review, 84*, 327–352.

Tversky, A., & Gati, I. (1982). Similarity, separability, and the triangle inequality. *Psychological Review, 89*, 123–154.

Tversky, A., & Kahneman, D. (1980). Causal schemas in judgments under uncertainty. In M. Fishbein (Ed.), *Progress in social psychology*. Hillsdale, NJ: Erlbaum.

Van Lehn, K., & Brown, J. S. (1980). Planning nets: A representation for formalizing analogies and semantic models of procedural skills. In R. E. Snow, P. A. Federico, & W. E. Montague (Eds.), *Aptitude, learning, and instruction: Cognitive process analogies* (Vol. 2, pp. 95–137). Hillsdale, NJ: Erlbaum.

Winston, P. H. (1982). Learning new principles from precedents and exercises. *Artificial Intelligence, 19*, 321–350.

Name index

Abelson, R. P., 115n1, 215
Achinstein, P., 52
Ackinclose, C. C., 229
Adams, J. A., 404
Adams, L., 477, 479
Adamson, L., 378
Alegria, J., 149
Alpert, A., 381, 382
Als, H., 378
Amarel, S., 346
Anderson, A., 316
Anderson, D., 13, 14, 15, 367, 490, 489–531, 532, 540, 559
Anderson, J. A., 299
Anderson, J. R., 7, 11, 13, 233, 243, 244, 245, 248, 249, 261, 267, 268, 269, 283, 284, 285, 347, 352–3, 357, 358, 360, 363, 364, 373, 415, 428, 429, 430, 438, 439, 444, 447, 452, 454, 455, 456, 457, 462, 463, 476–7, 484, 549, 552, 558, 559–60
Anderson, R. C., 77, 78, 125
Anglin, J. M., 159
Aristotle, 183, 194n1
Armstrong, R. C., 115n3
Armstrong, S. L., 54, 83, 85, 95, 115n1
Asch, S. E., 226, 473
Aschkenasy, J. R., 158

Bacon, F., 219
Bahrick, H. P., 88
Bahrick, P. O., 88
Baillargeon, R., 373, 378, 379, 381, 430
Ballato, S. M., 80–1, 82, 84, 85, 86, 87, 88, 89, 90, 91, 97, 114, 115n3
Balzac, H., 470
Banerji, R., 228, 473
Barclay, J. R., 77
Bargh, J. A., 97
Barsalou, L. W., 5, 19, 27, 73n2, 77, 78, 79–81, 82, 83, 84, 85, 86, 87, 88, 89, 90, 91, 93, 94, 95, 96, 97, 98, 103, 105, 107, 113, 114, 115n3, 137, 173, 181, 182, 187, 191–2, 193, 347, 348, 400, 435n3, 551, 556
Bartlett, F. C., 450
Batterman, N. A., 174, 226
Beach, L. R., 61
Bellezza, F. S., 82, 84–5, 87, 88
Benedict, H., 155, 167
Benningsfield, S. E., 476
Bereiter, C., 386, 472, 477
Berlin, B. D., 173
Berliner, D. C., 489
Bernstein, A., 418
Bertelson, P., 149
Bertenthal, B. I., 378
Billman, D. O., 226, 372, 395, 423
Billow, R. M., 223, 226
Binford, T. O., 293, 295–6
Birch, H. G., 399
Black, J. B., 395
Blewitt, P., 146
Boerger, A., 500, 503, 524, 528
Bohr, N., 433
Bond, R. N., 97
Bornstein, M. H., 149, 377
Bower, G. H., 95, 395
Bowerman, M., 161, 162
Boyes-Braem, P., 430
Boyle, C. F., 462
Brachman, R. J., 26
Bransford, J. D., 9, 14, 77, 367, 386, 405, 406, 423, 452, 455, 456, 463, 464, 471, 472, 473, 474, 475, 477, 478, 479, 482, 484, 487, 493, 532, 534, 535, 537, 540, 541, 542, 556, 561
Brazelton, T. B., 378
Brewer, W. F., 9, 367, 420, 426, 431, 435n4
Briggs, Henry, 472–3

567

Subject index

575

categorization, 49–50, 187, 546; development in, 191; effects of distributional properties on, 32–4, 35–8, 47; effects of variability on, 28–32, 35, 47; as explanation, 51–5; as form of inference, 53–4; independence of, from similarity, 23, 28–47; kinds of, 49–50; models of, 23–7, 24f; resemblance applied to, 21–3, 188; similarity theory of, 551; surface similarity in, 3; typicality, similarity and, 5–6, 19, 21–38, 48, 50–1, 181; unitary views of, 87–8

category judgments, 19, 34, 50–1, 374, 551, 555, 556; basis of, 5–6; in transformations of artifacts, 45–7; in transformations on natural kinds, 40–3

category membership, 21–3, 24, 25, 46, 47–8, 179–80, 188; children's judgments of, 374, 475; criteria for, 189, 534; goodness of, 27; judgments regarding, 85, 181, 188–9 (*see also* category judgments); similarity in, 26, 186–7, 193; stability of, 85, 87–8; typicality and, 35, 54

category representations: context-independent information in, 95–6; dynamic, 93–102; information incorporation into, 78; models of, 179; property generation in, 81–5; stability/instability of, 76–94, 114–15; vary across contexts, 77–8

causal explanation, 125, 370, 381, 386; infants' predisposition to seek, 4, 378, 428; search for, 376, 379, 385, 405

causal mechanisms, 13; children's sensitivity to, 371, 381–5, 407, 526–7

causal/relational network, 418

causal relations, 385, 558; hierarchies in, 337; primacy of, 259; in salient properties, 16; surface/deep properties, 434

causal structure: and transfer, 379–85, 407

causation, 318; mistreatment of, 507

change: experience of, 494

children, *see* development

choice problem(s), 60, 71–3, 223

chunking, 250; perceptual, 524

circularity, 511; in resemblance theory, 51, 52, 55n1

classical view, *see* concept representation

classification, 1, 53, 149, 184, 373

classification tasks, 146, 159, 161, 166; sameness relations, 163–5

cognition: analogy use in, 502–14; computational approach to, 243, 299; microstructure of, 298–312; models of, 243; multiple analogies in, 522–4; perception of similarities and analogies in, 1–2; role of similarity in, 180, 181; theories of, 242

cognitive architecture, 242, 243; design principles for, 243–9; general, 354; specialized, 357–8; subsystems in, 242–3

cognitive economy, 131, 135, 187; inference in, 123, 125, 127–8

cognitive embeddedness/disembedding, 371, 387, 397–9, 406, 556

cognitive flexibility, 135, 387, 406–7, 544; and encapsulation, 398–404, 406; factors affecting/impeding, 371, 386–406; functional, 15, 371, 387–8, 399–404, 406; in information retrieval, 95; and transfer, 15

cognitive skills: early learning of, 457; reminders in learning of, 438, 439, 440, 462, 465

cognitive system: dynamism of, 79; models of, 242; recency effect in, 97–8; use of analogies in, 218

color (dimension), 3, 170; organization of, 171–2, 173

color discrimination, 149, 158

color terms, 377–8

commonalities: abstract relational, 351; and access, 229; in analogy, 223; extraction of, 200, 226, 227–9, 230, 233; in goal structure, 395; of problem type, 455; relational, 222, 233, 334; source/target, 243, 248; structural/surface, 218–19, 220

comparisons, 222, 232; between domains, 318–19; double, 548; four-element, 554; framework for theory of mapping and, 546–65; in learning, 231–2; literal/metaphorical, 415; of problems, 457–8, 465; theory of, 554–62; three-element, 553–4, 555; two-element, 553

complexity: in advanced knowledge acquisition, 529–30; effect on cognition, 500; management of, 522–4; mastery of, 501–2; multiple analogies and, 528

component mapping, 549, 552, 553

composite images, 502, 522–4, 525, 529; as antidote for analogy-driven misconceptions, 514–28

composite imaging with selective contingent instantiation (CISCI), 499, 522–4, 529

comprehension, 300; of analogies, 427;

ments, 14, 16, 367, 470–1, 476–7,
493–4
problem schema(ta), 248, 262; new, 342,
356
problem solution(s), *see* problem solving
problem solving, 251, 268, 362; accessing prior material in, 228–9; analogy
in, 1, 9, 12–13, 214–17, 219, 267–8,
275–6, 294–5, 313–15, 333, 341–2,
424, 448 (*see also* analogical problem
solving); by children, 386, 539–60;
computational model of, 11, 242–66;
concepts and procedures as tools in,
479–80; context and, 15; creative,
282; flexible/inflexible, 244–5, 399–
404, 471, 478–9, 487–91, 492; formal
reasoning in, 307–11; imagination in,
306–7, 309–10; incorrect, 540–1;
models of, 246; by novices, 439, 443,
450, 455, 458–9, 483; old knowledge
in, 532–3, 536–7, 543; in PDP systems, 299–301; reduction of complex
problems to simple ones in, 309, 311;
remindings in, 438, 439, 537; search
processes in, 244–5; similarities and,
466; teaching, 471, 474–5, 493–4; use
of earlier problems in, 438, 439, 441,
443–5, 458–9, 460–2, 465
problem-solving: abilities, 300–1; aids,
teaching, 464–5; heuristics, 438;
mechanisms, 246; system, 242,
249–50
problem types, 456; ability to recognize,
452; learning, 463–4; reminding-
based generalizations in, 457
procedural knowledge, 249, 537
processes of induction (PI) program, 8,
243, 244, 248, 319–23; analogical
problem solving in, 250–61; architecture of, 249–50; bidirectional search
in, 244–5; comparison with previous
models of analogy, 257–61; computational framework for empirical findings, 261–4; creativity in, 328; critique
of, 354–7; and expository analogies,
323–4; in factual theory of analogy,
319–23; generalization in, 248; limitations of, 257, 260; spreading activation, 245–6
production rules, 124, 249, 286
production system architecture: analogy
use in, 11, 267–97
production systems, 319, 332, 341, 357
productive analogy, 14, 417–19; ability
to access, 428–32, 442

profound analogies, 12, 329–30; discovery of, 324–8
projection(s), 354; inductive, 369
prompts, prompting, 373, 473–4; and
transfer, 392, 394, 397, 405
properties: absolute, 78; accessibility of,
179–80, 189–90; combining judgments from different, 555–6; compar-
ison/mapping, 547, 551, 553, 554–5,
557–8, 559–60; of concepts, 123, 129–
30, 133, 134; context-independent,
73n2; deep, 179–80, 182, 185–6, 193–
4; descriptive, 420–1, 426, 427; extrinsic, 184; misleading, 503–4, 506–7,
508, 509; missing, 505; necessary and
sufficient, 184; in PI, 322; relational,
420–1, 427, 557; salient, 414, 419,
420–1, 423, 434; shared, 375; stability
of, 191–3; surface, 185–6, 188;
weighting of, 107–8; *see also* features
property correspondences, 547–9
property generation, 81–5, 97; and context-independent information, 95–6;
instability in, 90; within/between subject agreement, 84, 105, 107
property mapping, 548–9, 552, 553,
558; *see also* mapping
propositions: in PI, 319–23
prototype(s), 25–6, 27, 76, 115n1, 136,
302, 500; agreement in, in property generation, 83–5, 87; in concept meaning,
122; representations of, 186; similarity
to, and decision making, 60, 62, 63–5,
68–9; stability of, 73n2
prototype models, 5, 26, 27
prototypicality judgments, 188–9
psychological essentialism, 179–95, 376–7
PUPS (PenUltimᶜte Production System),
11, 13, 268–9, 354; analogical filling
of function slots, 278–80; analogy in,
271–8; compared with other work on
analogy, 291–6; critique of, 352–4;
discrimination learning in, 286–91;
knowledge compilation in, 285–6;
knowledge representation in, 269–71;
refinement in, 280–2
purpose-directed analogy, 292–3

quantitative relations, 168–70, 174

random choice(s), 325–6
realism, metaphysical, 181
reasoning: context in, 1, 215; developmental change in, 234n13, by example, 301; imagination in, 306–7, 309–